Code Blue

Bedside Procedures and Critical Information

Code Blue

Bedside Procedures and Critical Information

Rahul Jandial, MD, PhD

Assistant Professor, Division of Neurosurgery,
City of Hope Comprehensive Cancer Center,
Los Angeles, California

Danielle D. Jandial, MD

Gynecologic Oncology Fellow,
Division of Gynecologic Oncology,
University of California–Irvine,
Irvine, California

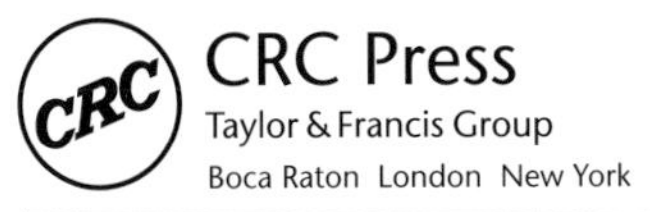

CRC Press is an imprint of the
Taylor & Francis Group, an **informa** business

CRC Press
Taylor & Francis Group
6000 Broken Sound Parkway NW, Suite 300
Boca Raton, FL 33487-2742

Printed on acid-free paper
Version Date: 20140327

Printed and bound in India by Replika Press Pvt. Ltd.

International Standard Book Number-13: 978-1-57626-253-5 (Paperback)

Library of Congress Cataloging-in-Publication Data

Jandial, Rahul.
Code blue / by Rahul Jandial and Danielle D. Jandial.
p. ; cm.
Includes bibliographical references.
ISBN 978-1-57626-253-5 (pbk.)
1. Emergency medicine--Handbooks, manuals, etc. 2. Emergency nursing--Handbooks, manuals, etc.
I. Jandial, Danielle D. II. Title.
[DNLM: 1. Cardiopulmonary Resuscitation--methods--Handbooks. WG 39 J33c 2009]

RC86.8.J36 2009
616.02'5—dc22 2008048466

Visit the Taylor & Francis Web site at
http://www.taylorandfrancis.com

and the CRC Press Web site at
http://www.crcpress.com

To our sons,
Ronak, Kai, and Zain,
with love

CONTRIBUTORS

Helene A. Duenas, BS
Physician Assistant Student, Oregon Health and Science University,
Portland, Oregon

Matthew J. Duenas
Stanford University, Stanford, California

Vincent J. Duenas, BS
City of Hope Cancer Center, Los Angeles, California

Melanie G. Gephart Hayden, MD, MAS
Resident, Department of Neurosurgery, Stanford University Hospital and Clinics,
Stanford, California

Amanda C. Hambrecht, BA
New York University School of Medicine, New York, New York

Allen Ho, BA
Harvard Medical School, Boston, Massachusetts

Danielle D. Jandial, MD
Gynecologic Oncology Fellow, Division of Gynecologic Oncology,
University of California–Irvine, Irvine, California

Rahul Jandial, MD, PhD
Assistant Professor, Division of Neurosurgery,
City of Hope Comprehensive Cancer Center,
Los Angeles, California

Rohit Mahajan, MD
Department of Anesthesiology, University of Michigan,
Ann Arbor, Michigan

PREFACE

Embarking on the first clinical rotation in a hospital is a daunting experience for all clinicians, whether physician's assistant, nurse, physician, technician, or student. Clearly, the foundation of medical textbook knowledge does not necessarily overlap with the know-how that makes one functional "in the trenches" at a hospital. The conventional remedy for this has been a deluge of handbooks, both large and small, that provide information, and sometimes reassurance, that can be readily retrieved from the coat pocket of an intimidated student clinician. Within this sea of clinical handbooks, few attack the body of knowledge that is commonly called on by all clinicians: bedside procedures and tabulations of high-yield values and measurements. *Code Blue* aspires to be that missing text.

This handbook is organized so that information is quickly and easily accessible. Divided into two sections, the first section contains 39 chapters divided into seven parts: Abdominal, Airway, Cardiothoracic, Neurosurgical, Vascular, Other, and Emergency Medical Management. These chapters provide information for performing different bedside procedures, many of them emergent in nature. Each chapter begins with a case scenario and includes details on indications, contraindications, and information about supplies and technique. Pearls and pitfalls have been incorporated into each chapter, providing additional insights and practical advice not always available in textbooks or articles. To convey the information without ambiguity, a consistent, bullet-point outline format with simple line drawings and radiographs displaying the technique nuances has been used. Finally, chapters conclude with reference to corresponding appendixes that are found in the second half of the text. The appendixes (also organized by organ systems) were chosen for being high yield. They contain the formulas, differentials, side effects, antibiotic sensitivities, and much more that clinicians use daily.

It is my hope that *Code Blue* will prove to be an accessible, exhaustive, and useful reference to students and practitioners alike, and that whether in print of digital format its proverbial worn corners and highlighted, tattered pages will be a testament to its ultimate utility.

Rahul Jandial

CONTENTS

APPENDIXES

Code Blue

Bedside Procedures and Critical Information

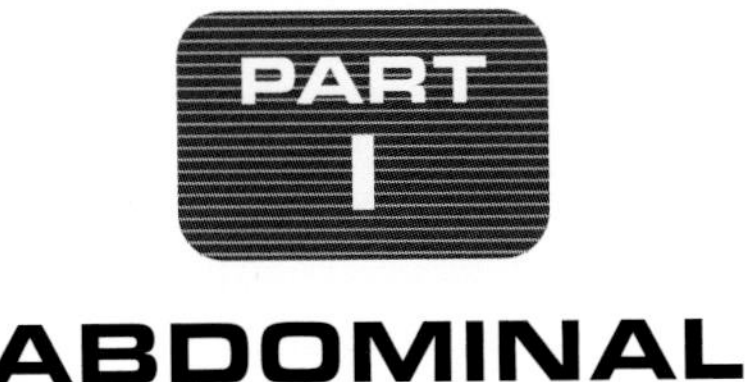

ABDOMINAL

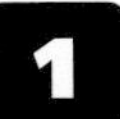

Diagnostic Peritoneal Lavage

A 32-year-old man is admitted following motor vehicle trauma. He has a history significant for known contrast allergy and is found to have a small amount of free fluid on abdominal ultrasound examination (Fig. 1-1).

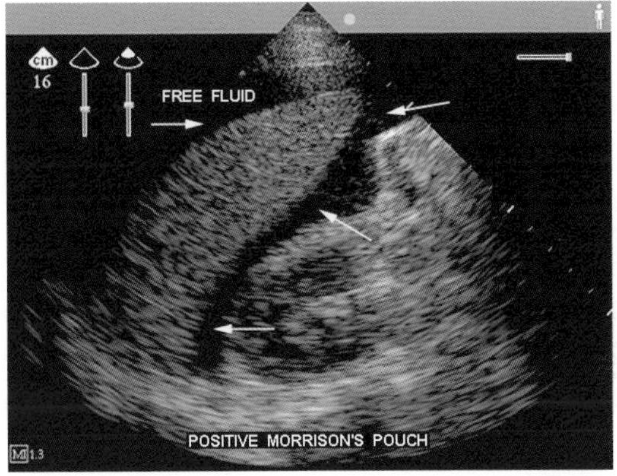

Fig. 1-1 Abdominal ultrasound showing free fluid.

INDICATIONS

- Blunt abdominal trauma with unreliable abdominal examination
- Mostly used to evaluate the abdomens of patients for whom CT scans are contraindicated (e.g., patients with known contrast allergy, too heavy for scanner, or unstable for transport)

CONTRAINDICATIONS

- Pregnancy
- When emergent exploratory laparotomy is indicated

SUPPLIES

- 1% lidocaine with 1:100,000 epinephrine
- Sterile gloves, towels, gown, cap, and mask
- Sterile preparation
- No. 10 blade
- 25-gauge needle
- 5 ml syringes
- Peritoneal dialysis catheter
- 1 L saline solution
- Tissue forceps
- Hemostats
- Self-retaining retractor
- Allis clamps
- 2-0 absorbable suture

POSITIONING

- Supine (Fig. 1-2)

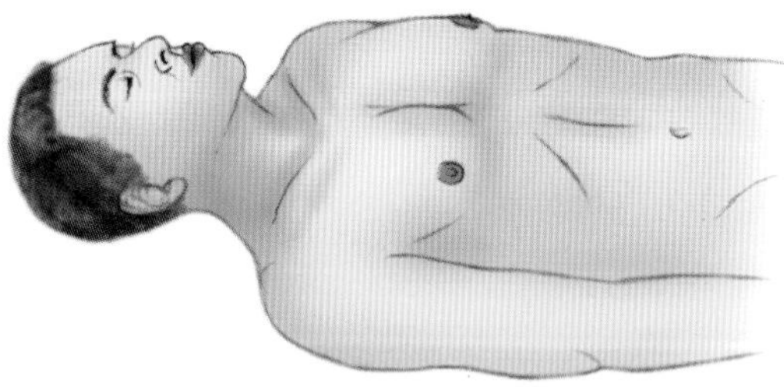

Fig. 1-2

TECHNIQUE

- Prepare and drape entire abdomen.
- The incision will be made at one-third the distance from the umbilicus to the pubic symphysis.
- In that area, raise a wheal under the skin with a 25-gauge needle using lidocaine with epinephrine.
- Incise the skin and carry the incision down to the linea alba (identified by its decussating fibers).
- Place the self-retaining retractor into the wound.
- Incise the fascia and peritoneum 1.5 cm longitudinally (Fig. 1-3), and grasp the edges with hemostats.
- Insert a peritoneal dialysis catheter into the pelvic cavity using an oblique downward trajectory.
- Attach the syringe to the catheter and aspirate. (Gross blood or bowel contents warrant emergent laparotomy.)
- Attach the peritoneal catheter to IV tubing and hang a bag of warmed saline solution.
- After 10 minutes, place the IV bag below the patient on the floor and allow the dialysate to drain out. Send a specimen from the drained fluid for a cell count and amylase.
- Close fascia and skin with interrupted absorbable suture.

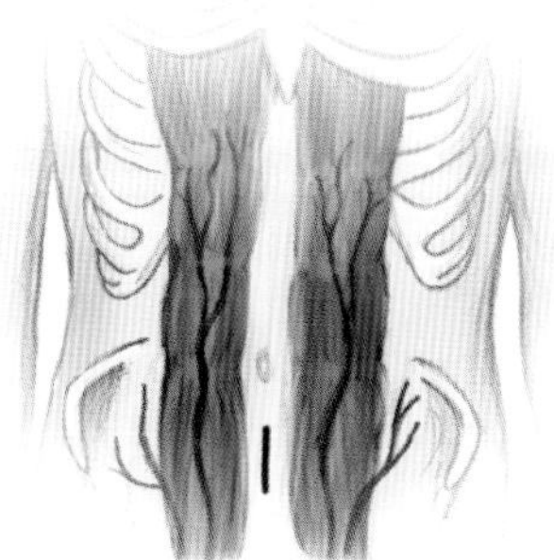

Fig. 1-3

PEARLS

- *Before an abdominal procedure, the stomach and bladder need to be decompressed with an NG tube and a Foley catheter, respectively.*
- *Epinephrine in the lidocaine decreases bleeding, thereby minimizing false-positive results.*
- *A preprocedure dose of gram-positive antibiotics decreases the risk of wound infection.*
- *During placement of saline solution into the abdomen, if any dialysate is found in a chest tube or Foley catheter, emergent laparotomy is indicated (diagnostic of perforated diaphragm or bladder, respectively).*
- *A diagnostic peritoneal lavage (DPL) specimen is considered positive with the following findings: amylase >175, red blood cell count >100,000/μl, or white cell count >500/μl.*

PITFALLS

- A DPL is not effective for a suspected retroperitoneal injury.
- Morbid obesity and a history of multiple abdominal surgeries raise the risk of bowel injury during an abdominal procedure.
- The presence of ascites can confound laboratory evaluation of a DPL specimen.
- The surgical approach can lead to bladder injury from the incision, bowel injury from an incision of fascia, hemorrhage from a vascular injury, peritonitis from poor aseptic technique, and wound infections.

✓ POSTPROCEDURE CHECK

❑ The operative wound site should receive routine wound care.

See Appendix A for additional helpful information.

2

Nasogastric Tube

A 45-year-old woman with a history of multiple abdominal surgeries presents with incessant vomiting.

INDICATIONS

- The need for enteral feeding
- Upper GI bleeding
- Ileus
- Small bowel obstruction
- Distended bowel loops (Fig. 2-1)
- Gastric outlet obstruction
- Acute gastric distention

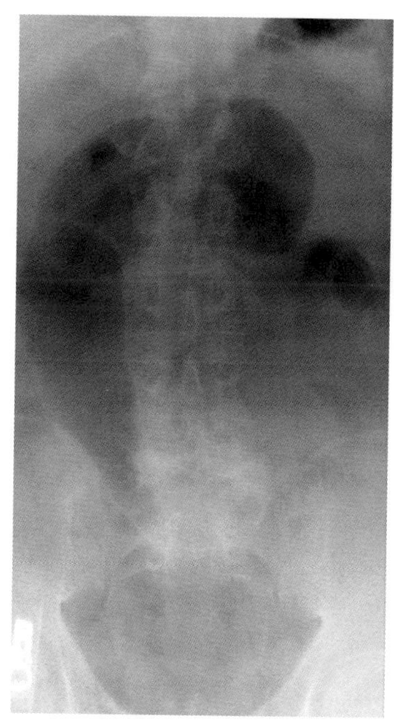

Fig. 2-1 Abdominal radiograph showing distended bowel loops.

CONTRAINDICATIONS

- Head trauma with any suspicion of basilar skull fracture
- Recent esophageal surgery

SUPPLIES

- Viscous lidocaine for the nose
- NG sump tube
- 60 ml syringe, catheter tip
- Stethoscope
- Water in cup with drinking straw

POSITIONING

- Sitting with head flexed (Fig. 2-2)

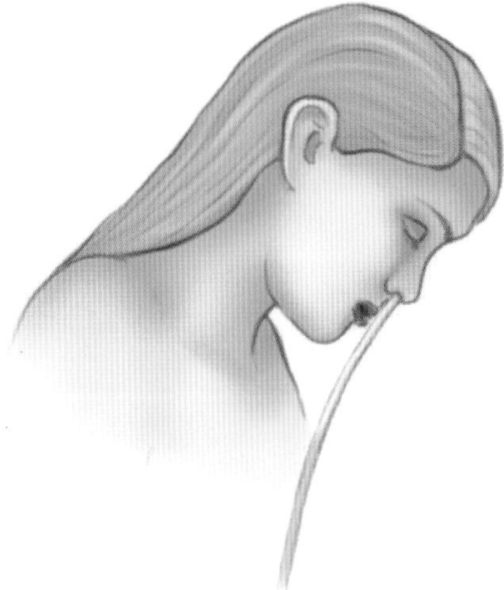

Fig. 2-2 Sitting with the head flexed.

TECHNIQUE

- Apply lubricant to an NG tube.
- Ask patient to flex the neck.
- Advance the NG tube into one naris, aiming posteriorly, and ask the patient to swallow.
- Advance the tube as the patient swallows.
- To verify proper position, inject 20 cc of air into the tube as you auscultate the epigastric region, listening for gurgling.
- Secure the tube with tape without applying pressure on the nose.

PEARLS

- *An orogastric tube should be placed when the patient has sustained a head trauma and a basilar skull fracture is suspected.*
- *Placing the tip of the NG tube in ice stiffens it and makes the tube easier to manipulate.*
- *Before any enteral feeding is initiated, correct placement of the NG tube should be verified by a chest radiograph.*
- *Measuring from the naris to the abdomen can help approximate the distance the NG tube needs to be advanced.*
- *Tape the NG tube without applying pressure on the naris to avoid erosion.*

PITFALLS

- While clamping the tube, keep in mind that the lower gastroesophageal sphincter is stented open and aspiration may occur.
- Long-term placement of NG tubes can lead to sinusitis. If this is suspected, remove the tube and place it in the other naris if still needed.
- Tracheal intubation with an NG tube in an awake patient leads to coughing and difficulty speaking.
- Complications include discomfort, alar erosion, gastritis, and epistaxis.

✓ POSTPROCEDURE CHECK

- ❑ Chest radiographs should be obtained immediately after placing the tube to verify placement below the diaphragm (Fig. 2-3).
- ❑ The NG tube should be irrigated with 30 ml of normal saline solution every 4 hours.

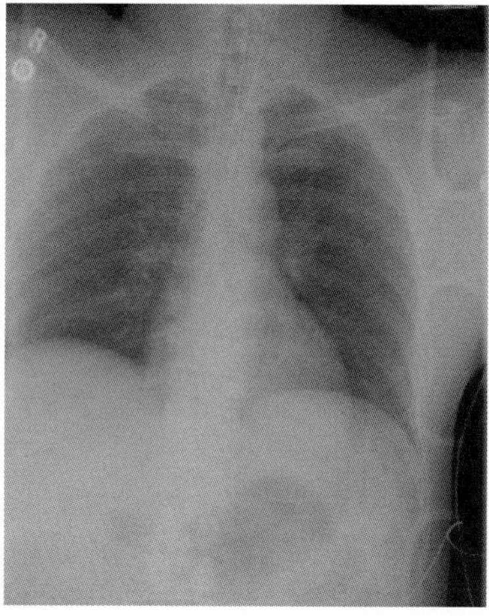

Fig. 2-3 Abdominal radiograph revealing the proper position for an NG tube in the fundus of the stomach.

See Appendix A for additional helpful information.

3

Sengstaken-Blakemore Tube

A 48-year-old woman with a history of alcohol abuse presents with profound hematemesis, hypotension, and tachycardia.

INDICATIONS

- Life-threatening hemoptosis from gastroesophageal varices (Fig. 3-1)

CONTRAINDICATIONS

- None

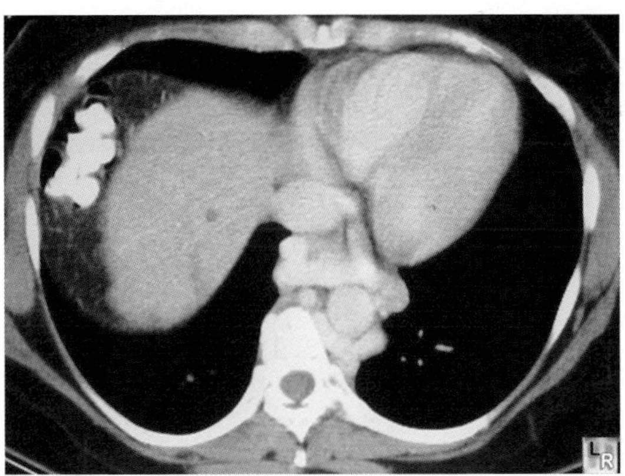

Fig. 3-1 Abdominal CT showing dilated esophageal varices.

SUPPLIES

- Viscous lidocaine (for the nose)
- Sengstaken-Blakemore (SB) tube
- Hemostat
- Heavy scissors
- 60 ml syringe for catheter
- NG tube
- Lubricant

POSITIONING

- Supine with neck slightly flexed

TECHNIQUE

- Place a large NG tube to evacuate the contents of the stomach (Fig. 3-2).
- Check both balloons on the SB tube for leaks.
- Flex the patient's neck, insert the SB tube into one naris, and advance into the pharynx.
- Ask the patient to swallow, and advance the tube approximately 45 cm (17.5 inches).
- Apply light intermittent suction to the gastric port to confirm placement with return of blood.
- If blood returns, inflate the gastric balloon slowly with 100 cc of air.
- Withdraw the tube until the gastroesophageal junction is obstructed by the balloon (see Fig. 3-2).
- Confirm placement with chest radiograph. If correctly placed, add another 150 cc of air to gastric balloon.

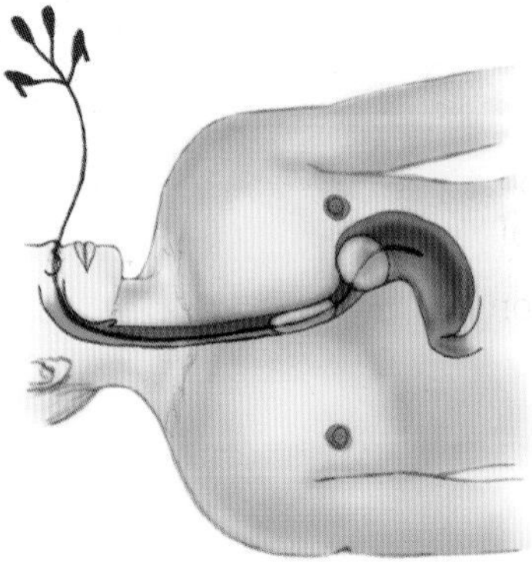

Fig. 3-2

- Irrigate the gastric port (not the gastric balloon) with saline solution to evaluate for persistence of hemorrhage. If hemorrhaging has ceased, deflate the balloon.
- If hemorrhage persists, attach the esophageal balloon port to a manometer and inflate to 30 to 40 mm Hg.
- Apply low intermittent suction to both ports.
- Every 4 hours, deflate the esophageal balloon to evaluate for persistence of hemorrhage and to prevent ischemic necrosis of the esophagus.
- Apply low intermittent suction to gastric and esophageal tubes.

TUBE REMOVAL

- Aspirate air from both balloons once bleeding has ceased for 24 hours.
- Remove the SB tube 48 hours after hemostasis is confirmed.

PEARLS

- *Intubation before performing this procedure can decrease aspiration risk.*
- *Placement of an SB tube should only be performed in an ICU setting in order to allow for close monitoring.*
- *After 24 hours of hemorrhage cessation, the balloons can be deflated. After an additional 24 hours, if no bleeding recurs, the SB tube can be removed.*

PITFALLS

- Even with intubation, the risk of aspiration remains a concern.
- If insufflation pressure is not monitored with a manometer during the initial inflation of the esophageal balloon, esophageal perforation can occur.
- Esophageal perforation can also occur after several hours to days of SB tube residence as a result of prolonged esophageal ischemia.
- Esophageal perforation requires an emergent surgical consultation.

✓ POSTPROCEDURE CHECK

- ❑ Check esophageal pressure at a minimum of every 4 hours.
- ❑ Order daily radiographs to verify proper placement.

See Appendix A for additional helpful information.

4

PARACENTESIS

A 21-year-old woman presents with liver failure and a distended, nontender abdomen.

INDICATIONS

- Ascites (Fig. 4-1)
- Spontaneous bacterial peritonitis
- Need to obtain diagnostic fluid
- Relief of abdominal discomfort or respiratory difficulty from abdominal fluid

CONTRAINDICATIONS

- Coagulopathy
- Bowel obstruction
- Distended bowel loops
- Pregnancy

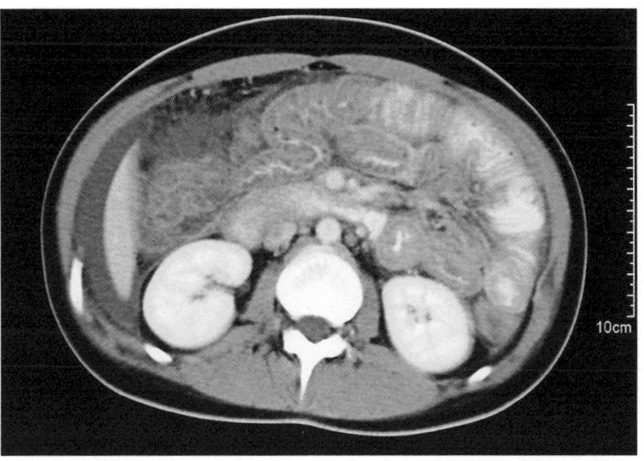

Fig. 4-1 Abdominal CT scan showing ascites.

SUPPLIES

- 1% lidocaine
- Sterile preparation
- Sterile gloves and solution
- 20- and 25-gauge needles
- 5 and 20 ml syringes
- No.10 blade scalpel
- Scissors
- 0.035-inch J-wire
- IV tubing
- Three-way stopcock
- 18- and 20-gauge IV catheter
- 16-gauge single-lumen central line catheter and dilator

POSITIONING

- Supine

TECHNIQUE

- Sites in which needle entry is safe take into consideration the course of the inferior epigastric vessels (Fig. 4-2).
- The bladder should be catheterized.

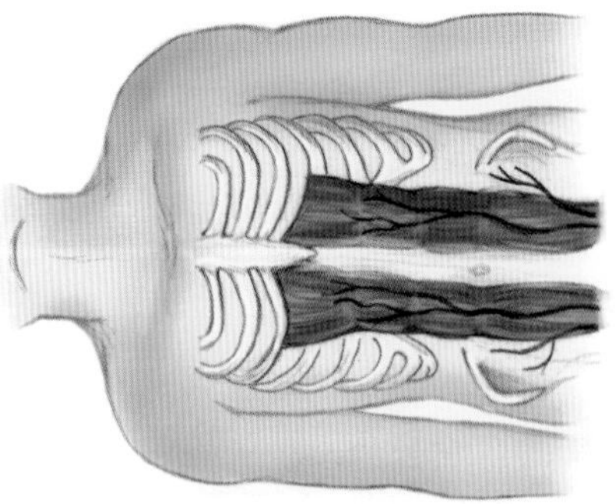

Fig. 4-2

- The insertion site should be free from infection.
- The insertion site should not be through or near any previous incision sites.
- The entry site can be either directly infraumbilical in the midline, directly lateral to the rectus abdominis on either side, or 2 cm medial to either anterior iliac spine.
- Prepare and drape the chosen site.
- Anesthetize the skin with 1% lidocaine using the 25-gauge needle, and anesthetize the abdominal wall (not past the peritoneum) using the 22-gauge needle.
- At an oblique angle, introduce the IV catheter into the abdominal cavity and maintain constant aspiration while advancing the catheter (Fig. 4-3).
- On entering the peritoneal space, you will encounter fluid egress. Advance the catheter and remove the needle.
- Remove 20 ml of fluid for laboratory evaluation.
- If persistent drainage is required, repeat the previous steps and insert a J-wire into the IV catheter.
- The J-wire will be in the peritoneal space and the IV catheter can be removed.
- Nick the skin adjacent to the entry point of the J-wire and dilate the skin, abdominal tissue, and peritoneum (do insert the dilator past the peritoneum) using the dilator over the J-wire.
- Remove the dilator and place a 16-gauge central line catheter over the J-wire and into the peritoneal space.
- Remove the J-wire and connect the central line catheter to IV tubing and to a vacuum or drainage bag.

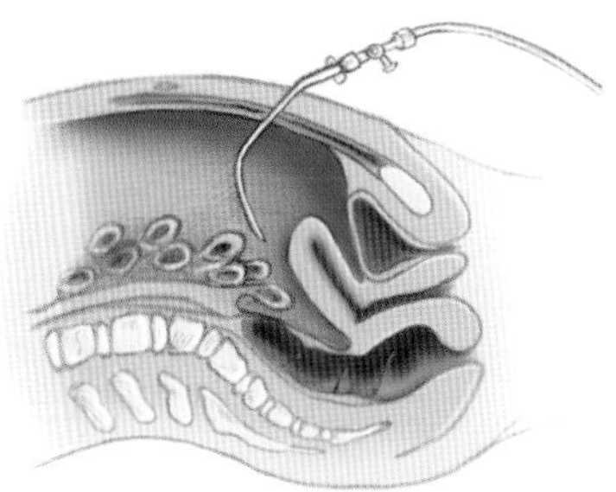

Fig. 4-3

PEARLS

- *Oblique needle entry allows the abdominal wall to collapse when the needle is removed. This helps prevent leakage after the procedure.*
- *If the catheter becomes occluded, drainage may improve if the patient is asked to rotate left and right in the bed several times.*

PITFALLS

- Manipulation of the catheter by reinserting a J-wire or needle can lead to bowel injury. It is preferable to begin the procedure anew at another site.
- After drainage of peritoneal fluid, a dramatic shift of intravascular fluid can occur into the newly emptied peritoneal space. This may result in hypotension, requiring volume support.
- Bowel perforation from needle insertion may only become apparent days after the procedure, in the form of clinically detectable peritonitis.
- Leakage of ascites from the needle insertion site can occur and is usually self-limited. Placing a suture can help occlude the tract.
- Bladder perforation during the procedure requires an immediate urology consultation.

✓ POSTPROCEDURE CHECK

- ❑ Monitor the patient's vital signs closely; hypotension can occur after the procedure from intravascular fluid shift and vagal response.

See Appendix A for additional helpful information.

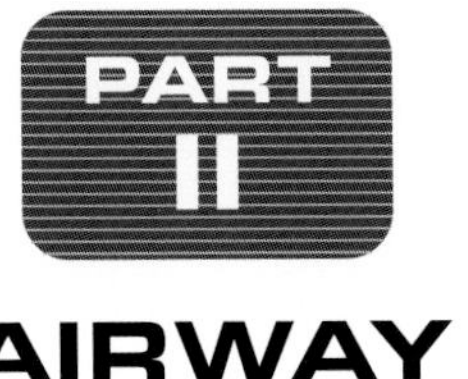

AIRWAY

5

Head Tilt and Jaw Thrust

A 59-year-old woman loses consciousness and falls to the ground in the hospital cafeteria; gurgling noises can be heard from the patient.

INDICATIONS

- Aid with mild upper airway obstruction
- Initial management of a compromised airway
- Preparation for intubation

CONTRAINDICATIONS

- Down syndrome
- Suspected cervical spine injury

SUPPLIES

- None

POSITIONING

- Supine

TECHNIQUE

- Place one hand on the patient's forehead and push down and posteriorly.
- Using two fingers of the other hand, lift the chin to elevate the mandible and hyoid bone (Fig. 5-1).
- Stand at the top of the patient's head.

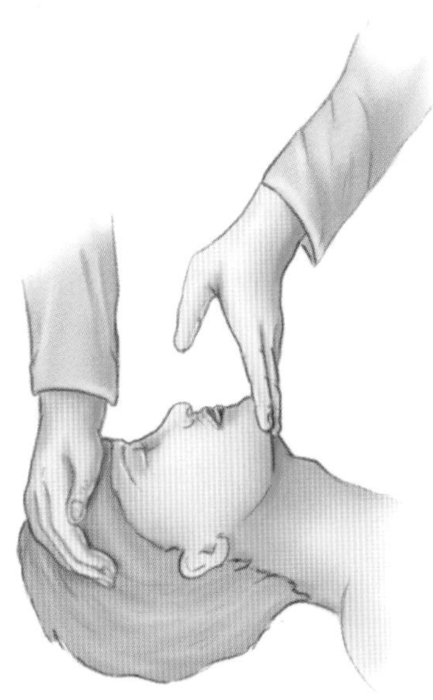

Fig. 5-1

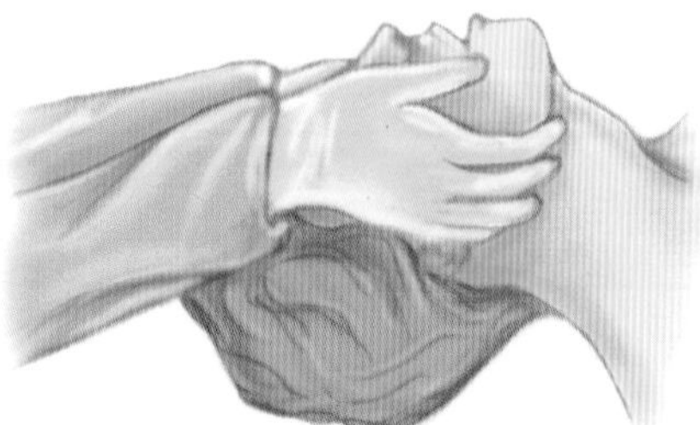

Fig. 5-2

- Open the patient's mouth and grasp the mandible with the fingers of both hands (Fig. 5-2).
- Lift the mandible over and above the maxilla.

PEARLS

- *Jaw thrust alone can be used if any cervical spine injury is suspected or if the patient has Down syndrome.*

PITFALLS

- In children less than 5 years of age, manual airway maneuvers can actually lead to further obstruction of the airway. The best airway patency is achieved with the head in a neutral position.

See Appendix B for additional helpful information.

6

Bag-Mask Ventilation

A 19-year-old man presents with upper airway obstruction after emergent crico-thyroidotomy.

INDICATIONS

- Preoxygenation before intubation
- Short-term oxygenation and ventilation when the patient is not respiring
- Transport of the patient when a ventilator is not available

CONTRAINDICATIONS

- Suspected cervical spine injury
- Tracheal fracture or laceration
- Tracheoesophageal fistula
- Hiatal hernia
- Facial fractures
- Facial degloving injury

SUPPLIES

- Face mask
- Respiratory bag
- Oxygen supply
- Suction device

POSITIONING

- Supine, with the neck in a neutral position. If a cervical spine injury has been excluded, mild neck extension can be helpful.

TECHNIQUE

- Place an oral or nasal airway.
- Grasp the mask with the thumb and index finger, allowing the remaining fingers to grasp the mandible (Fig. 6-1).
- Place the mask on the patient's face with its broader side on the chin area.
- Using the third, fourth, and fifth digits, pull the mandible up into the mask to create a good seal.
- Deliver breaths with the other hand.
- If you encounter difficulty with mask ventilation, an assistant can deliver breaths while you use both hands to grasp and place the mask securely (Fig. 6-2).

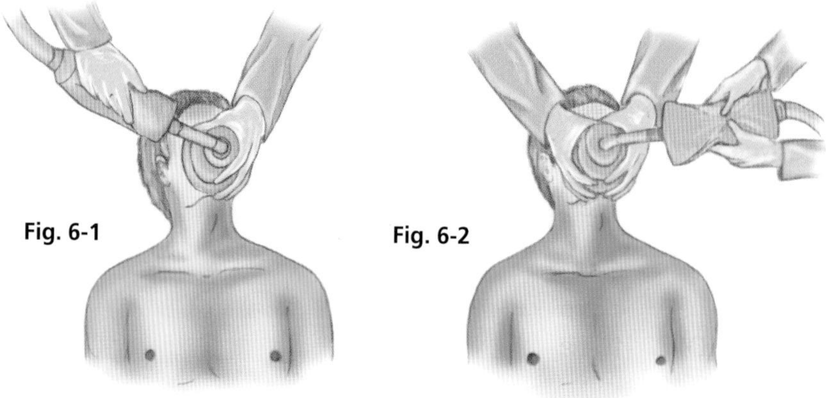

Fig. 6-1 **Fig. 6-2**

PEARLS

- *In a patient with spontaneous respirations, time the delivered breaths to coincide with spontaneous breaths.*
- *In a patient with tachypnea, allow for spontaneous breaths to occur in between delivered breaths.*

PITFALLS

- When securing the mask, avoid applying pressure on the patient's eyes.
- It is difficult to obtain a good facial seal with the mask on edentulous patients. Always consider using two hands to grasp the mask in these patients.

See Appendix B for additional helpful information.

7

Tracheal Intubation

A 38-year-old woman presents after a head injury with sudden neurologic deterioration; she is unresponsive to pain, mumbling, and her eyes are closed to pain.

INDICATIONS

- Inability to protect airway
- Inability to oxygenate adequately
- Inability to ventilate adequately
- Loss of consciousness or severely decreased mental status
- Anticipated fatigue from tachypnea
- Loss of or diminished respiratory drive
- During general anesthesia

CONTRAINDICATIONS

- Oral intubation should not be performed with tracheal fractures.
- Nasal intubation should not be performed if there is any coagulopathy or nasal injury.
- Nasal intubation should not be performed if basilar skull fracture is suspected.

SUPPLIES

- Anesthesia: induction agents (thiopental, etomidate, ketamine), neuromuscular blocking agents (succinylcholine or vecuronium), sedatives (diazepam or midazolam), resuscitation drugs (atropine, phenylephrine, ephedrine, and epinephrine), and topical lidocaine
- Laryngoscope handle and blade
- Macintosh blade
- Miller blade
- Respirator bag and mask
- Suction device
- Endotracheal (ET) tubes (with stylets)

POSITIONING

- Supine with neck slightly flexed

TECHNIQUE

- Check the ET tube cuff by inflating and deflating it. Check the blade and the handle to verify that its light is working.
- Preoxygenate the patient's lungs with the bag mask and instruct the patient to open the mouth.
- The assistant should apply cricoid pressure (Fig. 7-1).
- In an unconscious patient, use the dominant hand to open the mouth by applying a scissorlike motion of your finger to subluxate the jaw (Fig. 7-2).
- With your nondominant hand, place the laryngoscope blade in the right side of the mouth, and, avoiding contact with any teeth, aim the light toward the glottic opening.
- Using the MAC blade (shorter and slightly curved), place the tip under the epiglottis (Fig. 7-3).
- Using the Miller blade (longer and straight), place the tip in the vallecula so that the epiglottis cannot be seen (Fig. 7-4).

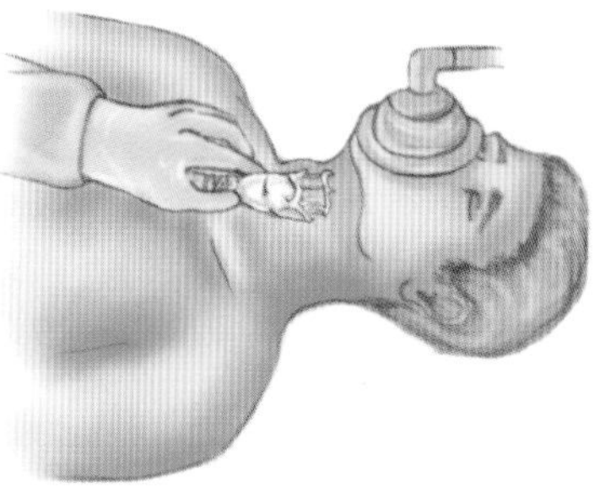

Fig. 7-1

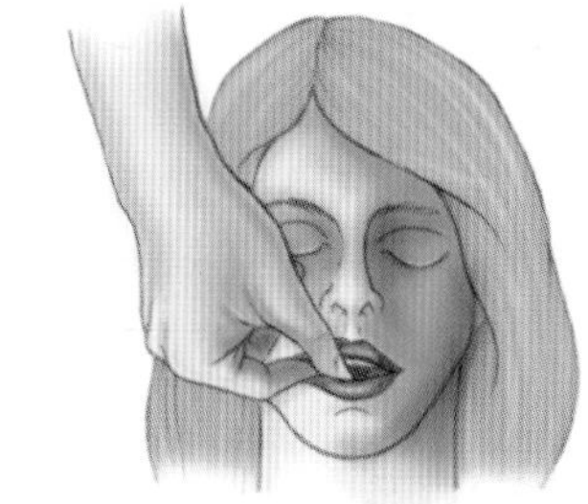

Fig. 7-2

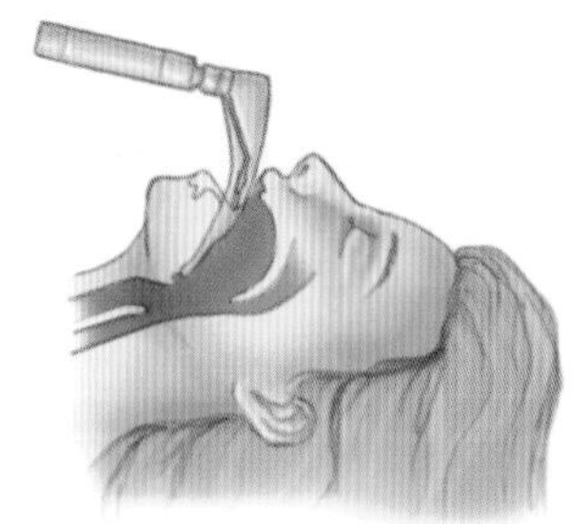

Fig. 7-3

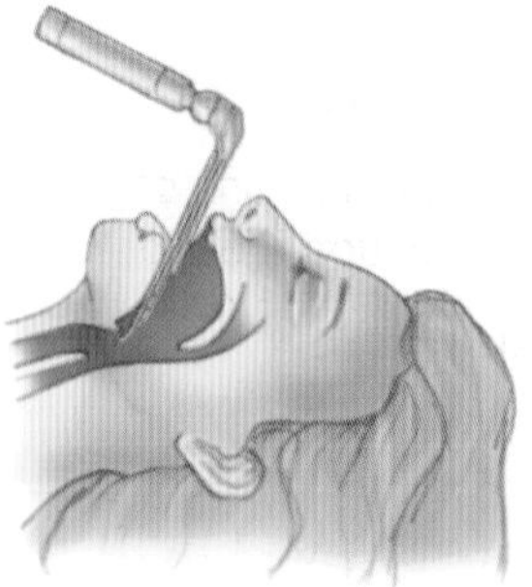

Fig. 7-4

- With your nondominant hand and wrist, lift the entire blade and handle up and down (aiming toward the patient's feet), exposing the vocal cords.
- Pass the styletted ET tube with your dominant hand into the side of the mouth and advance it between the vocal cords.
- Remove the stylet and inflate the ET tube cuff with 5 to 8 cc of air when the cuff is just distal to the vocal cords.
- Secure the ET tube to the mouth with your nondominant hand, and place the end-tidal CO_2 monitor in the breathing circuit.
- Examine the patient's chest for expansion and auscultate for the presence of breath sounds over lung fields and the absence of lung sounds over the gastric area.
- Secure the ET tube with tape and place a bite block or oral airway to prevent biting of the ET tube.

REMOVAL OF ENDOTRACHEAL TUBE

- Aspirate the mouth and oropharynx with a suction device, deflate the ET tube cuff, and remove the tube.

PEARLS

- *Between intubation attempts, bag-mask ventilation of the lungs should be performed.*
- *Generous opening of the mouth will aid in ET tube placement.*

PITFALLS

- Occasionally, air from the stomach can lead to a positive reading on the end-tidal CO_2 monitor. Always allow for several breaths before committing to successful placement of an ET tube.
- Repeated intubations can lead to laryngeal edema, making each subsequent intubation more difficult.
- Dislodged or broken teeth need to be recovered.

✓ POSTPROCEDURE CHECK

- ❑ Obtain chest radiographs to confirm proper placement (Fig. 7-5).
- ❑ Intubation of a left or right mainstem bronchus requires a 1 or 2 cm withdrawal of the tube and repeated chest radiographs.

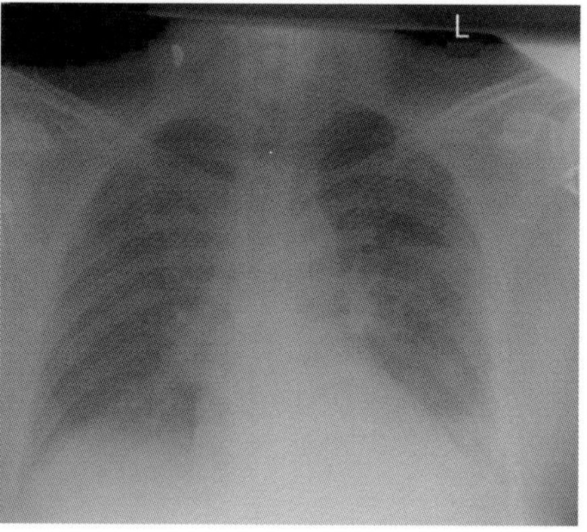

Fig. 7-5 Chest radiograph showing proper position of ET tube, 1 cm above the carina.

See Appendix B for additional helpful information.

8

Cricothyroidotomy

A 28-year-old man presents with a severe smoke inhalation injury and poor bag ventilation after failed intubation attempts by an emergency medicine physician.

INDICATIONS

- Unsuccessful endotracheal intubation and the need for pulmonary access
- Orofacial trauma precluding laryngoscopy
- Upper airway obstruction from any cause preventing ventilation

CONTRAINDICATIONS

- None

SUPPLIES

- Scalpel
- Sterile gloves and towels
- Sterile preparation
- Hemostats
- 3-0 silk ties
- Bag valve mask (Ambu bag)
- Tracheal spreader
- ETT, 6 or 8 Fr, or tracheostomy tube

POSITIONING

- Supine with the neck in a neutral position. If a cervical spine injury has been ruled out, mild neck extension can be helpful.

TECHNIQUE

- Prepare and drape the patient's neck in a sterile fashion (Fig. 8-1).
- Incise the skin in the midline, beginning at the inferior margin of the thyroid cartilage and extending to the cricoid cartilage.
- With the nondominant hand, stabilize the thyroid cartilage and palpate the cricothyroid membrane with the dominant hand.

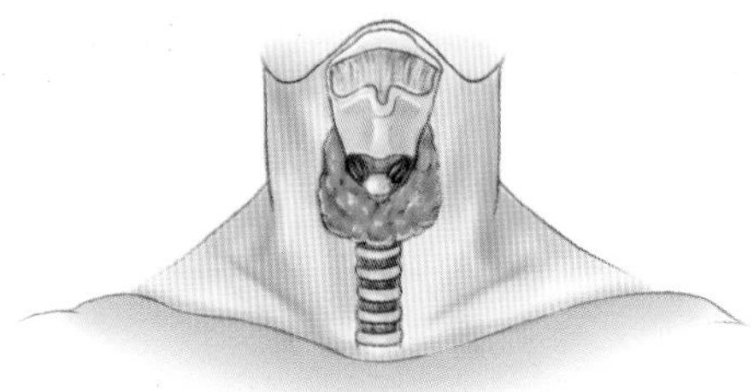

Fig. 8-1

- Maintaining the nondominant hand, incise the cricothyroid membrane with the scalpel. Incise horizontally approximately 2 to 3 cm (Fig. 8-2).
- Insert the tracheal spreader into the trachea and distract gently.
- Insert the tracheostomy tube and remove the spreader.
- Inflate the tracheostomy tube cuff and bag ventilate the patient's lungs with 100% oxygen.
- Auscultate the chest fields for clear breath sounds bilaterally.
- If the patient is less than 12 years of age, a needle cricothyroidotomy should be performed.

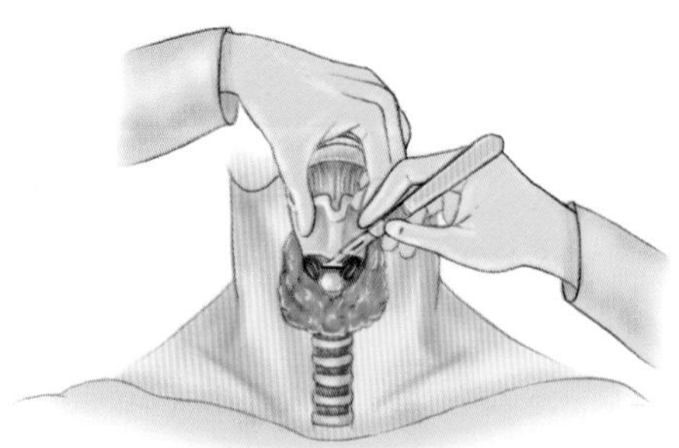

Fig. 8-2

- Insert a 12-gauge angiocatheter with a 5 ml syringe inferiorly at 45 degrees to the skin into the cricothyroid membrane (Fig. 8-3).
- Advance the catheter while aspirating with the syringe. Entry into the tracheal lumen will lead to aspiration of air.
- Advance the catheter over the needle and attach a pediatric ETT adapter.
- Ventilation can be performed through a needle cricothyroidotomy for only 30 to 45 minutes.

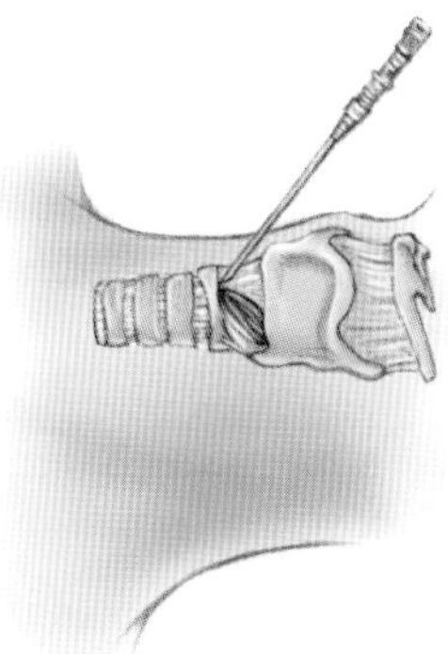

Fig. 8-3

PEARLS

- *Most centers recommend using needle cricothyroidotomy in children less than 12 years of age.*
- *If a tracheal spreader is unavailable, the heel of the scalpel handle can be inserted into the cricothyroid membrane to create the necessary opening.*
- *If a tracheostomy tube is unavailable, an ETT can be inserted into the trachea, and the cuff can then be inflated.*

PITFALLS

- If superficial bleeding occurs, vessels can be either tied off or clamped with hemostats.
- Deep incision of the cricothyroid membrane can injure the esophagus posterior to the posterior wall of the trachea. Consult with a general surgeon after securing the airway.
- Accidental extrusion of a tracheostomy tube within 5 days of original placement is an airway emergency, because tissues collapse and the lumen may not be easily recannulated.

✓ POSTPROCEDURE CHECK

- ❑ Chest radiographs should be taken to confirm proper placement of the ETT (with the end at 1 cm above the carina).
- ❑ Tracheostomy tubes should be securely sewn into the neck skin.

See Appendix B for additional helpful information.

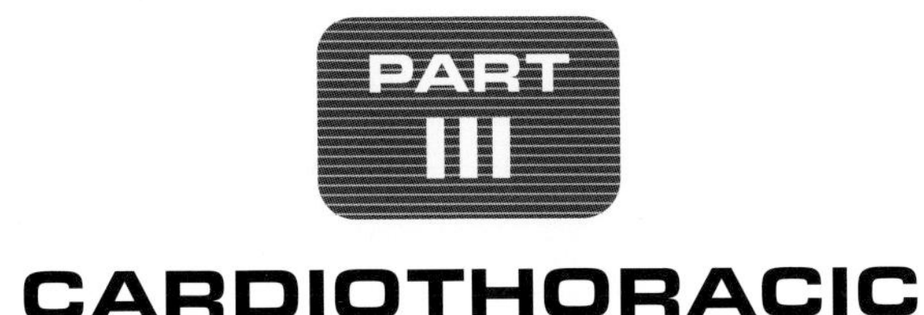

PART III

CARDIOTHORACIC

9

Pericardiocentesis

A 54-year-old man presents after a recent myocardial infarction with jugular venous distention, hypotension, tachycardia, and pulsus paradoxus. *Ultrasound reveals pericardial effusion (Fig. 9-1), equalization of pressures in all four cardiac chambers, decreased stroke volume, and reduced ventricular diastolic filling.*

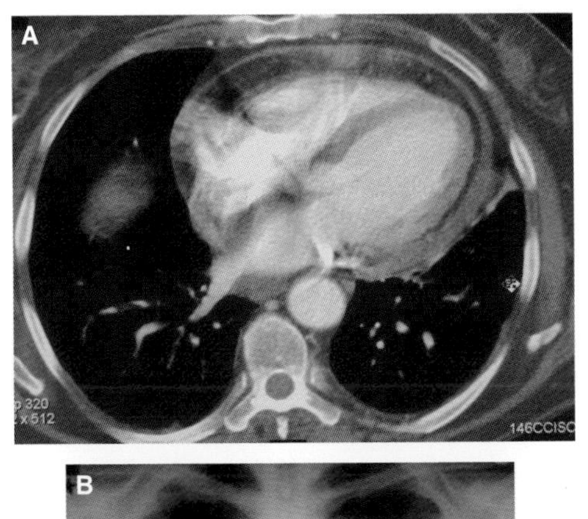

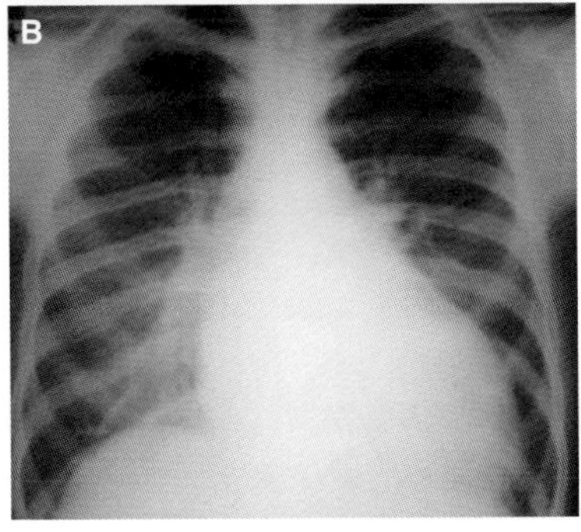

Fig. 9-1 Chest CT scan **(A)** and chest radiograph **(B)** showing pericardial effusion.

INDICATIONS

- To obtain pericardial fluid for laboratory evaluation
- To relieve cardiac tamponade (cardiac compression by fluid within the pericardial sac).

CONTRAINDICATIONS

- Coagulopathy
- After cardiac surgery
- Acute traumatic hemopericardium
- Pericardial effusion that is small (<200 ml) or located posterior or lateral to the heart

SUPPLIES

- 1% lidocaine without epinephrine
- Sterile gloves, towels
- Sterile preparation
- No.10 blade scalpel
- 30 ml syringe
- Alligator connector
- 16- or 18-gauge spinal needle (3 inches long)
- ECG monitor
- 2-0 nylon suture

POSITIONING

- Supine, with the head of the bed elevated 30 degrees above horizontal (Fig. 9-2)

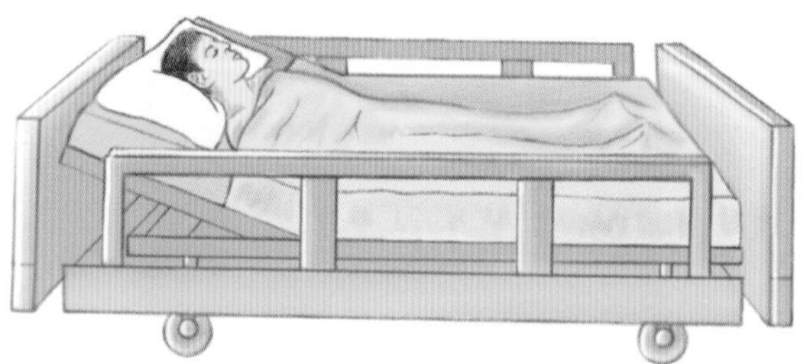

Fig. 9-2

TECHNIQUE

- Prepare and drape the patient's subxiphoid area in a sterile fashion (Fig. 9-3).
- Anesthetize the skin 0.5 cm to the left of the xiphoid tip with 1% lidocaine.
- Attach a precordial limb lead of the ECG machine to the spinal needle with an alligator clamp.
- Connect the 30 ml syringe to the needle and advance (Fig. 9-4).
- Advance the needle below the thorax, aiming toward the left shoulder at a 45-degree angle to the skin.
- Apply constant, gentle aspiration pressure to the needle while advancing it.
- When you encounter the pericardial sac, a negative deflection of the QRS complex will be seen on the ECG (Fig. 9-5).
- Continue to advance the needle past the pericardium; blood or effusion should be encountered.
- If ST-segment elevation is seen, the tip of the needle is in the myocardium. (Withdraw the needle until no ST-segment elevations occur.)

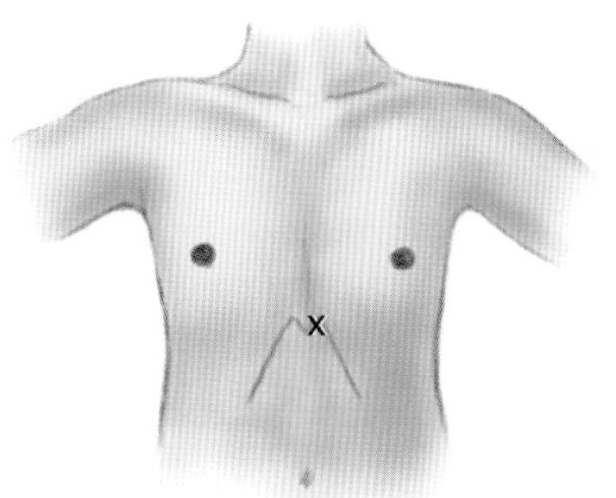

Fig. 9-3

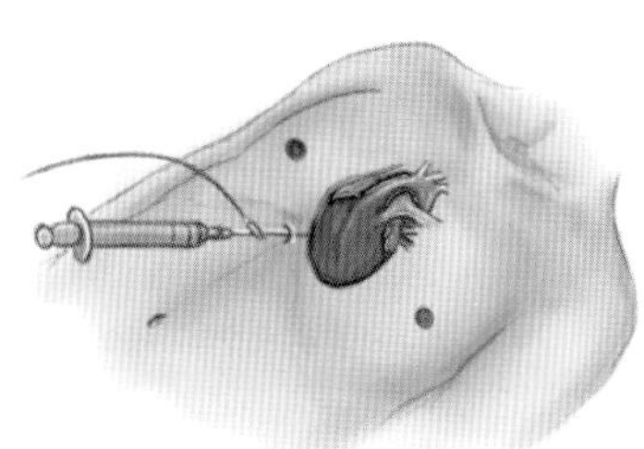

Fig. 9-4

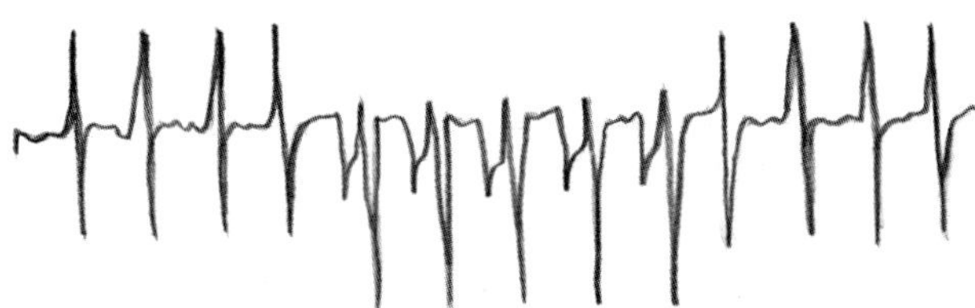

Fig. 9-5 Negative deflection of the QRS complex.

PEARLS

- *Pericardiocentesis should be performed in a monitored setting.*
- *For continuous drainage of fluid, a 16-gauge catheter can be inserted into the pericardial space using the Seldinger technique. The Seldinger technique uses the temporary insertion of a J-tip wire through the insertion needle to maintain a pathway into the pericardial space or vessel lumen. The insertion needle is removed and exchanged with the 16-gauge catheter over the J-tip wire, and the wire is subsequently removed.*
- *Relief of cardiac tamponade leads to a decrease in right atrial pressure and an increase in cardiac output.*

PITFALLS

- A hemothorax or pneumothorax should be monitored with serial chest radiographs and may require tube thoracostomy.
- Arrhythmias can occur, and the needle should be withdrawn if they do. Follow Advanced Cardiac Life Support protocols.
- If an air embolus occurs during the procedure, withdraw air from needle if possible. Then place the patient in a combined left lateral decubitus and Trendelenburg position to trap the air in the right ventricle. Treat with serial chest radiographs to evaluate for absorption, or consider placing a central line and withdrawing the air.

✓ POSTPROCEDURE CHECK

- ❑ The patient should receive cardiac monitoring.

See Appendix C for additional helpful information.

10

THORACENTESIS

A 61-year-old female smoker with a right pulmonary nodule presents with dyspnea and orthopnea. A chest radiograph reveals opacification of the right costophrenic recess.

INDICATIONS

- Pleural effusion leading to dyspnea (Fig. 10-1)
- Diagnostic removal of pleural fluid to determine cause of pleural effusion

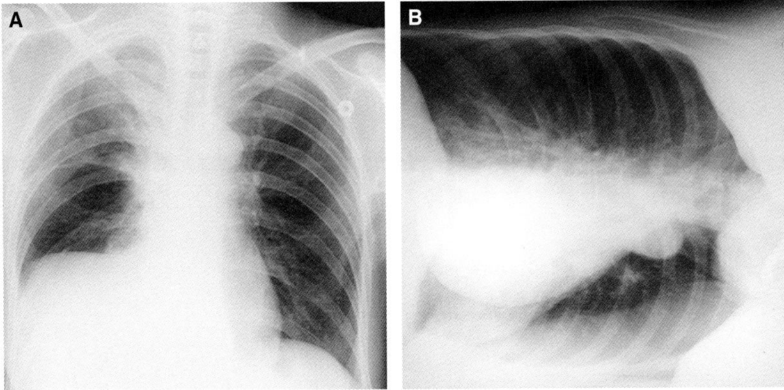

Fig. 10-1 **A,** Chest radiograph showing right pleural effusion. **B,** Chest radiograph with patient in the left lateral decubitus position reveals left pleural effusion layering on the lateral chest wall.

CONTRAINDICATIONS
- Coagulopathy

SUPPLIES
- 1% lidocaine
- Sterile preparation
- Sterile gloves and solution
- 22- and 25-gauge needles
- Long 18-gauge needle for insertion
- 10 ml and 30 ml syringes
- No.10 blade
- Scissors
- 0.035 inch diameter J-wire
- IV tubing
- Three-way stopcock
- Vacuum bottles
- 16-gauge single-lumen central line and dilator

POSITIONING
- Awake patients should be seated at the edge of the bed with arms and head resting on a bedside table. Intubated patients should be in the lateral decubitus position (Fig. 10-2).

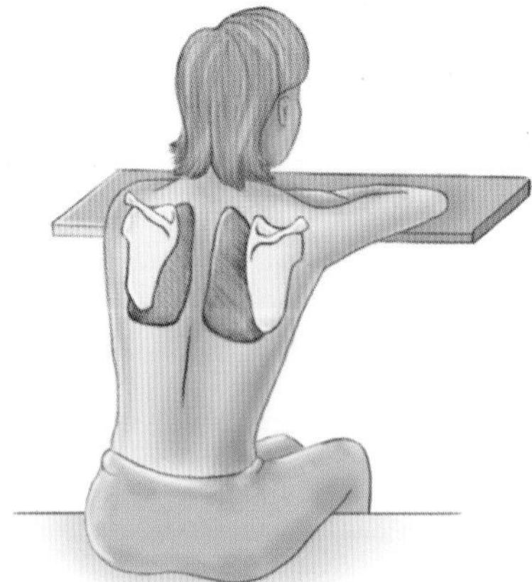

Fig. 10-2

TECHNIQUE

- Attempt to identify the upper and lower margins of the pleural effusion by percussion. Marking with a sterile marker may be helpful.
- Prepare and drape in sterile fashion.
- Locate the rib two interspaces below the top of the effusion—but not below the eighth rib.
- In the midclavicular line on the identified rib, anesthetize the skin with 1% lidocaine using the 25-gauge needle.
- Using the 22-gauge needle, anesthetize the deeper subcutaneous tissue and periosteum of the rib (Fig. 10-3).
- Using the same needle, "walk" along the rib until the needle can be advanced over the rib into the pleural space.
- This should be done with the needle under constant, gentle aspiration until pleural fluid is encountered.
- Withdraw the 22-gauge needle.
- Attach a 10 ml syringe to the 18-gauge needle and insert it into the pleural space in the same manner as for the 22-gauge needle (Fig. 10-4).
- Once pleural fluid is encountered, stabilize the needle shaft on the skin with one hand and remove the syringe with the other hand.
- Immediately cover the needle head with a finger to prevent air from entering.

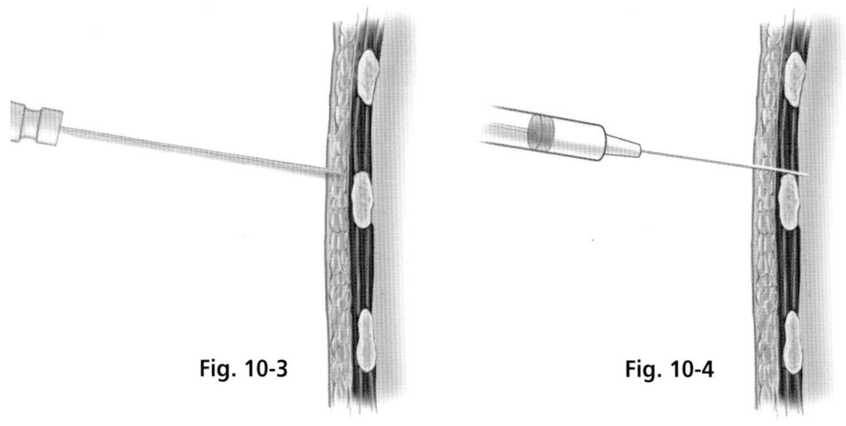

Fig. 10-3

Fig. 10-4

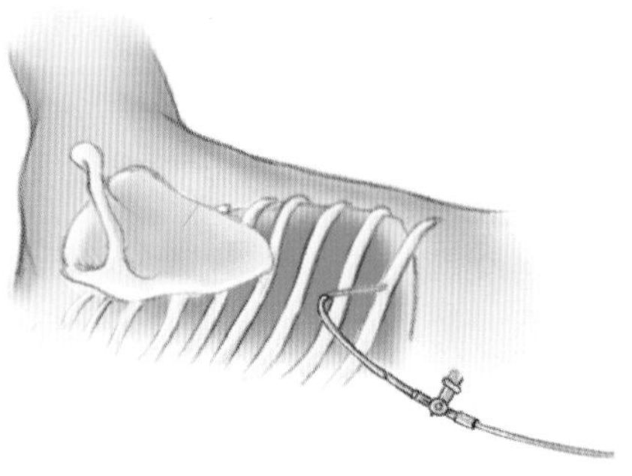

Fig. 10-5

- With the hand that removed the syringe, place a J-wire into the needle and direct it inferiorly into the pleural space using the Seldinger technique (Fig. 10-5) (see Chapter 9).
- Remove the needle, leaving the wire in place.
- Using the scalpel, nick the skin adjacent to the entry site of the J-wire and introduce the dilator over the wire into the subcutaneous tissue.
- Remove the dilator and introduce the 16-gauge catheter over the wire into the pleural space.
- Remove the wire and connect IV tubing, the three-way stopcock, and the suction apparatus to the catheter.
- Draw back from a syringe attached to the stopcock to confirm that the catheter tip remains in the pleural space.
- Apply antibiotic ointment and a heavy occlusive dressing.

PEARLS

- *Percussion is difficult to perform in intubated patients who are in the lateral decubitus position; identifying pleural effusion can be aided with the use of ultrasound.*
- *Aiming the needle in a slightly inferior direction can help guide the J-wire inferiorly as well. With the patient in the sitting position, the effusion should take a dependent, inferior position.*
- *Entering the interspace directly above the rib avoids injury to the intercostal neurovascular bundle that is located directly beneath each rib.*

PITFALLS

- Injury to the intercostal vein or artery during needle insertion may lead to hemothorax. Serial chest radiographs should be obtained, and a tube thoracostomy may be necessary if hemothorax is significant.
- If pleural effusion cannot be drained well because of loculations, a tube thoracostomy may be necessary.
- A small pneumothorax after thoracocentesis can be followed with serial chest radiographs. A large, growing, or symptomatic pneumothorax requires management with tube thoracostomy.
- Entry below the eighth rib risks inadvertent entry into the abdominal cavity.

✓ POSTPROCEDURE CHECK

- ❑ A chest radiograph should be obtained immediately after the procedure to evaluate improvement of pleural effusion and rule out pneumothorax.

See Appendix C for additional helpful information.

11

Tube Thoracostomy: Chest Tube

A 21-year-old man presents with sudden-onset left thoracic pain after a fall and shortness of breath. Chest radiograph reveals loss of lung markings in the left lung and mediastinal shift to the right.

INDICATIONS

- Hemothorax
- Pneumothorax (>15%)
- Pneumothorax (symptomatic, regardless of size) (Fig. 11-1)
- Pleural effusion (persistent)
- Empyema

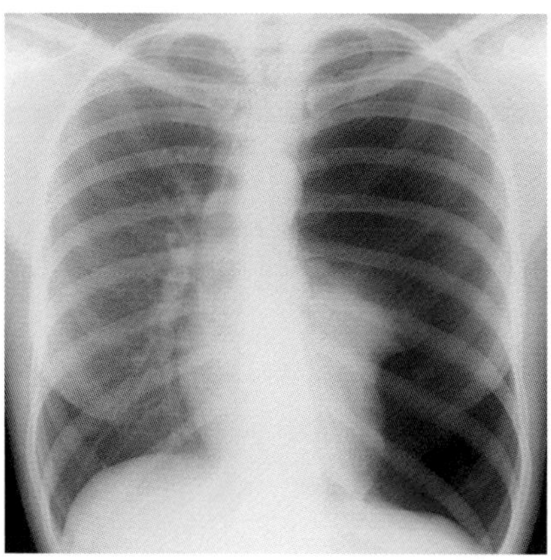

Fig. 11-1 Chest radiograph showing a tension pneumothorax with mediastinal shift.

CONTRAINDICATIONS

- None

SUPPLIES

- Lidocaine; IV sedation optional
- Sterile gloves and towels
- Sterile preparation
- Chest tubes: 12 to 28 Fr for pneumothoraces and 34 to 40 Fr for fluid drainage
- 0 sutures (2)
- No. 15 blade
- Long Kelly clamps (2)
- Long tonsillar clamp
- Heavy scissors
- Chest drainage equipment with water
- Xeroform gauze
- Sterile dressing
- Cloth tape

POSITIONING

- Supine with ipsilateral arm raised above the head (and secured) to expose and widen intercostal spaces (Fig. 11-2)

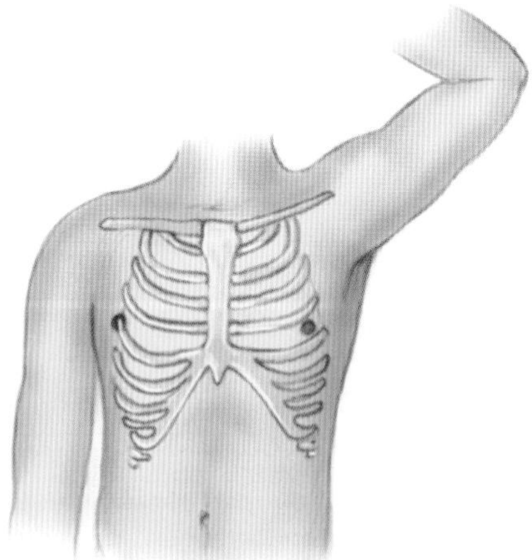

Fig. 11-2

TECHNIQUE

- Identify the fifth intercostal space.
- Mark the space and the sixth rib anterior axillary line.
- Prepare and drape the patient's chest.
- Raise a skin wheal and infiltrate down to the periosteum of the sixth rib.
- Incise 2 to 3 cm parallel to the axis of the ribs over the sixth rib to penetrate the pleura slightly superiorly into the fifth intercostal space (Fig. 11-3).
- Measure the chest tube on the outside of the chest to determine the needed length; remember the needed length on the calibrated tube.
- With a tonsillar clamp, create a tract from the incision to the pleural space (Fig. 11-4).
- Enter the pleural space by rolling over the sixth rib. This avoids the neurovascular bundle on the inferior aspect of the ribs.
- When a rush of air is encountered, the clamp should not be advanced any farther.
- Spread the clamp to widen the tract, allowing for sufficient space to advance the tonsillar clamp and chest tube.
- Insert your index finger into the tract and pleural space. Rotate a flexed finger tip circumferentially to free up any adhesions.

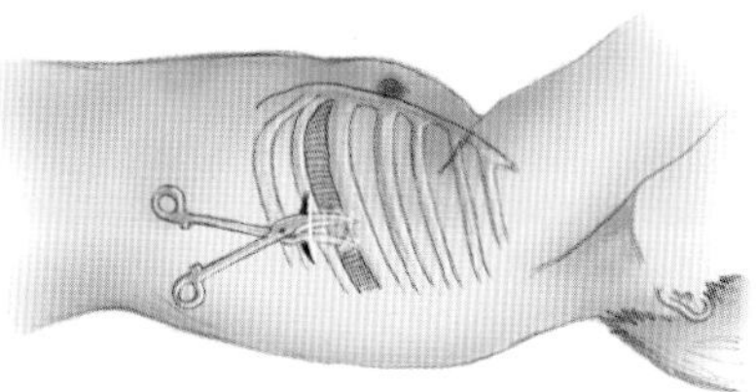

Fig. 11-3

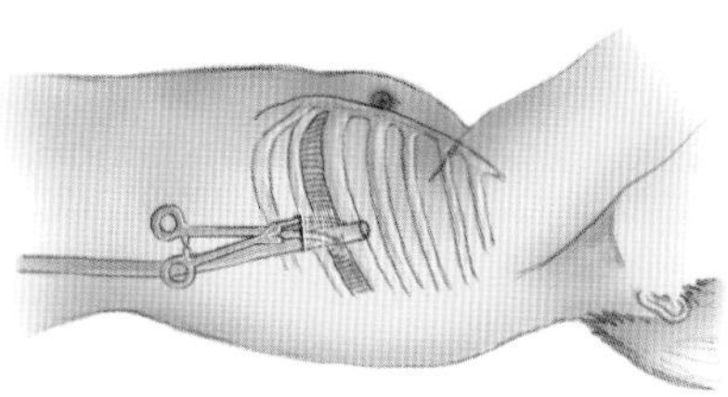

Fig. 11-4

- Place one Kelly clamp on the distal end of the chest tube.
- Insert both through the subcutaneous tract into the pleural cavity (Fig. 11-5).
- Direct the tube posteriorly for fluid drainage or anteriorly for air drainage.
- Open the clamp and insert the tube farther to the premeasured length.
- Place two vertical mattress sutures on each side of the chest tube. One anchors the tube and the other will close the skin when the tube is eventually removed.
- Position Xeroform gauze and a large sterile dressing.

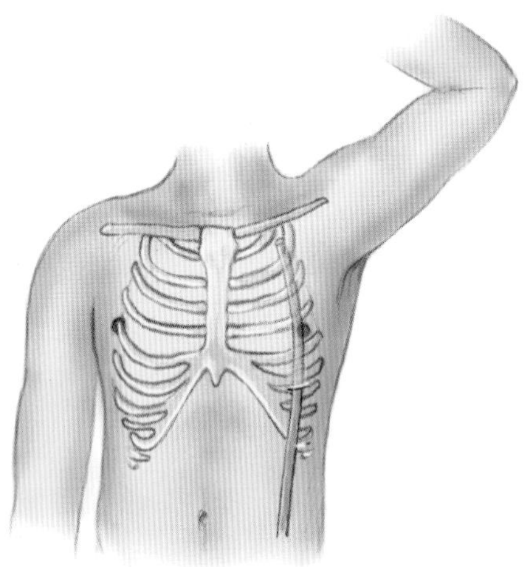

Fig. 11-5

CHEST TUBE REMOVAL

- Cut the suture anchoring tube (do not cut the suture that will reapproximate the skin).
- Place Xeroform gauze and a sterile dressing over the insertion site.
- Ask the patient to take a deep breath and hold it; this prevents further inhalation during tube removal, preventing a pneumothorax.
- Remove the tube during peak inspiration.
- Have an assistant place pressure over the skin while you tie the skin suture.
- Apply a sterile dressing.
- Obtain chest radiographs to rule out a pneumothorax.

PEARLS

- *Secure the patient's arm above his or her head to expand the intercostal spaces.*
- *Err one intercostal space higher if you are unsure of rib spacing. Avoid making the incision below the diaphragm because of the potential for risk to the spleen or liver.*
- *When you are placing the two vertical mattress sutures, place the anchoring suture at the edge of the incision and the skin suture in the middle of the incision.*
- *A large well-taped Xeroform dressing prevents air leakage.*

PITFALLS

- Persistent pneumothorax should be confirmed with serial chest radiographs and treated with additional chest tubes as needed.
- If the abdomen is entered, contact a general surgeon.
- If there is a hemorrhage or lung injury, monitor chest tube output and follow with chest radiographs. If output is >200 ml/hr or a total of 1.5 L, an emergent thoracotomy is indicated.
- In the presence of cardiac arrhythmias, withdraw the chest tube 1 to 4 cm, maintaining proximal chest tube holes in the pleural space.

✓ POSTPROCEDURE CHECK

- ❑ Immediately check the patient's vital signs.
- ❑ Order a chest radiograph immediately after the tube thoracostomy to confirm proper location. Check whether the proximal hole (marked with a break in the radiopaque line) is inside the pleural space (Fig. 11-6).

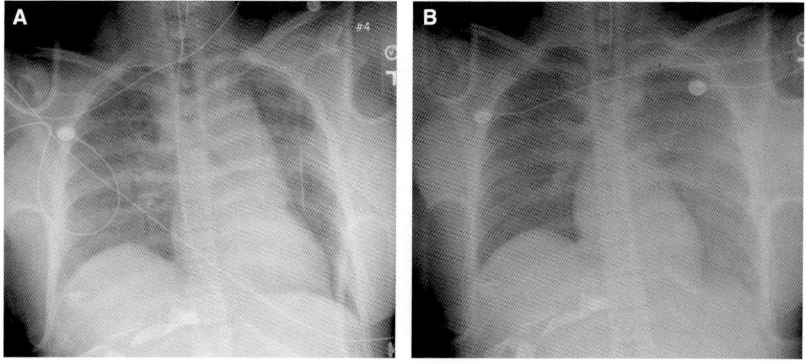

Fig. 11-6 Chest radiographs showing kinked placement **(A)** and proper placement **(B)** of a left chest tube.

See Appendix C for additional helpful information.

12

Emergency Thoracotomy

An 18-year-old man presents with severe hypotension after a gunshot wound to the chest.

INDICATIONS

- Cardiac arrest with penetrating thoracic trauma
- Severe hypotension and penetrating vascular injury

CONTRAINDICATIONS

- Cardiac arrest from blunt trauma

SUPPLIES

- Sterile gloves and towels
- Sterile preparation
- No. 10 blade
- Thoracic wall retractor
- Mayo scissors
- Forceps
- Suction device
- Aortic clamp

POSITIONING

- Supine, with the ipsilateral arm raised above the head (and secured) to expose and widen the intercostal spaces (Fig. 12-1)

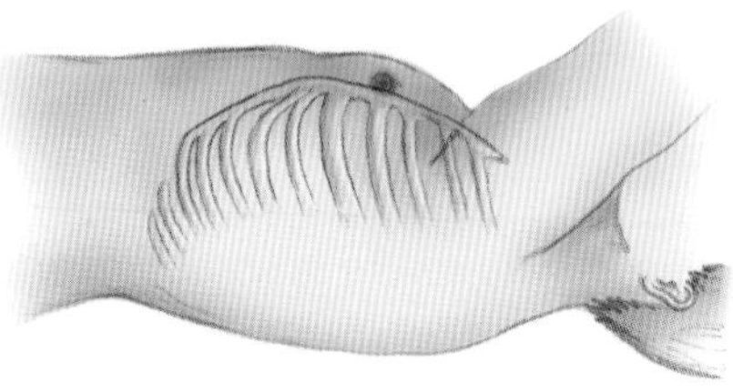

Fig. 12-1

TECHNIQUE

- Identify the left fifth intercostal space (Fig. 12-2).
- Prepare and drape the patient's chest.
- Incise from the level of the midclavicular line, down on the fifth rib as far around the thorax as possible.
- Using the Mayo scissors, open the pleural space above the fifth rib. Keep the scissors partially open while performing this step to avoid pulmonary injury.

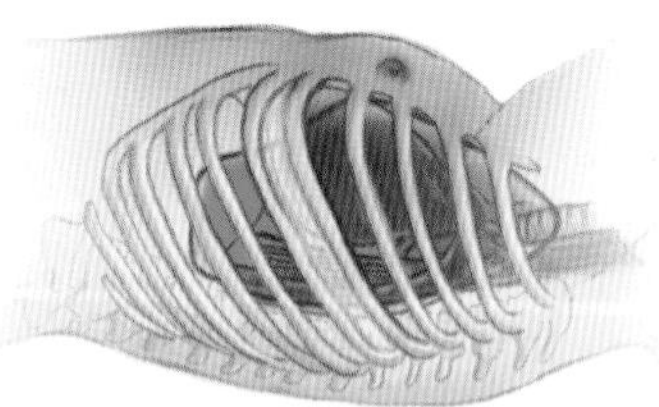

Fig. 12-2

- Insert the thoracic wall retractor (Fig. 12-3).
- Identify the descending aorta by manually elevating the left lung.
- Using blunt dissection with your finger, separate the descending aorta from the posterior mediastinum.
- Place an aortic clamp on the aorta in the region of blunt dissection, taking care to avoid other structures, including the esophagus (anterior to aorta), within your clamp (Fig. 12-4).
- Manually retract the left lung inferiorly to expose the pericardial sac.
- Using Mayo scissors or Metzenbaum scissors, open the pericardial sac with a longitudinal incision.
- The longitudinal incision will prevent injury to the phrenic nerve.
- Suction any clots and deliver the heart into the left hemithorax to evaluate.
- The heart can receive epinephrine injection and/or cardiac massage.
- Take patient emergently to operating room to complete the operation.

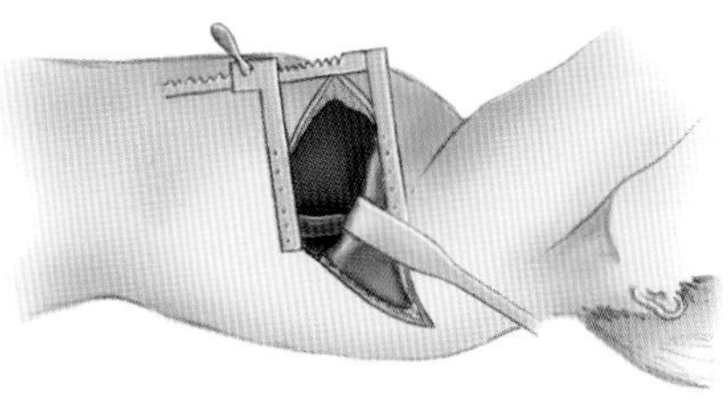

Fig. 12-3

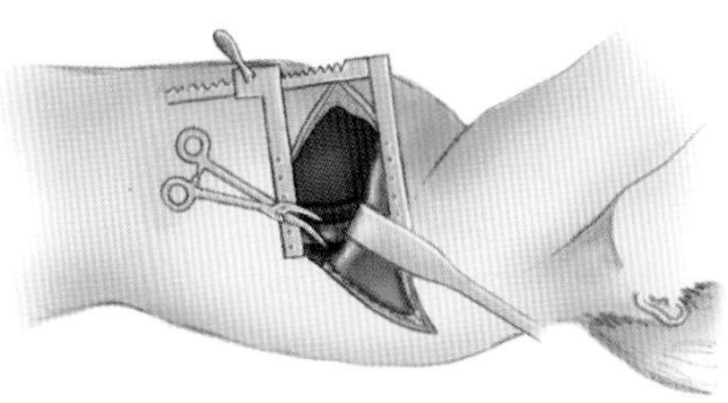

Fig. 12-4

PEARLS

- *Secure the patient's arm above the head for expansion of intercostal spaces.*
- *Err one intercostal space higher if unsure of rib spacing. Avoid making the incision below the diaphragm to minimize risk to the patient's spleen or liver.*
- *An NG tube can be placed and palpated in the esophagus to help distinguish it from the aorta.*
- *The aorta will be pulsatile, whereas the esophagus will not be.*
- *Tears in the heart can be repaired with nonabsorbable sutures.*

PITFALLS

- Failure to make a generous incision limits the ability to manipulate the lungs and heart.
- Beginning the incision too close to the sternum may lead to internal mammary artery injury—necessitating repair in the operating room.

✓ POSTPROCEDURE CHECK

- ❑ This bedside procedure is completed in the operating room with standard postoperative checks.

See Appendix C for additional helpful information.

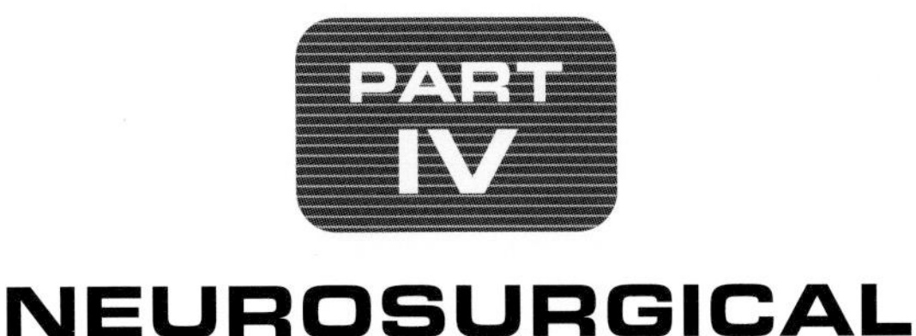

PART IV
NEUROSURGICAL

13

Intracranial Pressure Monitor: Bolt

An 18-year-old man presents with a moderate head injury and requires emergent open tibial fracture washout.

INDICATIONS (Fig. 13-1)

- Severe head injury
- Intracranial pressure (ICP) monitoring required

CONTRAINDICATIONS

- Coagulopathy (INR >1.3 or platelets <80,000/ml)

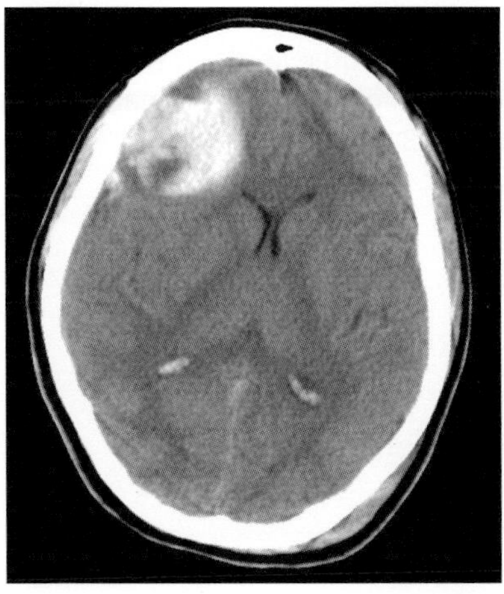

Fig. 13-1 Head CT scan revealing left frontal intracerebral hemorrhage.

SUPPLIES

- 1% lidocaine
- Sterile towels, gloves, gown
- Sterile preparation
- Razor
- Scalpel
- Cranial twist drill
- Intracranial pressure monitor
- Sterile dressing

POSITIONING

- Supine with head of the bed at 30 degrees

TECHNIQUE

- Shave a 2 cm circular area in the right frontal region of the patient's scalp (Fig. 13-2).
- The procedure is performed with the clinician at the head of the patient's bed.
- Prepare and drape the entire site. Place one towel parallel to and on top of the sagittal sinus as a marker for the course of this large vein.
- Kocher's point is 12 cm posteriorly in the midpupillary line and 2.5 cm lateral to midline.
- Make a 0.5 cm parasagittal stab incision with Kocher's point in the middle of the incision.
- Using the twist drill at a 90-degree angle to the skull, make a hole in the skull; the bit for placing the Camino monitor is smaller than the bit for ventricular catheter placement (Fig. 13-3).

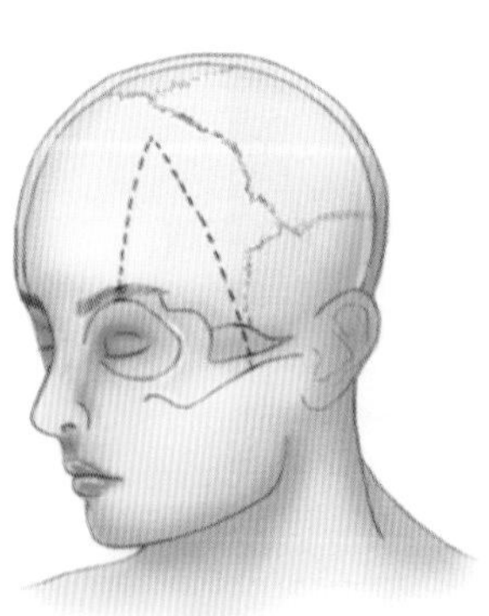

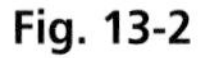

Fig. 13-2

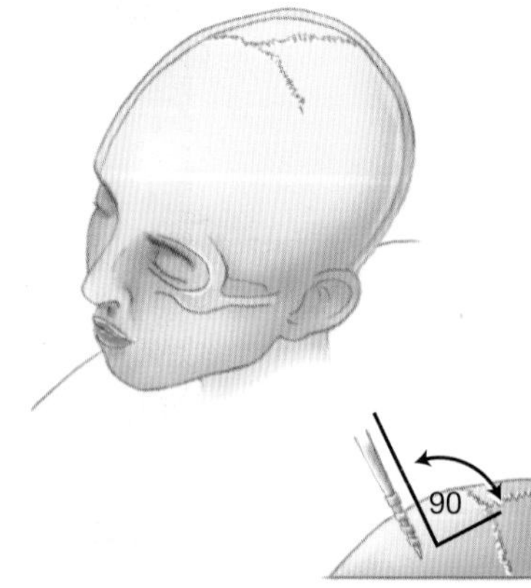

Fig. 13-3

- Take care not to plunge into the brain as you drill past the inner table of the calvaria.
- Irrigate the wound and penetrate the dura (if not opened by the drill) with a needle or stylet.
- With your left hand, palpate the patient's nose to establish midline.
- Screw a bolt into the calvaria (nearly to the hub of the bolt) (Figs. 13-4 and 13-5).
- Loosen cap and insert the ICP monitor probe 5 cm into the bolt and lock the cap (this grasps the monitor probe and prevents migration into the brain).
- Calibrate the ICP monitor and confirm ICP waveform.
- Place a clear plastic hub over the bolt and monitor.
- Apply sterile dressing.

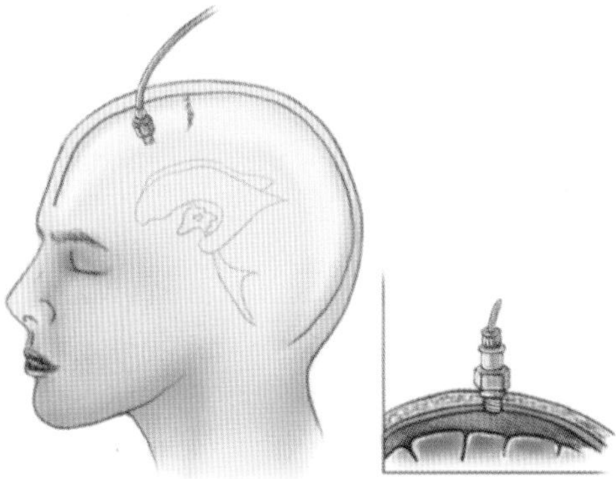

Fig. 13-4

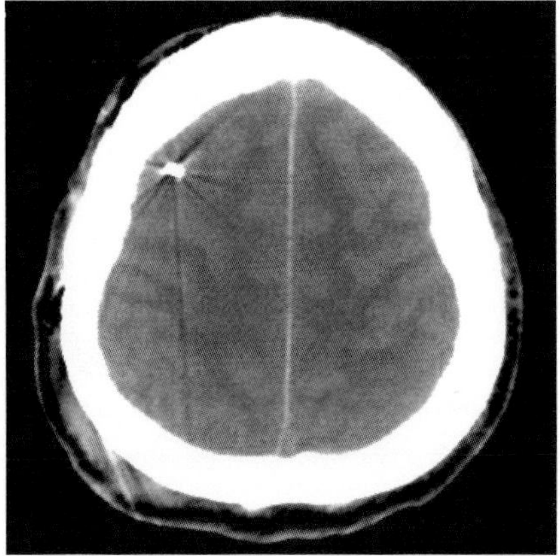

Fig. 13-5 Head CT image. The position of the right ICP monitor probe is adequate in the superficial cortex; it should be placed no deeper than 1 cm.

PEARLS

- *Placing the Camino monitor on the side of maximum injury provides the most accurate ICP measurements.*
- *It is helpful to mark Kocher's point with a measuring tape.*
- *Rotating the drill handle while removing the drill bit from the skull helps clear out bone debris.*
- *If there is a potential need for ventricular drainage, insert bolt 2 cm anterior to Kocher's point for ventricular catheter placement.*

PITFALLS

- The Camino monitor does not measure ICP changes from temporal lobe masses very well.
- If the patient has a seizure or sudden deterioration during neurologic examination, or if frank blood exits the catheter, an intracerebral hemorrhage may have occurred. Abort the procedure and order a *stat* CT scan of the head to evaluate for hemorrhage. Large hemorrhages with midline shift may need to be evacuated in the operating room.

✓ POSTPROCEDURE CHECK

- ☐ Patients with Camino monitors need to have neurologic checks every hour and should be in the ICU.

See Appendix D for additional helpful information.

14

Lumbar Puncture: Spinal Tap

A 31-year-old man presents with neck stiffness and photophobia. Head CT scan does not reveal any intracranial mass lesion.

INDICATIONS

- To obtain a cerebrospinal fluid (CSF) specimen
- To drain CSF for communicating hydrocephalus or pseudotumor cerebri
- Administer intrathecal antibiotics, chemotherapeutic agents, or contrast medium

CONTRAINDICATIONS

- Any patient without intracranial imaging
- Obstructive hydrocephalus
- Intracranial tumor, abscess, or hematoma
- Coagulopathy
- Skin infection over insertion site
- Tethered cord

SUPPLIES

- 1% lidocaine
- Sterile gloves and towels
- Sterile preparation
- 22- and 25-gauge needles
- 5 ml syringe
- 18- or 22-gauge spinal needle (long needle with stylet)
- Manometer
- CSF collection tubes
- Dressings

POSITIONING

- Left lateral decubitus in the fetal position at the edge of the bed (Fig. 14-1)

Alternate Positioning

- Sitting with arms and shoulders on a table (Fig. 14-2)

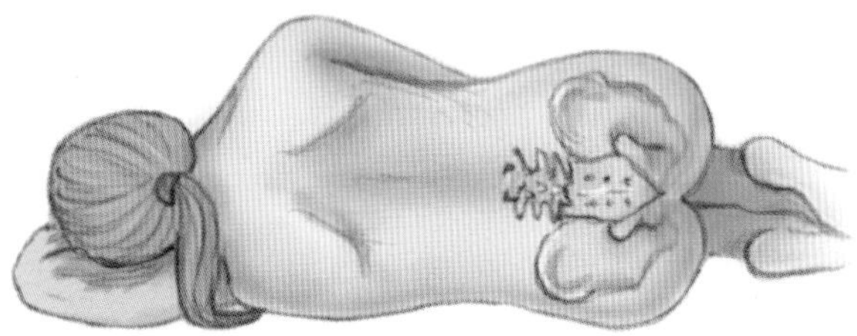

Fig. 14-1

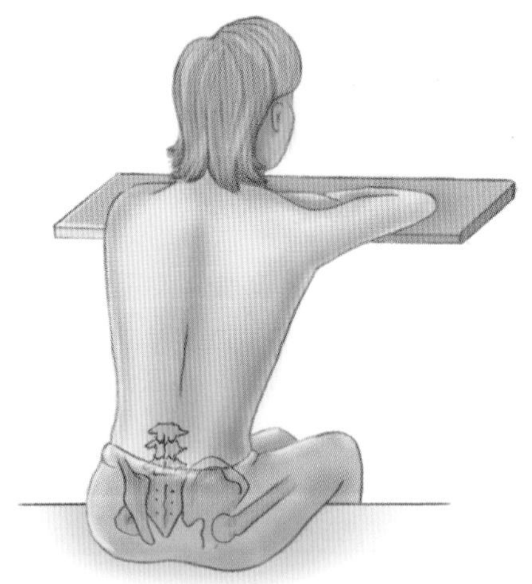

Fig. 14-2

TECHNIQUE

- Prepare and drape the entire lower back.
- The insertion site is the L4-5 interspace, which can be approximated by a horizontal line across the superior iliac crests.
- Using the 25-gauge needle and 1% lidocaine, anesthetize the skin over the insertion site.
- Anesthetize the deeper subcutaneous tissue with 1% lidocaine and a 22-gauge needle.
- Insert the spinal needle with a stylet along the anesthetized tract toward the spinal canal (Fig. 14-3).
- Never insert the spinal needle without the stylet in place.
- The trajectory is approximately 30 degrees to the skin in a cranial direction. Aim between the spinous processes (which can be palpated) in the midline toward the interspace created by the lamina above and below (Fig. 14-4).
- Degenerative spine disease can lead to bony overgrowth and decreased interspace size.
- The ligamentum flavum is a point of resistance encountered before entering the spinal canal and thecal sac.
- If bone is encountered, withdraw the spinal needle and stylet to the skin and change the trajectory to slightly more or less oblique.
- If the needle is in the spinal column, remove the stylet and observe for CSF egress.

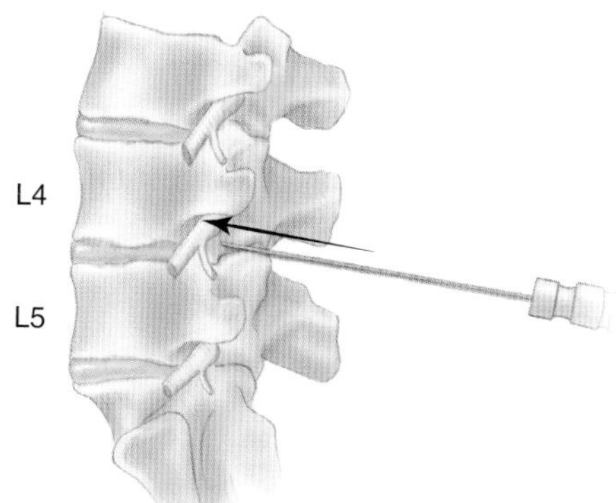

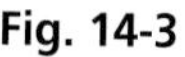

Fig. 14-3

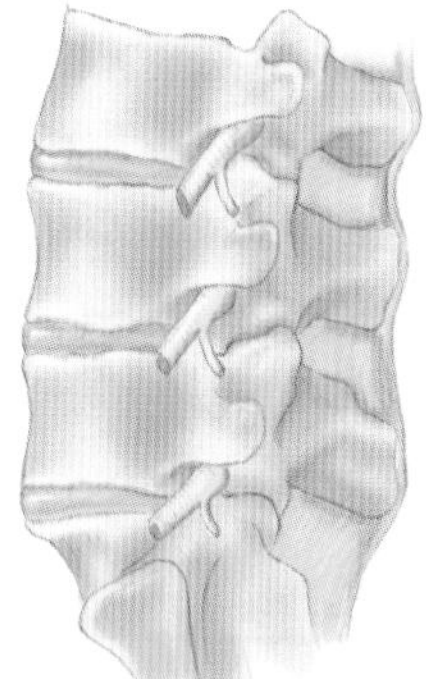

Fig. 14-4

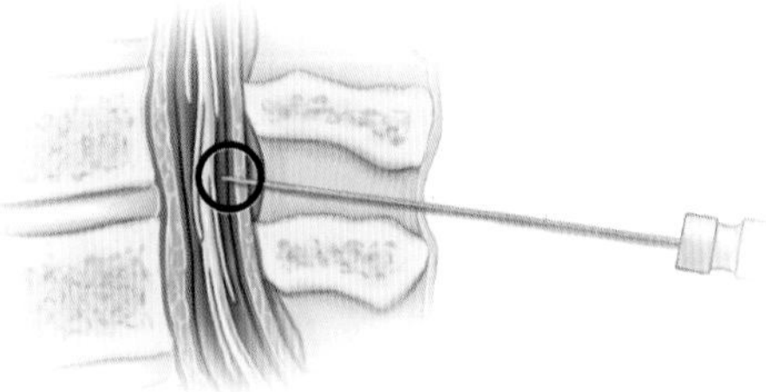

Fig. 14-5

- The needle can be withdrawn 1 cm without removing the stylet, and occasionally the needle tip will reenter the thecal sac and CSF egress will occur. This occurs if the needle has penetrated both walls of the thecal sac (Fig. 14-5).
- Attach manometer and obtain pressure measurement.
- Collect CSF in four collection tubes.
- Replace the stylet and remove the needle.
- Apply sterile dressing.

PEARLS

- *Hyperflexion of the patient's spine provides the greatest access to the spinal interspace.*
- *If unsuccessful at L4-5, proceed to the space below, and, if still unsuccessful, proceed to the space above L4-5.*
- *If the clinician is left-handed, it is easier for the patient to be in the right lateral decubitus position.*
- *Raising the patient's head can help deliver more CSF to the lumbar thecal sac.*
- *Blood-tinged CSF is not uncommon; the blood usually abates as more CSF is removed.*

PITFALLS

- The conus medullaris is at approximately L2, and needle insertion at this level or above can lead to spinal cord injury.
- Inserting the spinal needle can lead to nerve root injury (awake patients report numbness or tingling). If this occurs, the needle should be withdrawn and a different insertion site chosen.
- Rare cases of aortic or vascular puncture have been reported. If this occurs, withdraw the needle and consult with vascular surgery.
- Removal of spinal fluid can lead to headaches. This is usually self-limiting, but keep the patient supine.
- If the patient experiences rapid neurologic deterioration, it is a neurosurgical emergency. The patient may have herniated or developed a subdural hematoma. Stop the procedure, elevate the head of the bed, intubate, and call neurosurgery.

✓ POSTPROCEDURE CHECK

- ❑ Neurologic checks should be obtained for several hours after lumbar puncture.

See Appendix D for additional helpful information.

15

Lumbar Drain

A 44-year-old woman presents with a 1-week history of CSF rhinorrhea after head trauma and known cribriform fracture.

INDICATIONS

- Treatment of CSF leaks or fistulas after neurologic surgery or trauma
- Temporary CSF diversion for communicating hydrocephalus

CONTRAINDICATIONS

- Any patient without intracranial imaging
- Obstructive hydrocephalus
- Intracranial tumor, abscess, or hematoma
- Coagulopathy (platelets <50,000/ml)
- Skin infection over insertion site
- Tethered cord

SUPPLIES

- 1% lidocaine
- Sterile gloves and towels
- Sterile preparation
- 22- and 25-gauge needles
- 5 ml syringe
- 14-gauge Touhy needle
- Lumbar drain and bag
- Manometer
- CSF collection tubes
- Large transparent dressing

POSITIONING

- Left lateral decubitus in the fetal position at the edge of the bed (see Fig. 14-1 on p. 62)

TECHNIQUE

- Prepare and drape the entire lower back.
- The insertion site is the L4-5 interspace, which can be approximated by a horizontal line across the superior iliac crests.
- Using the 25-gauge needle and 1% lidocaine, anesthetize the skin over the insertion site.
- Anesthetize the deeper subcutaneous tissue with 1% lidocaine and a 22-gauge needle.
- Insert the Touhy needle with the stylet along the anesthetized tract toward the spinal canal (Fig. 15-1).
- Never insert the spinal needle without the stylet in place.
- The bevel of the needle should be facing the ceiling for this part of the procedure.
- The trajectory is approximately 30 degrees to the skin in a cranial direction. Aim between the spinous processes (which can be palpated) in the midline toward the interspace created by the lamina above and below (Fig. 15-2).
- Degenerative spine disease can lead to bony overgrowth and decreased interspace size.

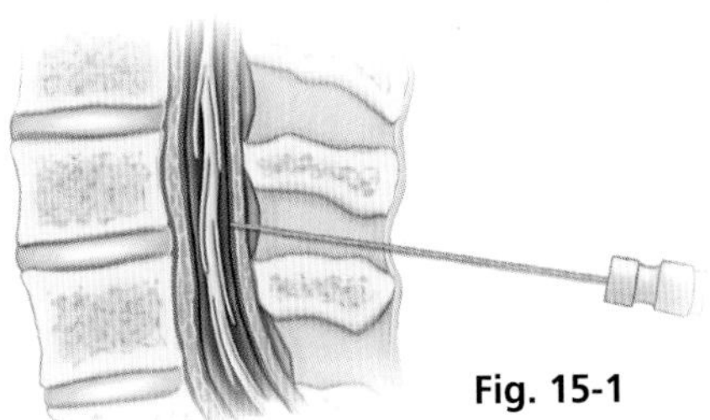

Fig. 15-1

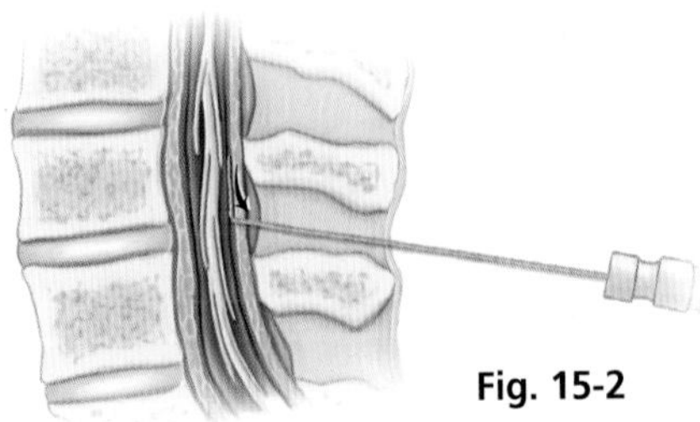

Fig. 15-2

- The ligamentum flavum is a point of resistance encountered before entering the spinal canal and thecal sac.
- If bone is encountered, withdraw the Touhy needle and stylet to the skin and change the trajectory to slightly more or less oblique.
- If the needle is in the spinal column, remove the stylet and observe for CSF egress.
- The needle can be withdrawn 1 cm without removing the stylet, and occasionally the needle tip will reenter the thecal sac and CSF egress will occur. This occurs if the needle has penetrated both walls of the thecal sac.
- If good CSF flow is observed, turn the bevel of the needle toward the patient's head to help introduce the catheter into the thecal sac.
- Insert the lumbar drain into the needle to approximately 10 to 25 cm.
- Confirm that CSF can be seen percolating from the distal external end of the lumbar drain. This confirms that the drain is in the thecal sac.
- Remove the Touhy needle without withdrawing the lumbar drainage catheter.
- Secure the drain to the patient's back and have the distal end extend to the patient's flank or trapezius area. The entire course of the drain should be covered with a sterile dressing.
- Connect the hub to the drain and attach IV tubing to the hub.

PEARLS

- *Hyperflexion of the patient's spine provides the greatest access to the spinal interspace.*
- *If unsuccessful at L4-5, proceed to the space below, and, if still unsuccessful, proceed to the space above L4-5.*
- *If the clinician is left-handed, the procedure is easier if the patient is in the right lateral decubitus position.*
- *Raising the patient's head can help deliver more CSF to the lumbar thecal sac.*
- *Blood-tinged CSF in not uncommon; the blood usually abates as more CSF is removed.*
- *Patients should be on antibiotics with gram-positive coverage while the lumbar drain is in place.*
- *If difficulty is encountered when feeding the drain into the lumbar space, it may help to depress the needle toward the legs to create a less acute angle of entry into the thecal sac.*

PITFALLS

- The conus medullaris is at approximately L2, and needle insertion at this level or above can lead to spinal cord injury.
- Insertion of a spinal needle can lead to nerve root injury (awake patients report numbness or tingling). If this occurs, the needle should be withdrawn and a different insertion site chosen.
- Rare cases of aortic or vascular puncture have been reported. If this occurs, withdraw the needle and consult vascular surgery.
- Removal of spinal fluid can lead to headaches. This is usually self-limiting, but keep the patient supine.
- If the patient experiences rapid neurologic decline, it is a neurosurgical emergency. The patient may have herniated or developed a subdural hematoma. Stop the procedure, elevate the head of the bed, intubate the patient, and call neurosurgery.

✓ POSTPROCEDURE CHECK

- ❑ Neurologic checks should be obtained for several hours after lumbar puncture.
- ❑ The lumbar drain should be clamped while the patient is ambulating.
- ❑ CSF drainage should not exceed 350 ml/day.

See Appendix D for additional helpful information.

16

Shunt Tap

A 23-year-old woman with a history of hydrocephalus treated with a right ventriculoperitoneal shunt presents with persistent headache and vomiting. A CT scan of her head reveals ventricular dilation.

INDICATIONS

- Obtain sample of CSF
- Emergent CSF removal in patients with neurologic deterioration from hydrocephalus
- Evaluate shunt function or intraventricular pressure (Fig. 16-1)
- Injection of antibiotics, chemotherapeutic agents, or contrast medium

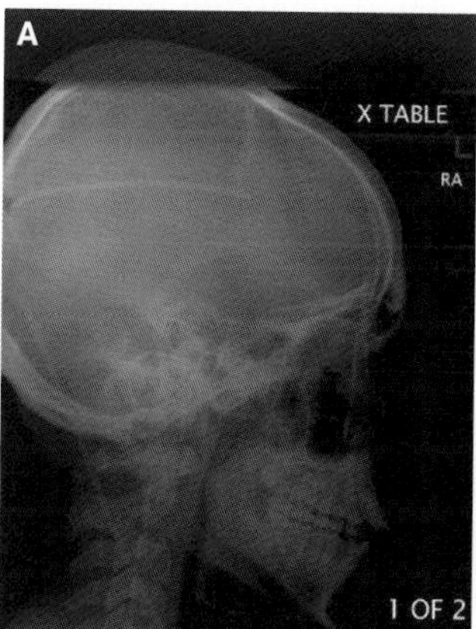

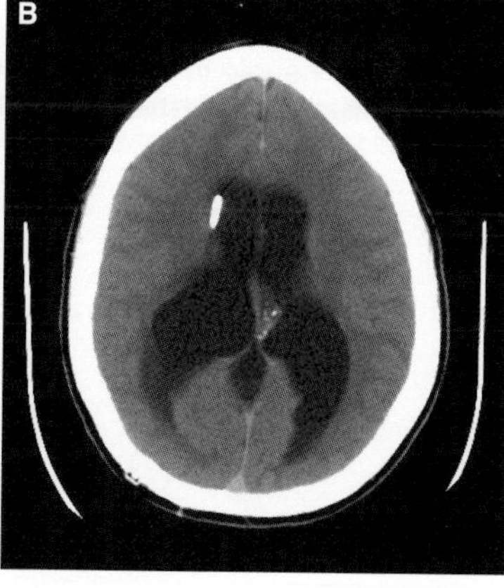

Fig. 16-1 **A,** Skull radiograph. The path of the shunt apparatus should be evaluated for a break or disconnection; neither is present here. **B,** CT scan of the head. Patient has hydrocephalus (ventriculomegaly), and the proximal tip of the shunt is in an adequate position in the right frontal ventricle. The diagnosis is shunt malfunction.

CONTRAINDICATIONS

- Skin infection over shunt bubble
- Collapsed ventricles

SUPPLIES

- Sterile gloves and towels
- Sterile preparation
- 23- or 25-gauge butterfly needle
- 10 ml syringes
- Manometer

POSITIONING

- Supine for frontal bubbles or sitting for occipital bubbles

TECHNIQUE

- Shunt bubbles (Fig. 16-2) are located near the incision sites into which the shunts are inserted, typically in the frontal or occipital region.
- Palpate the scalp and locate the shunt bubble, keeping in mind that some patients have multiple shunts.
- Prepare and drape the shunt bubble area.
- Palpate the shunt bubble of interest, keeping in mind that patients may have several shunts.
- Holding a butterfly needle in one hand and aspirating the syringe with the other hand, insert the needle into the center of the bubble at a slightly oblique angle (Fig. 16-3).

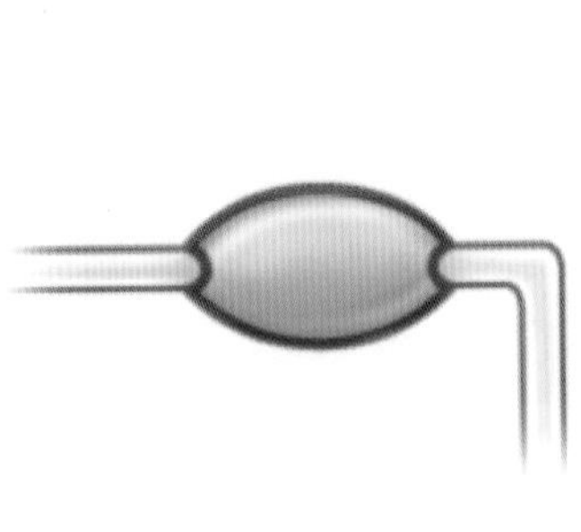

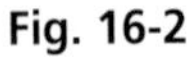

Fig. 16-2

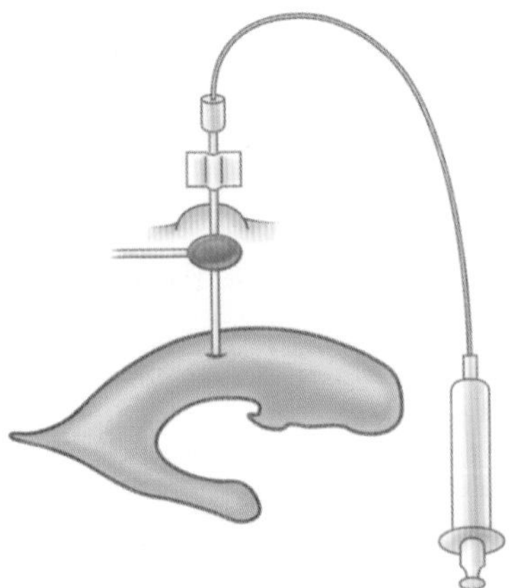

Fig. 16-3

- Once the needle is inside the bubble, CSF should flow into the syringe.
- If unable to obtain CSF, attempt to insert the needle deeper, or withdraw the needle and attempt insertion into other areas of the shunt bubble.
- If unable to aspirate CSF and you are confident of entry into the bubble, proximal shunt (ventricular catheter) obstruction is likely.

PEARLS

- *Numerous shunt types exist, and if you are not confident of the location of the shunt bubble, do not insert the needle into the scalp above the shunt apparatus*
- *Always obtain a CT scan of the head to evaluate ventricular size, and always obtain a series of shunt radiographs to exclude a broken shunt.*
- *If the patient experiences sudden neurologic deterioration, consult neurosurgery. Emergent ventricular decompression can be achieved by bedside externalization of the shunt or ventriculostomy.*
- *A lumbar puncture can be performed to obtain CSF and does not risk seeding the shunt apparatus.*

PITFALLS

- Shunt tap is not a benign procedure. Each attempt can inoculate the cerebrospinal space and the shunt apparatus. If performing a shunt tap for infectious workup, definitively exclude all other sources of infection.
- Removing more than 20 ml of CSF can lead to subdural hematomas if the ventricle is decompressed too rapidly.

✓ POSTPROCEDURE CHECK

- ❑ Neurologic checks should be performed after a shunt tap.

See Appendix D for additional helpful information.

17

Fontanelle Tap

A 4-week-old male infant presents with germinal matrix hemorrhage and ventricular dilation.

INDICATIONS

- Infant younger than 18 months with an open fontanelle (unfused cranial sutures)
- Severe hydrocephalus requiring urgent decompression
- Life-threatening ventriculoperitoneal shunt obstruction and removal of CSF is required.

CONTRAINDICATIONS

- Coagulopathy

SUPPLIES

- Sterile gloves and towels
- Sterile preparation
- Sterile marking pen
- 22-gauge spinal needle
- 22-gauge butterfly needle
- 5 ml syringe

POSITIONING

- Supine with the head slightly raised

TECHNIQUE

- Prepare and drape the patient's forehead and anterior skull.
- Palpate the anterior fontanelle and mark the midline (the course of the superior sagittal sinus) with a marking pen.
- The insertion site should be as lateral as possible but still within the fontanelle opening.
- With one hand, grasp the butterfly needle and insert it perpendicularly into the scalp immediately adjacent to the coronal suture.
- Insert the needle up to 2 to 3 cm until CSF egress is encountered; if no CSF is encountered, remove the needle and redirect.

PEARLS

- *Marking the midline helps orient the clinician to the course of the superior sagittal sinus.*
- *Reviewing ultrasound images helps the clinician visualize the size of the ventricles.*

PITFALLS

- Hemorrhage during needle insertion should lead to immediate cessation of the procedure and emergent CT scan of the head or emergent ultrasound imaging to evaluate the size of the hemorrhage and mass effect.
- Any changes in mental status, pupils, or motor examination findings should be evaluated by ultrasound or CT scans; if mass effect is seen from hemorrhage or herniation, neurosurgery should be consulted emergently.

✓ POSTPROCEDURE CHECK

- ❑ Neurologic checks should be performed every hour for at least the first 4 hours after fontanelle tap.

See Appendix D for additional helpful information.

18

VENTRICULOSTOMY

A 48-year-old man presents with severe headache, and a head CT scan reveals dense subarachnoid hemorrhage.

INDICATIONS

- Severe head injury
- Subarachnoid hemorrhage (Fig. 18-1)
- Intraventricular hemorrhage
- Need of ICP monitoring and treatment of elevated intracranial pressures

CONTRAINDICATIONS

- Coagulopathy (INR >1.3 or platelets <80,000/ml)

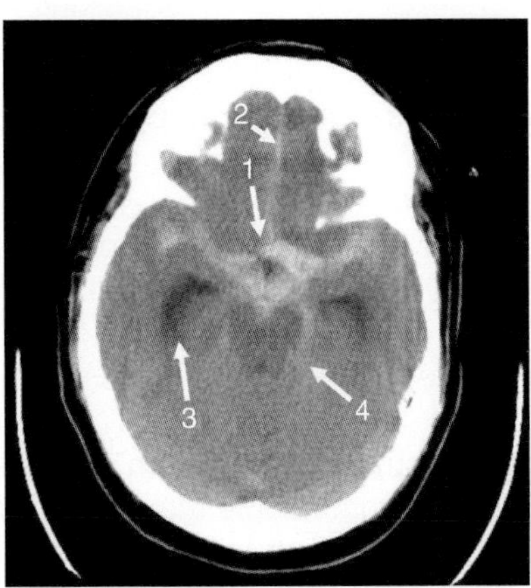

Fig. 18-1 CT scan of the head. Subarachnoid hemorrhage (*1, 2,* and *4*) and dilated temporal horn of the ventricle *(3)*.

SUPPLIES

- 1% lidocaine
- Sterile towels, gloves, and gown
- Sterile preparation
- Razor
- Scalpel
- Cranial twist drill
- Ventricular catheter and IV tubing with ICP monitor
- 2-0 nylon suture and needle driver
- Sterile dressing

POSITIONING

- Supine with the head of the bed at 30 degrees

TECHNIQUE

- Shave the right frontal region of the patient's scalp (see Fig. 13-2 on p. 58).
- The procedure is performed with the neurosurgeon at the head of the patient's bed.
- Prepare and drape the entire site. Place one towel parallel to and on top of the sagittal sinus as a marker for the course of this large vein.
- Drape the patient's face as well, allowing for palpation of the nose during catheter placement.
- Open the ventricular catheter kit and use measuring tape to locate Kocher's point.
- Kocher's point is 12 cm posteriorly in the midpupillary line and 2.5 cm lateral to the midline.
- Make a 2 cm parasagittal incision, with Kocher's point in the middle of the incision.
- Insert a self-retaining retractor.
- Using the heel of the scalpel handle, scrape the periosteum off the cranium.
- Using the twist drill at a 90-degree angle to the skull, make a hole in the skull (see Fig. 13-3 on p. 58).
- Take care not to plunge the drill into the brain as you drill past the inner table of the calvaria.
- Irrigate the wound and penetrate the dura with a needle (if not opened by the drill), and widen slightly to accommodate the ventricular catheter.
- Insert a tunneler through the scalp from within the wound, and exit 3 cm lateral to the wound near the temporalis region.
- Maintain the heel of the introducer within the wound.

- With the left hand, palpate the patient's nose to establish the midline.
- Grasp the catheter and stylet as one apparatus, and position it inside the skull hole (Fig. 18-2).
- The trajectory of insertion is 90 degrees to the skull, aiming toward the medial canthus of the ipsilateral eye and never deeper than 7 cm (Fig. 18-3).
- Insert the catheter and observe for CSF egress after removing the stylet.
- If no CSF is encountered, remove the catheter (without reinserting the stylet) and repeat attempted insertion.

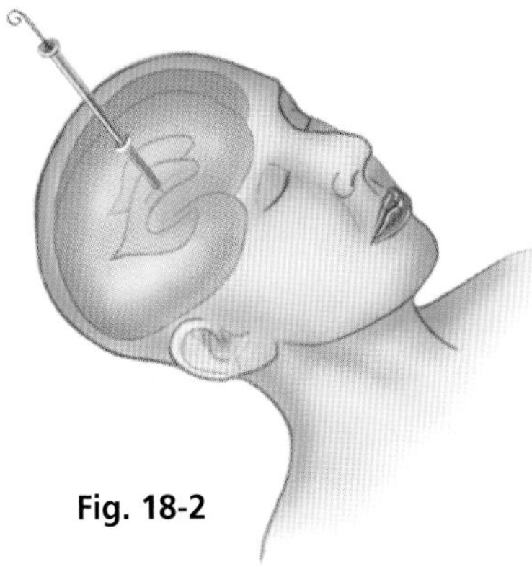

Fig. 18-2

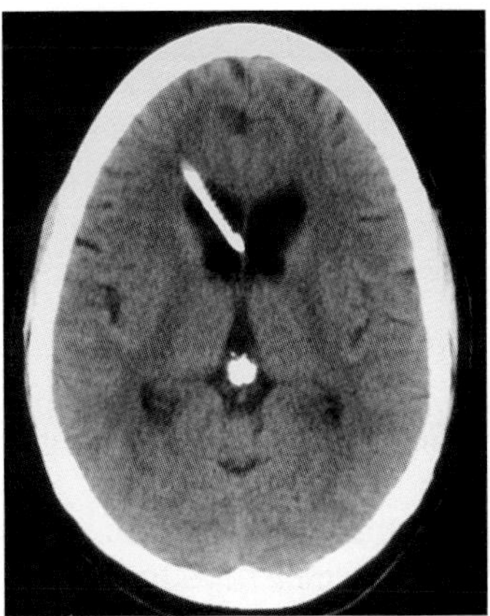

Fig. 18-3 CT scan of the head. Adequate placement of ventriculostomy catheter in the right lateral ventricle (frontal horn); optimal placement is in the third ventricle.

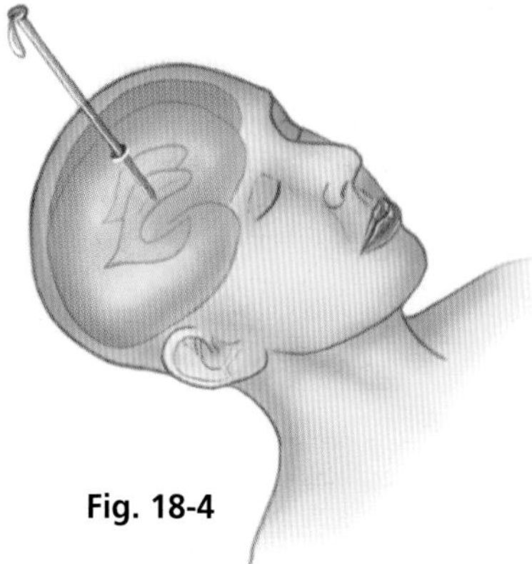

Fig. 18-4

- If CSF egress is seen from the catheter, attach the catheter to the hub of the tunneler and tunnel under the scalp to exit near the temporalis region (Fig. 18-4).
- Care must be taken during tunneling of the catheter to not withdraw or introduce the catheter any further into the brain and ventricle.
- Remove the tunneler from the catheter and check again for CSF egress.
- Connect the catheter to the hub and IV tubing and to the drainage bag.
- Close the incision with a running 2-0 nylon suture, taking care to not injure the catheter below in the wound.
- Anchoring sutures can be placed around the catheter that has been tunneled.
- Apply sterile dressing.

PEARLS

- *If the patient has a tumor, intracerebral hemorrhage, arteriovenous malformation (AVM), or significant ventricular hemorrhage on the right side, a left frontal ventriculostomy should be performed.*
- *It is helpful to use a measuring tape to mark Kocher's point.*
- *Rotating the drill handle while removing the drill bit from the skull helps clear out bone debris.*
- *Mass effect from the trauma of tumors can shift the ventricular system, and the trajectory of insertion may have to be altered slightly.*
- *Irrigate the IV tubing with saline solution to remove air bubbles that may limit CSF egress through the drainage system.*
- *Suspected ventriculitis should be managed with vancomycin and a third-generation cephalosporin.*

PITFALLS

- There is a 1 in 70 risk of intracerebral hemorrhage from placing a ventricular catheter.
- If the patient has a seizure or sudden onset of neurologic deterioration, or if frank blood egresses from the catheter, an intracerebral hemorrhage may have occurred. Abort the procedure and immediately obtain CT scans of the head to evaluate for hemorrhage. Large hemorrhages with a midline shift may need to be evacuated in the operating room.
- Never insert the ventricular catheter more than 7 cm (there is a potential for penetrating vascular structures).
- If the ventricular catheter cannot be placed into the frontal horn of the ventricle after three attempts, abort the procedure and place a Camino monitor.
- Patients should be on gram-positive antibiotics while the catheter is in place. CSF samples can be obtained from the hub every 3 days to evaluate for ventriculitis.

✓ POSTPROCEDURE CHECK

- ☐ Patients with ventricular catheters need to have neurologic checks every hour and should be in the ICU.

See Appendix D for additional helpful information.

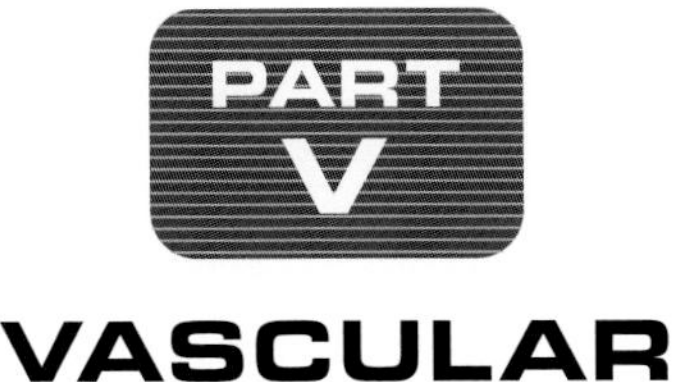

VASCULAR

19

Saphenous Vein Cutdown

A 38-year-old woman presents with severe burn injury and dehydration. Attempts to obtain central venous access have been unsuccessful.

INDICATIONS

- Inability to gain percutaneous venous access

CONTRAINDICATIONS

- Coagulopathy
- Venous thrombosis in the leg

SUPPLIES

- 1% lidocaine
- Tourniquet
- Sterile gloves and towels
- Sterile preparation
- No. 10 blade
- Forceps, hemostat, and small scissors
- 5 ml syringe
- 25-gauge needle
- IV angiocatheter and catheter
- Gauze and silk ties

POSITIONING

- Supine with leg turned slightly outward

TECHNIQUE

- The most superficial and most consistent location of the greater saphenous vein is 1 cm superior and 1 cm anterior to the medial malleolus (Fig. 19-1).
- Prepare and drape in sterile fashion.
- Using 1% lidocaine and a 25-gauge needle, anesthetize the skin over the intended incision site.
- Make a transverse incision, with the expected saphenous vein site in the middle of the incision (Fig. 19-2).
- Using the forceps and hemostat, dissect down and identify the vein.
- Dissect around the vein and free it from its adhesions and the saphenous nerve
- Successful dissection of the vein allows circumferential access for a length of 2 cm.

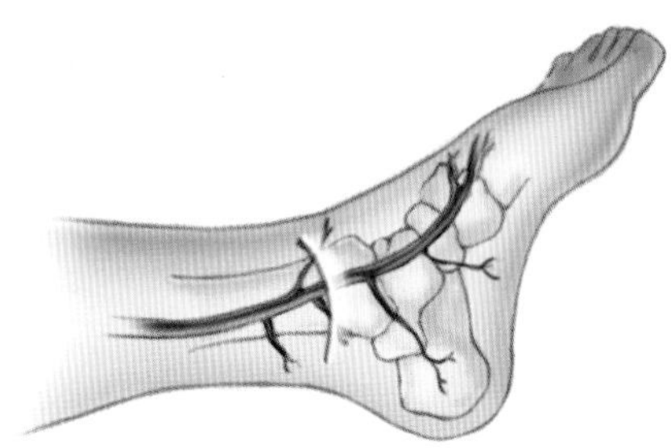

Fig. 19-1

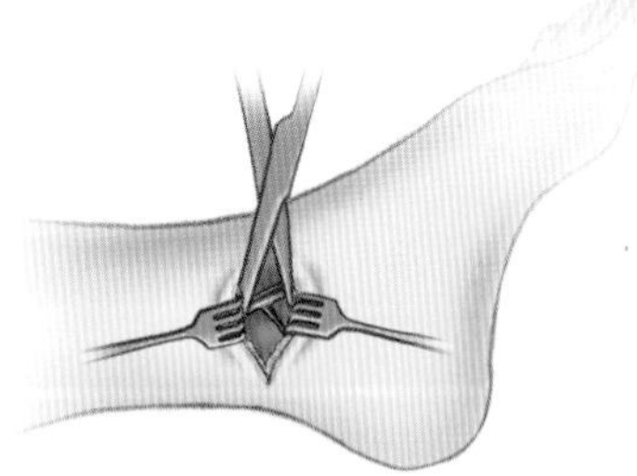

Fig. 19-2

- Place silk ties around the vein, one at its proximal end and one at its distal end.
- Place a surgical knot on the distal tie and leave the proximal tie untied.
- In the middle of the exposed vein, make a small venotomy and dilate the hole with the hemostat (Fig. 19-3).
- Place the angiocatheter into the vein and advance proximally (Fig. 19-4).
- Tie the proximal silk suture around the vein and angiocatheter without kinking the angiocatheter.
- Secure the portion of the catheter and IV tubing that is outside the wound to the skin with sutures.
- Close the wound with simple interrupted nylon sutures.

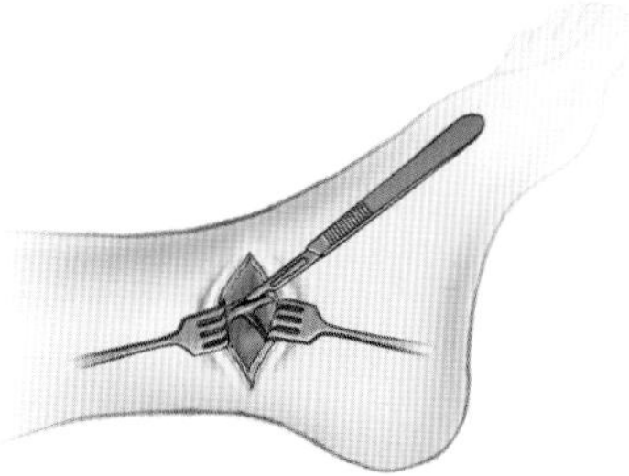

Fig. 19-3

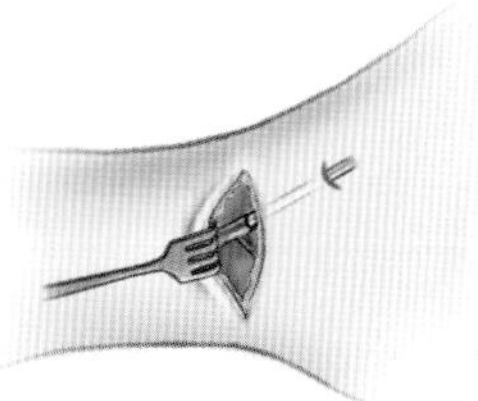

Fig. 19-4

PEARLS

- *Cutting the saphenous vein should not be painful in an awake patient.*
- *Hemorrhage can be stopped with gauze and gentle pressure.*

PITFALLS

- If the patient is awake and the saphenous vein is cut, the patient will experience pain.
- Infection at the site of cutdown is usually superficial phlebitis and can be treated with catheter removal and warm compresses.

20

Central Venous Access: Subclavian Vein

A 33-year-old man presents with a closed head injury requiring barbiturate coma.

INDICATIONS

- Multiple or long-term drug infusion
- Central venous pressure (CVP) monitoring
- Parenteral nutrition
- Central venous access in the setting of head injury

CONTRAINDICATIONS

- Coagulopathy
- Venous thrombosis

SUPPLIES

- 1% lidocaine
- Sterile gloves, towels, gown, and mask
- Sterile preparation
- Shoulder roll
- Scalpel
- 22- and 25-gauge needles
- 5 ml syringes
- 18-gauge needle (long for insertion)
- 0.035-inch J-wire
- 2-0 silk suture

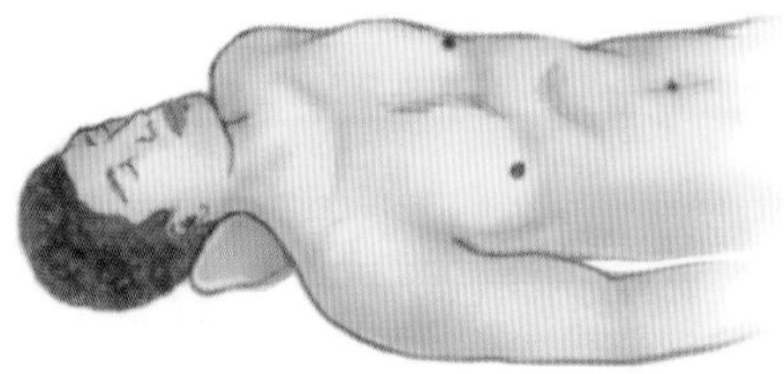

Fig. 20-1

POSITIONING

- Supine and in the Trendelenburg position; place a shoulder roll between the scapulas, and have the patient's head turned away from the insertion site (Fig. 20-1)

TECHNIQUE

- Prepare and drape the patient's neck from the ipsilateral shoulder to across the sternum, including the ipsilateral internal jugular vein.
- The insertion site is 1 cm below the clavicle at one third the distance of the clavicle, measuring from the shoulder (Fig. 20-2).
- Anesthetize the skin with 1% lidocaine using the 25-gauge needle.
- Anesthetize the tissue beneath the skin and toward the clavicle; always aspirate the syringe before injection to prevent intravascular infusion.
- The periosteum of the clavicle should be anesthetized as well.
- Attach a 5 ml syringe to the 18-gauge needle, and grasp the syringe with your dominant hand.
- Place the index finger of the other hand on the suprasternal notch as a target toward which the needle will be directed.
- Insert the needle and draw back on the syringe plunger to create negative pressure.
- With the syringe slightly drawn, advance the needle toward the suprasternal notch and below the clavicle (Fig. 20-3).
- The angle of insertion is very low and should parallel the floor; the bevel should be toward the patient's heart.
- Entry into the subclavian vein results in a flush of venous blood into the syringe (venous blood is darker than arterial blood).
- If air or arterial blood (lighter than venous blood and pulsatile) is encountered, abort the procedure.

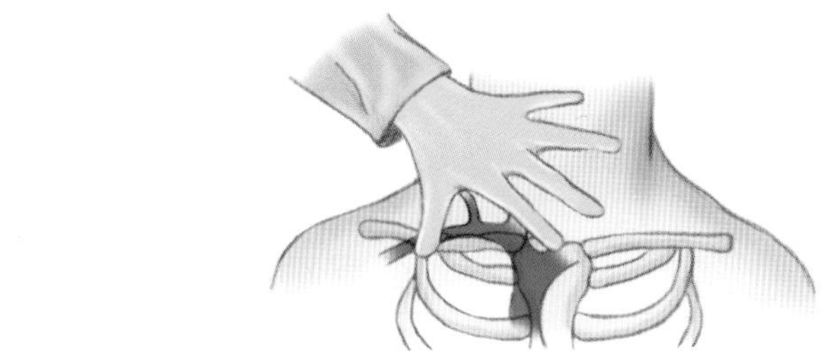

Fig. 20-2

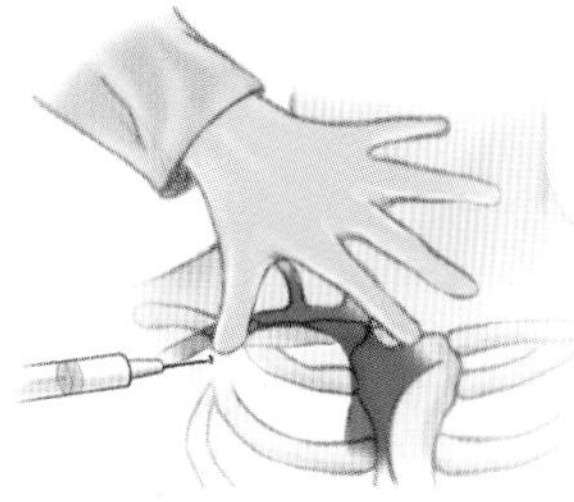

Fig. 20-3

Fig. 20-4

- When convinced of good venous access with the insertion needle, remove the syringe and introduce the J-wire through the needle while maintaining the position of the needle with the other hand (Fig. 20-4).
- The wire should insert with minimal resistance. If it does not, remove the wire and confirm intravenous access by reattaching the syringe and drawing back the plunger on to obtain good venous flow.
- Insert the wire again.
- Once the wire is inserted, remove the needle over the wire while maintaining your grasp of the wire at all times to prevent inadvertent wire embolism in the patient.
- Nick the skin adjacent to the wire with the scalpel to allow the dilator to be inserted.
- Insert the dilator over the wire approximately 3 cm to dilate subcutaneous tissue; maintain grasp of the wire at all times to prevent inadvertent wire embolism in the patient.
- Remove the dilator and advance the central venous catheter over the J-wire to a length of 15 cm (right-sided approach) or 18 cm (left-sided approach).
- Remove the wire and confirm proper placement by aspirating from all ports.

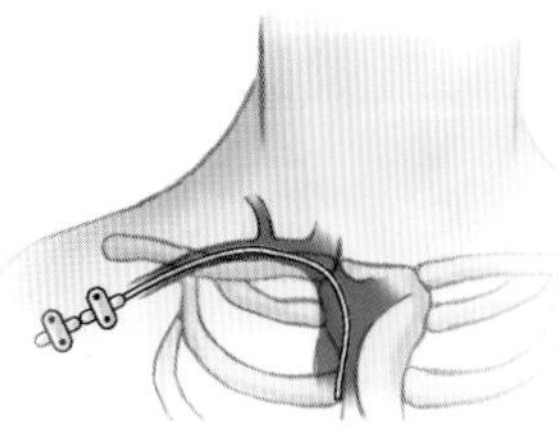

Fig. 20-5

- Flush ports with saline solution and cap all ports.
- Suture both hubs on the catheter to the skin and apply sterile dressing (Fig. 20-5).
- Obtain a chest radiograph to confirm placement and exclude pneumothorax.

PEARLS

- *Preparing the ipsilateral internal jugular vein allows for an alternative venous access route without having to redrape.*
- *After a failed subclavian venous access attempt, do not try to access the contralateral side without first examining a chest radiograph to exclude pneumothorax on the original insertion site. This avoids the possibility of bilateral pneumothoraces.*
- *Having the bevel of the needle facing the patient's heart can help direct the guidewire away from the internal jugular vein and toward the superior vena cava (SVC).*
- *Turning the patient's head to the ipsilateral side during insertion of the J-wire can decrease the chances of advancing the wire into the ipsilateral internal jugular vein.*
- *If the patient is hypotensive and you are unsure whether the subclavian vein or artery has been entered, compare the color of the withdrawn blood with a specimen from an arterial line, or attach a pressure transducer and IV tubing to the needle to obtain pressure (arterial versus venous).*
- *On a chest radiograph, the distal catheter tip should be at the junction of the SVC and right atrium.*

PITFALLS

- Advancing too far beneath the clavicle increases the risk of pneumothorax; some suggest using your nondominant thumb to press the needle under the clavicle while advancing.
- Advancing the dilator past 3 to 4 cm can dilate the vessel and is not necessary.
- Inserting the needle into an artery should lead to temporary cessation of the procedure. Withdraw the needle and apply manual pressure for 10 minutes; monitor the patient's vital signs.
- An apparent pneumothorax in a chest radiograph should be managed by tube thoracostomy if it is more than 10% of ipsilateral lung volume.
- Air embolus can be deadly and should be managed by immediate aspiration of air from the needle or catheter, if possible. If the patient is unstable, initiate ACLS; if stable, place the patient in the left lateral decubitus and Trendelenburg position to trap air in the right ventricle.
- Arrhythmias usually resolve as the catheter or wire is pulled out of the right atrium or ventricle; the proper placement of the catheter is in the SVC.

✓ POSTPROCEDURE CHECK

- ☐ Obtain an immediate chest radiograph to confirm proper placement and to exclude pneumothorax (Fig. 20-6).

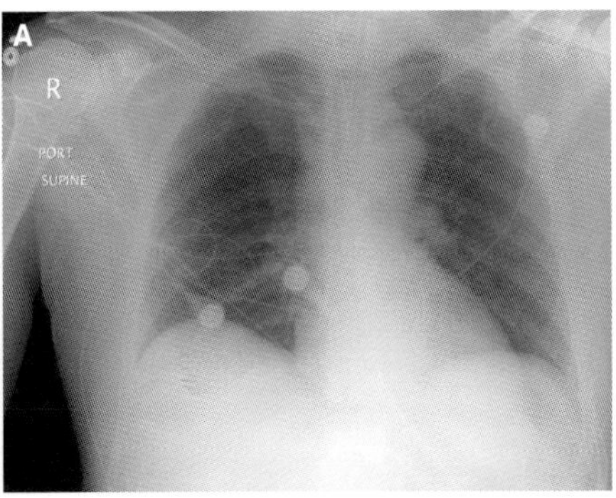

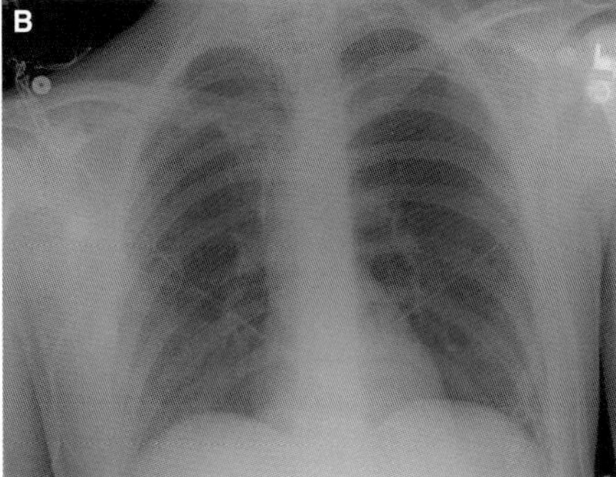

Fig. 20-6 **A,** Chest radiograph. Right subclavian line with proximal tip at the junction of the vena cava and atrium. **B,** Chest radiograph. Left subclavian line with proximal tip at the junction of the vena cava and atrium.

21

Central Venous Access: Internal Jugular Vein

A 59-year-old woman in the ICU with bacteremia and hypotension requires continuous infusion of multiple medications.

INDICATIONS

- Multiple or long-term drug infusion
- CVP monitoring
- Parenteral nutrition
- Central venous access without head injury
- Hemodialysis

CONTRAINDICATIONS

- Coagulopathy
- Venous thrombosis
- Previous ipsilateral neck surgery

SUPPLIES

- 1% lidocaine
- Sterile gloves, towels, gown, and mask
- Sterile preparation
- Shoulder roll
- Scalpel
- 22- and 25-gauge needles
- 5 ml syringes
- 18-gauge needle (long for insertion)
- 0.035-inch J-wire
- 2-0 silk suture

POSITIONING

- Supine and in the Trendelenburg position, with the head turned away from the insertion site to expose the neck

TECHNIQUE

- Prepare and drape the patient's neck from the ear to the clavicle and from the ipsilateral shoulder to across the sternum.
- The insertion site is at the apex created by the heads of the sternocleidomastoid muscles (Fig. 21-1).
- Anesthetize the skin with 1% lidocaine using the 25-gauge needle.
- Anesthetize the tissue beneath the skin; always aspirate the syringe before injection to prevent intravascular infusion.
- Palpate the carotid pulse; the insertion site is lateral to that in the apex of the sternocleidomastoid heads.
- Attach a 5 ml syringe to the 22-gauge needle and grasp the syringe with your dominant hand.

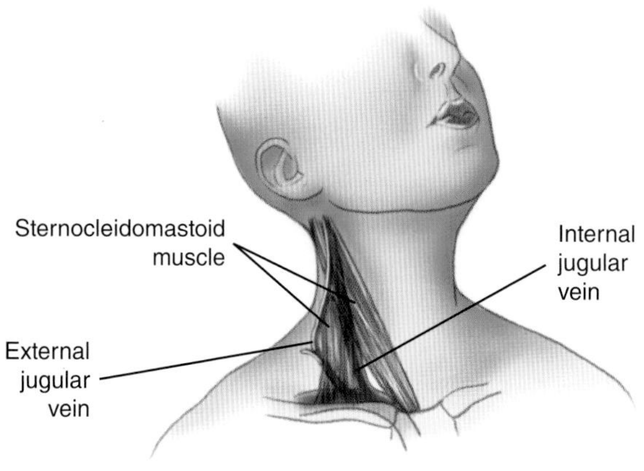

Fig. 21-1

- Insert the needle and draw back on the syringe plunger to create negative pressure (Fig. 21-2).
- Advance with the syringe slightly drawn toward the ipsilateral nipple at a 45-degree angle.
- Entry into the subclavian vein results in a flush of venous blood into the syringe (darker than arterial blood).
- If no venous blood is encountered after inserting the needle 3 cm, withdraw the needle and through the same puncture site redirect the trajectory slightly more laterally.
- If air or arterial blood (lighter red and pulsatile) is encountered, stop the procedure.
- When convinced of good venous access with the 22-gauge needle, repeat the steps with the 18-gauge needle using the 22-gauge needle's trajectory for guidance.
- If good venous access is obtained with the 18-gauge needle, remove the syringe and insert the J-wire.
- The wire should insert with minimal resistance. If it does not, remove the wire and confirm intravenous access by reattaching the syringe and drawing back on the plunger to get good venous flow.
- Insert the wire again.
- Once the wire is inserted, remove the needle over the wire. Maintain grasp of the wire at all times to prevent inadvertent wire embolism in the patient.

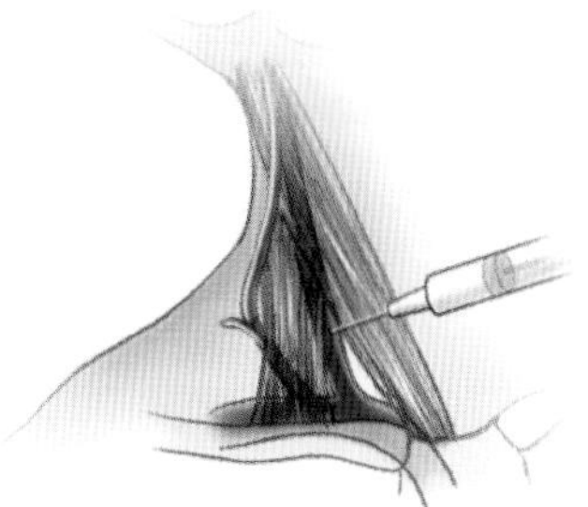

Fig. 21-2

- Nick the skin adjacent to the wire with a scalpel to allow insertion of the dilator.
- Insert the dilator over the wire approximately 1 to 2 cm to dilate subcutaneous tissue, maintaining grasp of the wire at all times to prevent inadvertent wire embolism in the patient.
- Remove the dilator and advance the central venous catheter over the J-wire to a length of 9 cm (right-sided approach) or 12 cm (left-sided approach).
- Remove the wire and confirm proper placement by aspirating from all ports.
- Flush ports with saline solution and cap all ports.
- Suture both hubs on the catheter to the skin, and apply sterile dressing.
- Obtain a chest radiograph to confirm placement and rule out pneumothorax.

PEARLS

- *Subclavian venous access is preferred in patients with head injuries, because it does not impede cerebral venous drainage.*
- *Preparing the ipsilateral internal jugular vein provides an alternative route for venous access without having to redrape.*
- *If a patient is hypotensive and you are unsure whether the internal jugular vein or carotid artery is entered, compare the color of the withdrawn blood with a specimen from an arterial line, or attach a pressure transducer and IV tubing to the needle to obtain pressure (arterial versus venous).*
- *Never insert an 18-gauge needle without having some sense of where the vessel is by first finding it with the smaller 22-gauge needle; a carotid puncture with a 22-gauge needle is usually controllable with compression.*
- *Advancing the dilator more than 1 or 2 cm can dilate the vessel and is not necessary.*
- *On the chest radiograph, the distal catheter tip should be at the SVC/right atrial junction.*

PITFALLS

- Carotid artery puncture from needle insertion should lead to temporary cessation of the procedure. Withdraw the needle and apply manual pressure for 10 minutes; monitor vital signs. Consult surgery if unable to obtain hemostasis.
- Pneumothorax on a chest radiograph should be managed by tube thoracostomy if it is more than 10% of the ipsilateral lung volume.
- Air embolus can be deadly and should be managed by immediate aspiration of air from the needle or catheter, if possible. If the patient is unstable, initiate ACLS; if stable, place the patient in the left lateral decubitus and Trendelenburg position to trap air in the right ventricle.
- Arrhythmias usually resolve as the catheter or wire is pulled out of the right atrium or ventricle; proper placement of the catheter is in the SVC.
- Rarely, temporary Horner's syndrome can result from puncture of the carotid sheath.

✓ POSTPROCEDURE CHECK

- ❑ Obtain an immediate chest radiograph to confirm proper placement and exclude pneumothorax (Fig. 21-3).

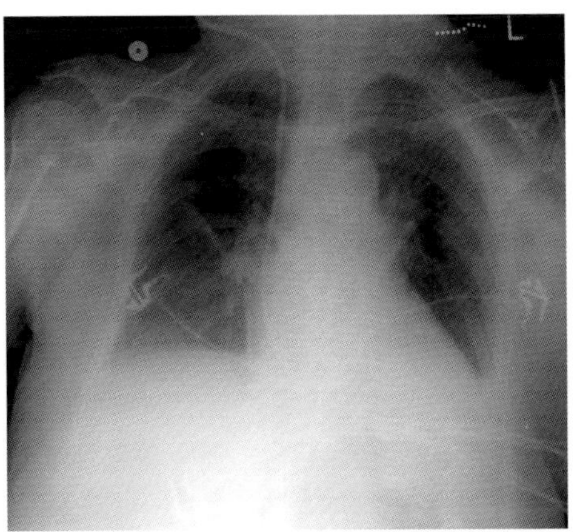

Fig. 21-3 Chest radiograph. The right internal jugular line can be seen extending from the neck to the clavicle. Through this internal jugular access, a pulmonary artery catheter has been inserted into the heart.

22

Femoral Venous Access

A 59-year-old woman in the ICU with bacteremia and hypotension requires continuous infusion of multiple medications.

INDICATIONS

- Emergent central access
- Hemodialysis
- Unable to obtain subclavian or internal jugular venous access

CONTRAINDICATIONS

- Coagulopathy
- Venous thrombosis
- Previous surgery in the ipsilateral inguinal area
- Unable to lay flat

SUPPLIES

- 1% lidocaine
- Sterile gloves, towels, gown, and mask
- Sterile preparation
- Scalpel
- 22- and 25-gauge needles
- 5 ml syringes
- 18-gauge needle (long for insertion)
- 0.035-inch J-wire
- 2-0 silk suture

POSITIONING

- Supine with the inguinal area exposed

TECHNIQUE

- Prepare and drape the patient's groin from the midline to the lateral thigh and from the lower abdomen to the upper thigh.
- The insertion site is 1 cm below the inguinal ligament and lateral to the femoral artery (Fig. 22-1).
- If a pulse cannot be palpated, the insertion point is at the midpoint of the anterior superior iliac spine and pubic symphysis.
- Anesthetize the skin with 1% lidocaine using the 25-gauge needle.
- Anesthetize the tissue beneath the skin; always aspirate the syringe before injecting to prevent intravascular infusion.
- Palpate the femoral artery pulse with your nondominant hand; the insertion site is just medial to the artery.
- Attach a 5 ml syringe to the 18-gauge needle and grasp the syringe with your dominant hand (Fig. 22-2).
- Insert the needle and draw back on the syringe plunger to create negative pressure.

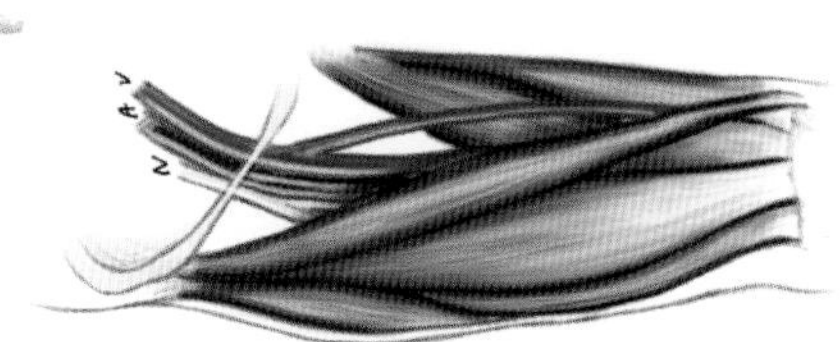

Fig. 22-1

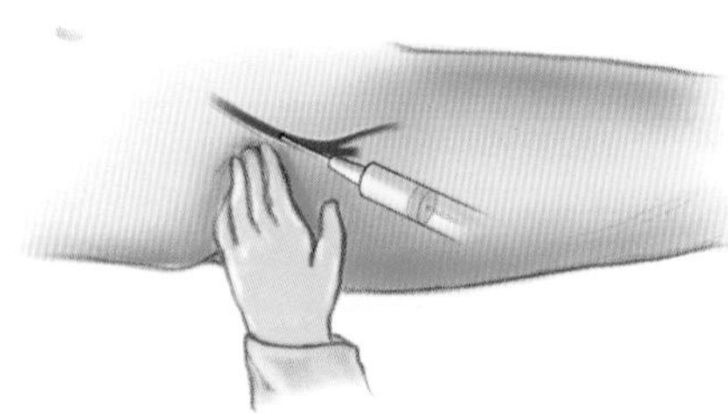

Fig. 22-2

- Advance the needle with the syringe slightly drawn, parallel to the pulse, and at a 45-degree angle.
- Entry into the femoral vein results in a flush of venous blood into the syringe (darker than arterial blood).
- If no venous blood is encountered after inserting the needle 5 cm, withdraw the needle and, through the same puncture site, redirect the trajectory slightly more medial.
- If arterial blood (redder and pulsatile) is encountered, stop the procedure.
- If good venous access is obtained with the 18-gauge needle, remove the syringe and insert the J-wire.
- The wire should insert with minimal resistance. If it does not, remove the wire and confirm intravenous access by reattaching the syringe and drawing back on the plunger to get good venous flow.
- Insert the wire again.
- Once the wire is inserted, remove the needle over the wire. Maintain grasp of the wire at all times to prevent inadvertent wire embolism in the patient.
- Nick the skin adjacent to the wire with the scalpel to allow insertion of the dilator.
- Insert the dilator over the wire approximately 3 to 4 cm to dilate the subcutaneous tissue; maintain grasp of the wire at all times to prevent inadvertent wire embolism.
- Remove the dilator and advance the central venous catheter over the J-wire to a length of 15 cm.
- Remove the wire and confirm proper placement by aspirating from all ports.
- Flush ports with saline solution and cap all ports.
- Suture both hubs on the catheter to the skin and apply sterile dressing.

PEARLS

- *If the patient is hypotensive, and you are unsure whether the femoral vein or artery is entered, compare the color of the withdrawn blood with a specimen from an arterial line or attach a pressure transducer and IV tubing to the needle to obtain pressure (arterial versus venous).*
- *Advancing the dilator more than 3 or 4 cm can dilate the vessel and is not necessary.*

PITFALLS

- A femoral artery puncture resulting from needle insertion should lead to temporary cessation of the procedure. Withdraw the needle and apply manual pressure for 20 minutes, and then place a sandbag over the site for 30 minutes. Monitor ipsilateral pulses in the foot (dorsalis pedis).

✓ POSTPROCEDURE CHECK

- ☐ Check the patient's foot pulse on the ipsilateral side (dorsalis pedis artery).

23

Pulmonary Artery Catheter

A 69-year-old man has cardiac decompensation after coronary artery bypass.

INDICATIONS

- Need to monitor hemodynamic parameters (vasomotor instability, after cardiac surgery or congestive heart failure)
- Evaluation of volume status to guide management

CONTRAINDICATIONS

- Subclavian vein thrombosis
- Coagulopathy
- Severe pulmonary hypertension

SUPPLIES

- 1% lidocaine
- Sterile gloves and towels
- Sterile preparation
- No.10 blade
- 22- and 25-gauge needles
- 5 ml syringe
- Cordis catheter and dilator
- Long 18-gauge needle to access the vein
- 0.035-inch J-wire
- Swan-Ganz catheter kit

POSITIONING

- Supine in the Trendelenburg position, with a shoulder roll under the scapula of the procedure side

TECHNIQUE

- The patient should have a central venous Cordis catheter in place and be prepared and draped in sterile fashion.
- Open the Swan-Ganz kit and evaluate the balloon tip for proper inflation and deflation (Fig. 23-1).
- Flush all ports with saline solution, and connect the pressure-monitoring line to the transducer to confirm the waveform as you wiggle the tip.
- Encase the Swan-Ganz catheter in the plastic sheath provided, and insert the encased catheter into the Cordis catheter to 20 cm (using the markings on the Swan-Ganz catheter).
- At 20 cm, inflate the balloon and ensure that there is a CVP waveform.
- Continue to advance the catheter with the balloon inflated to 40 cm (right ventricle) and 50 cm (pulmonary artery). Verify progression from the SVC/right atrium to the right ventricle to the pulmonary artery with corresponding waveform changes (Figs. 23-2 and 23-3).

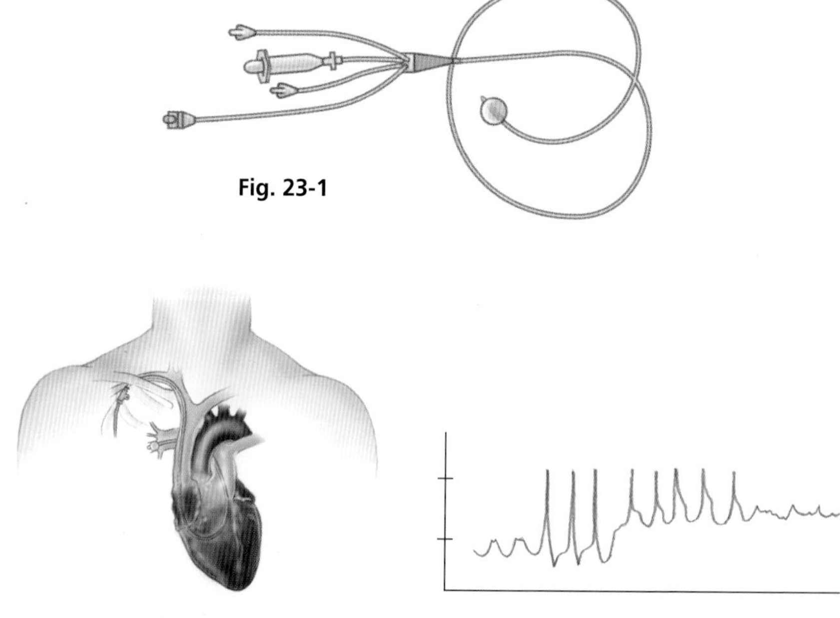

Fig. 23-1

Fig. 23-2

Fig. 23-3

- Continue inserting (no more than 70 cm) until the waveform dampens.
- This occurs because of wedging and can be confirmed by return of PA waveform when the balloon is deflated.
- Never withdraw with the balloon inflated.

PEARLS

- *The right internal jugular and left subclavian veins are the best sites for placing a pulmonary catheter, because they provide the least tortuous courses for entering the left ventricle of the heart.*
- *If unable to wedge the PA catheter, and 70 cm of tubing has been inserted, deflate the balloon and withdraw 20 cm. Reinflate the balloon and attempt to wedge again.*
- *Never inflate the balloon for more than 1 or 2 minutes.*
- *Once the catheter is wedged, some clinicians withdraw the tip 0.5 cm and confirm the ability to wedge. This may help prevent overwedging and pulmonary artery and parenchymal injury.*
- *A catheter in place for more than 3 days is associated with a higher risk of infection.*
- *If any resistance is encountered during withdrawal of the catheter, make sure the balloon is deflated. If resistance persists, assume the catheter is knotted and obtain a chest radiograph; fluoroscopic guidance by interventional radiology may be needed to uncoil a knotted catheter.*

PITFALLS

- Placing a PA catheter can lead to arrhythmias. Typically they arise when the catheter tip passes through or unintentionally becomes coiled within the right ventricle. Short runs of ventricular tachycardia or premature ventricular contractions that are asymptomatic are well tolerated; however, any persistence or hemodynamic instability should be treated with ACLS protocols.
- Overwedging can lead to pulmonary infarction.
- In the rare event of pulmonary artery rupture, consult cardiac surgery emergently.
- Inflation of the balloon can lead to balloon rupture, leading to an air embolus. This can lead to pulmonary infarction or myocardial infarction if the patient has a patent foramen ovale. Place the patient in the left lateral decubitus and Trendelenburg position to trap air in the right ventricle. An attempt can be made to withdraw air through a triple-lumen catheter, or if the air collection is small it can be followed and allowed to absorb.

✓ POSTPROCEDURE CHECK

- ☐ A chest radiograph should be obtained after PA catheter placement, and daily radiographs should be obtained for as long as the catheter is in place (Fig. 23-4).

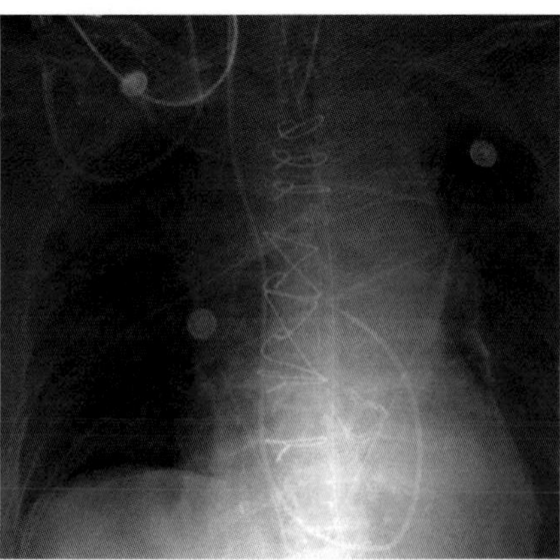

Fig. 23-4 Chest radiograph showing properly placed pulmonary artery catheter inserted through the right internal jugular vein access. Note the sternal wires from cardiac surgery.

24

Arterial Line: Radial Artery

A 58-year-old woman is on a ventilator and has labile blood pressures.

INDICATIONS

- Frequent need for arterial blood gas (ABG)
- Need for continuous blood pressure monitoring

CONTRAINDICATIONS

- Failed Allen test

SUPPLIES

- 1% lidocaine
- Sterile gloves and towels
- Sterile preparation
- 25-gauge needle
- 5 ml syringe
- 16- or 18-gauge angiographic catheters
- Silk suture
- Pressure bag and IV tubing
- Heparinized flush

POSITIONING

- Place a rolled towel under the wrist to expose the ventral surface of the forearm. Tape down the fingers with the wrist in dorsiflexion (Fig. 24-1).

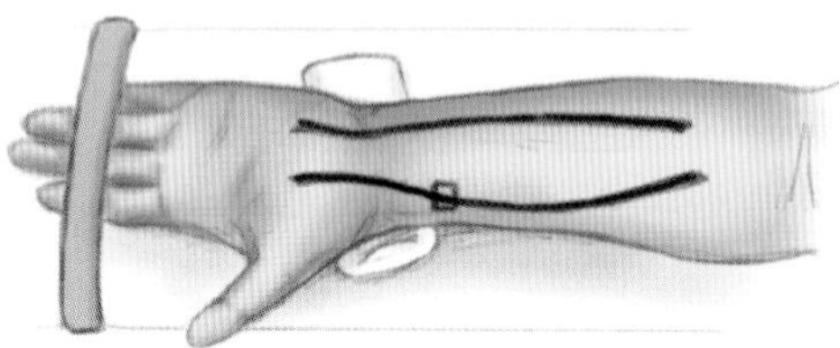

Fig. 24-1

TECHNIQUE

- Always perform an Allen test before performing radial artery cannulation.
- Compress both the ulnar and radial arteries, and allow the blood in the hand to drain out of the veins (Fig. 24-2).

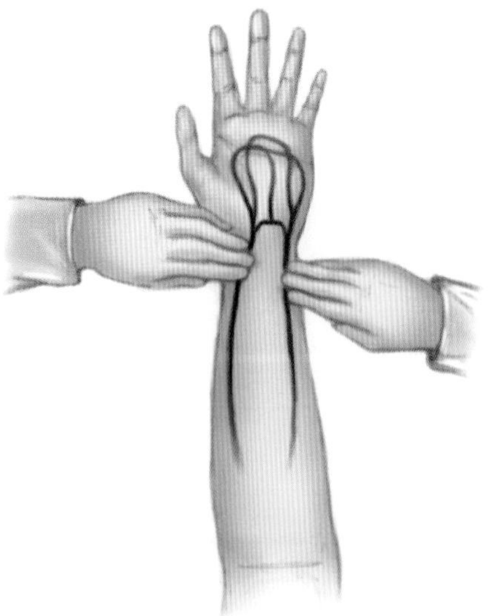

Fig. 24-2

- Release the ulnar artery and keep the radial artery depressed.
- If hand color does not return within 5 seconds, the Allen test is positive and the ulnar artery does not provide sufficient collateral flow in case the radial artery is damaged.
- Prepare and drape the wrist.
- Using the 25-gauge needle, anesthetize the skin over the radial pulse in the distal forearm.
- Insert the angiocatheter at a 45-degree angle into the radial artery until a flush of blood is seen in the hub of the angiocatheter (Fig. 24-3).
- If blood is not encountered, slowly withdraw the needle; this may place the needle tip back into the arterial lumen if the needle had penetrated both walls of the artery.
- If still unable to obtain blood, modify the trajectory and move the needle tip several millimeters proximal on the wrist.
- Once confident of entry into the radial artery, advance the angiocatheter or guidewire into the lumen.
- Slowly advance the catheter into the artery while holding the needle steady.
- Remove the needle and look for pulsatile blood flow.
- Attach the flush system and IV tubing.
- Suture the catheter to the skin and apply sterile dressing.

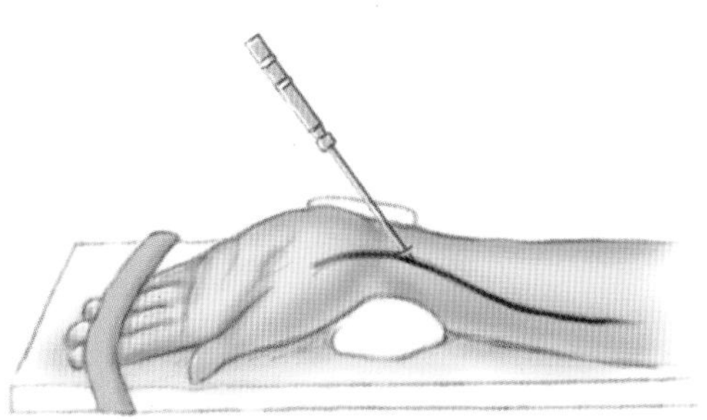

Fig. 24-3

PEARLS

- *Secure the hand firmly with tape.*
- *The actual location of the artery tends to be slightly medial to the palpated pulse.*
- *Make sure a blood pressure cuff is not on the same arm as your intended radial artery cannulation.*

PITFALLS

- If any ischemia of the fingers is suspected, abort the procedure and remove the catheter.
- Bleeding from failed attempts can be controlled with compression.

25

Arterial Line: Dorsalis Pedis Artery

A 58-year-old woman is on a ventilator with labile blood pressures. Neither a radial nor a femoral arterial line can be placed.

INDICATIONS

- Frequent need for ABG
- Need for continuous blood pressure monitoring

CONTRAINDICATIONS

- Unable to palpate dorsalis pedis artery pulse

SUPPLIES

- 1% lidocaine
- Sterile gloves and towels
- Sterile preparation
- 25-gauge needle
- 5 ml syringe
- 16- or 18-gauge angiographic catheter
- Silk suture
- Pressure bag and IV tubing
- Heparinized flush

POSITIONING

- Supine with the dorsal foot in the neutral position (Fig. 25-1)

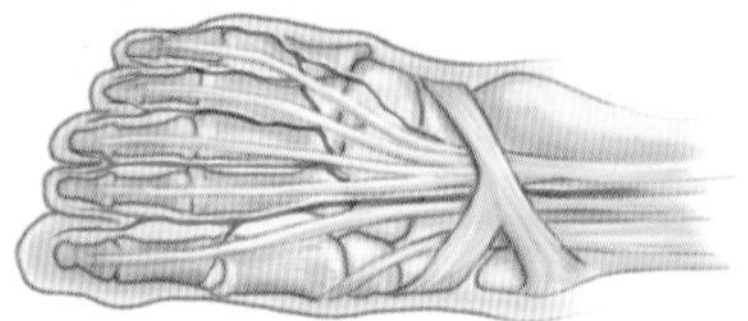

Fig. 25-1

TECHNIQUE

- Prepare and drape the dorsal foot.
- Palpate the dorsalis pedis pulse at the level of the metatarsal-cuneiform joint; the pulse at this level will be just lateral to the extensor hallucis longus tendon.
- Using a 25-gauge needle, anesthetize the skin over the insertion site.
- Insert the angiocatheter at a 45-degree angle and with the bevel up until blood is seen in the hub of the angiocatheter (Fig. 25-2).
- If blood is not encountered, slowly withdraw the needle, which may place the needle tip back into the arterial lumen if the needle penetrated both walls of the artery.
- If still unable to obtain blood, modify the trajectory toward 60 degrees.
- Once you are confident of entry into the radial artery, advance the angiocatheter or guidewire into the lumen.
- Slowly advance the catheter into the artery while holding the needle steady.
- Remove the needle and look for pulsatile blood flow.
- Attach the flush system and IV tubing.
- Suture the catheter to the skin and apply sterile dressing.

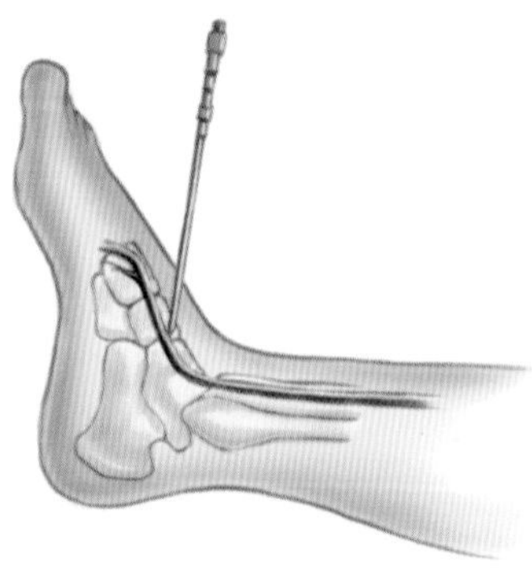

Fig. 25-2

PEARLS

- *Excessive plantar flexion of the foot can dampen the arterial pulse.*
- *Radial and femoral arterial lines are preferred over dorsalis pedis arterial lines because of slightly higher rates of ischemia encountered with the dorsalis pedis approach.*

PITFALLS

- If any ischemia of the toes is suspected, abort the procedure and remove the catheter.
- Bleeding from failed attempts can be controlled with compression.

✓ POSTPROCEDURE CHECK

- ❑ Examine the toes for ischemia while the dorsalis pedis arterial lines are in place.

26

Arterial Line: Femoral Artery

A 58-year-old woman is on a ventilator with labile blood pressures. A radial arterial line cannot be placed.

INDICATIONS

- Continuous blood pressure monitoring
- Need for frequent ABG
- Access for angiographic studies or intraaortic balloon pump

CONTRAINDICATIONS

- Coagulopathy
- Previous inguinal surgery
- Unable to lay flat when a femoral line is in place

SUPPLIES

- 1% lidocaine
- Sterile gloves, towels, gown, and mask
- Sterile preparation
- Scalpel
- 25-gauge needle
- 5 ml syringes
- 18-gauge needle (long for insertion)
- 0.035-inch J wire
- 2-0 silk suture
- Pressure bag and IV tubing
- Heparinized flush

POSITIONING

- Supine with groin area exposed

TECHNIQUE

- Prepare and drape the patient's groin from midline to lateral thigh and from lower abdomen to upper thigh.
- The insertion site is 1 to 2 cm below the inguinal ligament and medial to the femoral artery (Fig. 26-1).
- If a pulse cannot be palpated, the insertion point is at the midpoint of the anterior superior iliac spine and pubic symphysis.
- Anesthetize the skin with 1% lidocaine using a 25-gauge needle.
- Anesthetize the tissue beneath the skin; always draw back the syringe plunger before injection to prevent intravascular infusion.
- Palpate the femoral artery pulse with the nondominant hand at the insertion site.
- Attach a 5 ml syringe to an 18-gauge needle and grasp the syringe with the dominant hand.
- Insert the needle and draw back on the syringe plunger to create negative pressure (Fig. 26-2).

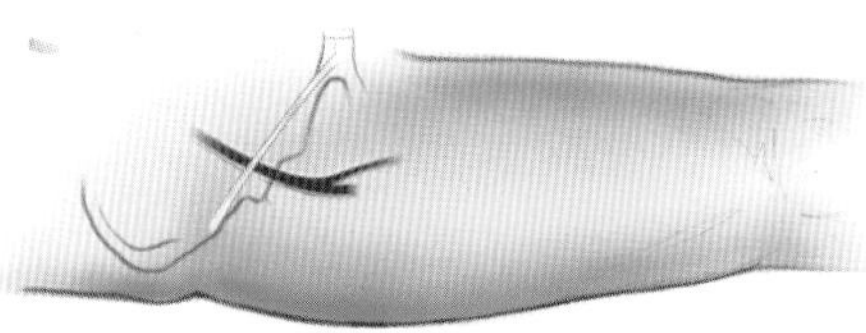

Fig. 26-1

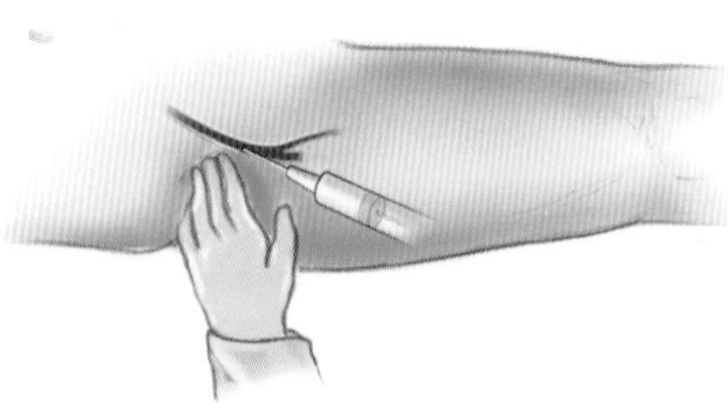

Fig. 26-2

- Advance the needle, with the syringe slightly drawn, parallel to the pulse and at a 45-degree angle.
- Entry into the femoral artery results in a flush of blood in the syringe (a brighter red than venous blood).
- If no arterial blood is encountered after inserting the needle 5 cm, withdraw the needle and, through the same puncture site, redirect the trajectory slightly more medial.
- If venous blood is encountered, withdraw the needle and apply pressure.
- If good arterial access is obtained with the 18-gauge needle, remove the syringe and insert a J-wire.
- The wire should insert with minimal resistance. If it does not, remove the wire and confirm intravenous access by reattaching the syringe and drawing back on the plunger to get good arterial flow.
- Insert the wire again.
- Once the wire is inserted, remove the needle over the wire while maintaining your grasp of the wire at all times to prevent inadvertent wire embolism.
- Nick the skin adjacent to the wire with a scalpel to allow insertion of the dilator.
- Insert the dilator over the wire approximately 1 to 2 cm to dilate subcutaneous tissue; maintain your grasp of the wire at all times to prevent inadvertent wire embolism.
- Remove the dilator and advance the central venous catheter over the J-wire to a length of 15 cm.
- Remove the wire and confirm proper placement by aspirating from all ports.
- Flush ports with saline solution and cap all ports.
- Suture both hubs on the catheter to the skin and apply sterile dressing.

PEARLS

- *If the patient is hypotensive, and you are unsure whether the femoral vein or artery is entered, compare the color of the withdrawn blood with a specimen from an arterial line, or attach a pressure transducer and IV tubing to the needle to obtain pressure (arterial versus venous).*
- *Advancing the dilator more than 1 or 2 cm can dilate the vessel and is not necessary.*

PITFALLS

- Femoral venous puncture from needle insertion should lead to temporary cessation of the procedure. Withdraw the needle and apply manual pressure for 5 minutes. Placing the arterial line can then be attempted again.

✓ POSTPROCEDURE CHECK

- ☐ Examine the arterial pulses in the foot (dorsalis pedis and posterior tibialis) while the femoral arterial line is in place.

27

Pediatric Intraosseous Access

Two young boys present with severe dehydration after 3 days with gastroenteritis.

INDICATIONS

- Children less than 3 years of age
- Unable to gain percutaneous venous access
- Insufficient time for venous cutdown

CONTRAINDICATIONS

- Coagulopathy
- If the extremity has a fracture, place the needle distal to the fracture

SUPPLIES

- Sterile gloves and towels
- Sterile preparation
- No. 10 blade
- 16- or 18-gauge bone marrow aspiration needle

POSITIONING

- Supine

TECHNIQUE

- The needle insertion site is on the medial side of the lower leg, 3 cm inferior to the tibial tuberosity, aiming for the tibial head (Fig. 27-1).
- Alternatively, the femoral head can be used; in this case the insertion site is the medial leg.
- Prepare and drape the anticipated insertion site.
- Insert the needle (bevel up) into the marrow of the selected site (Fig. 27-2).
- Proper insertion is confirmed by aspiration of bone marrow.
- Secure the needle with tape and begin a slow infusion of fluid.

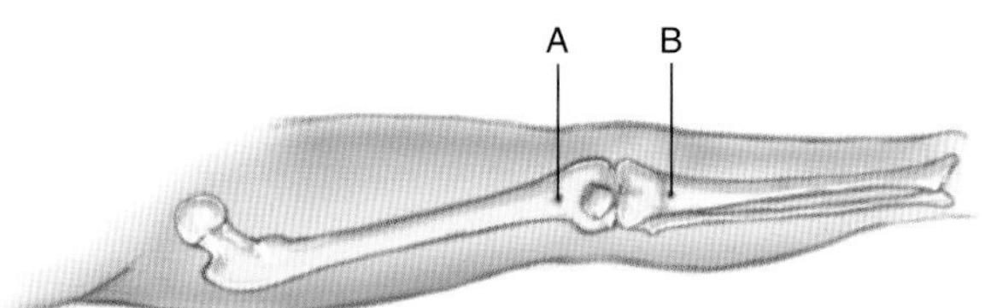

Fig. 27-1 Femoral head *(A)*. Tibial tuberosity *(B)*.

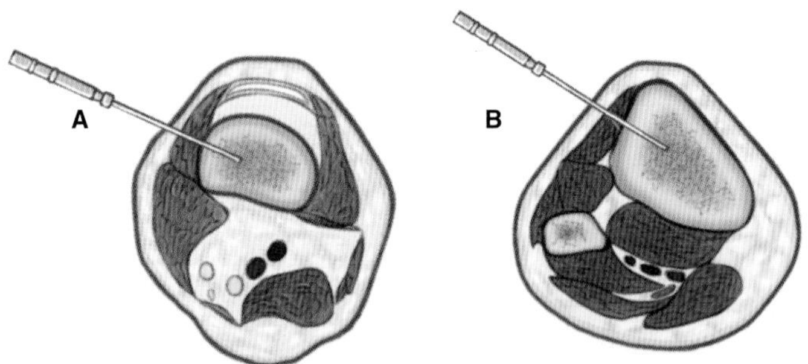

Fig. 27-2 **A,** Femoral head. **B,** Tibial tuberosity.

PEARLS

- *Intraosseous access is for emergency use only; once the patient is stabilized, other access should be obtained.*
- *In case the distal femur is needed for bone marrow access, it is best to prepare and drape the entire medial leg near the knee.*

PITFALLS

- If 5 ml of fluid cannot be easily infused into the marrow, the needle may not be in the proper place and should be reinserted.
- Osteomyelitis and compartment syndrome can occur rarely. Treat these with long-term antibiotics or fasciotomy, respectively.

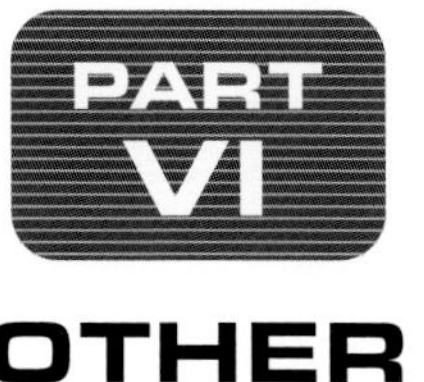

OTHER

28

Epistaxis: Nasal Packs and Foley Catheters

A 24-year-old man with a known vascular nasal tumor presents with unrelenting nasal bleeding.

INDICATIONS

- Recalcitrant nasal bleeding

CONTRAINDICATIONS

- None

SUPPLIES

- 1% lidocaine with 1:1000 epinephrine
- Forceps
- Foley catheter and 10 ml syringe
- Suction device
- Lubricated gauze
- Silver nitrate sticks

POSITIONING

- Sitting

TECHNIQUE

- Insert two cotton swabs soaked in 2% lidocaine with epinephrine into the bleeding nare.
- Search for the bleeding point, and attempt to cauterize it with silver nitrate sticks.
- If bleeding continues, place lubricated gauze into the nare, layering it from the nasal floor to the nasal roof (Fig. 28-1).
- If bleeding still persists, a Foley catheter needs to be placed (Fig. 28-2).
- Remove the nasal packs and insert a Foley catheter into the nasopharynx.
- Inflate the Foley balloon with 10 cc of air, and slowly withdraw the catheter until the balloon obstructs the posterior choana.
- Tape the catheter to the nose to prevent migration.
- If bleeding persists, surgical or endovascular occlusion of the maxillary and anterior ethmoidal arteries is necessary; obtain ear, nose, and throat (ENT) consultation.

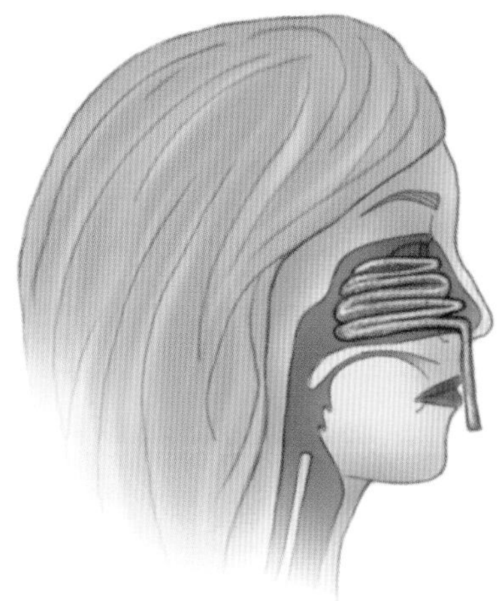

Fig. 28-1

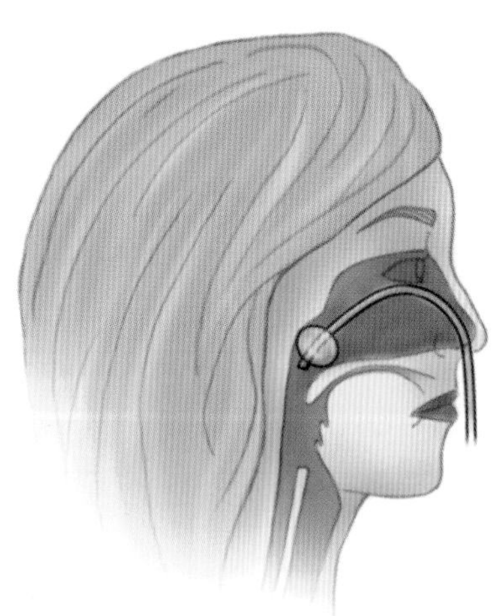

Fig. 28-2

PEARLS

- *Patients should receive antibiotics when they have nasal packs.*
- *Patients with Foley catheters in place for epistaxis should be admitted to the hospital and receive antibiotics.*

PITFALLS

- Some patients with nasal packs may have difficulty breathing; these patients require observation.
- If infection is suspected, the nasal packs must be removed.

✓ POSTPROCEDURE CHECK

- ❑ Nasal packs should be removed by ENT several days after being placed.

See Appendix E for additional helpful information.

29

Suprapubic Aspiration/ Catheterization

A 59-year-old man presents with benign prostatic hypertrophy and failed urinary catheterization with a coudé catheter.

INDICATIONS

- Inability to catheterize the bladder
- False passage into the penis
- Urethral stricture
- Acute prostatitis
- Urethral trauma

CONTRAINDICATIONS

- Pregnancy
- Coagulopathy
- Nondistended bladder
- Adhesions at the insertion site (previous operations below the umbilicus or pelvic radiation)
- Bladder cancer

SUPPLIES

- 1% lidocaine
- Sterile gloves and towels
- Sterile preparation
- Percutaneous suprapubic catheter set (10 Fr and 14 Fr)
- Urinary drainage bag
- No. 10 blade
- 20-gauge spinal needle
- 22- and 25-gauge needles

- 10 ml syringes
- Forceps
- Suction device
- 3-0 nylon suture and needle driver

POSITIONING

- Supine

TECHNIQUE

- Depending on the suprapubic catheter set, it may have its own needle, or you may have to use a separate 20-gauge needle (Figs. 29-1 and 29-2).
- Prepare the patient for the procedure by percussing for a distended bladder in the suprapubic region.
- Prepare and drape in a sterile fashion.
- Assemble the catheter kit (never insert the needle tip past the length of the catheter sleeve, or the drainage catheter may be punctured).
- The insertion site can be either 4 cm above the pubic symphysis (if there is no previous midline incision) or 4 cm above and 2 cm lateral on either side (Fig. 29-3).
- The spinal needle is used to locate the bladder and provide a tract for the suprapubic catheter to follow.

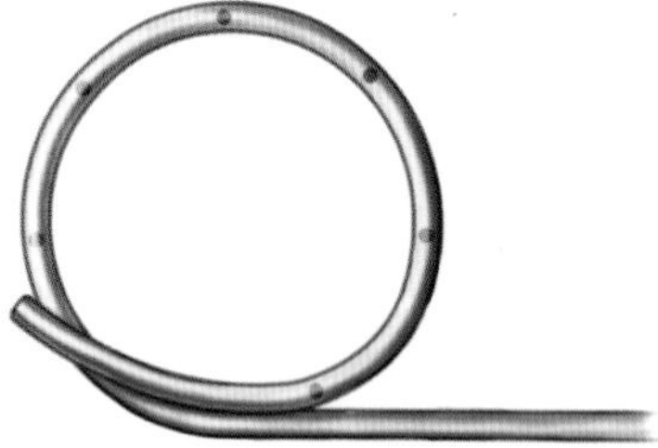

Fig. 29-1

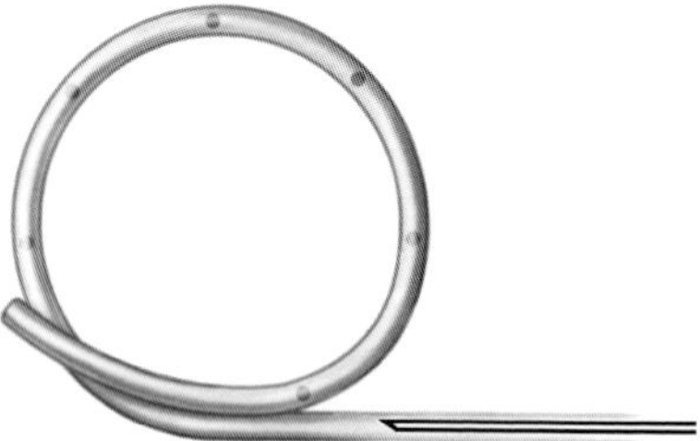

Fig. 29-2

- Insert the spinal needle (with obturator) into the anesthetized area chosen at a 45- to 60-degree angle, aiming toward the pubic symphysis (Fig. 29-4).
- After advancing 3 to 5 cm, remove the obturator of the spinal needle and attach a 10 ml syringe.
- Attempt to aspirate urine; if unable, advance the needle and obturator 1 cm farther and reaspirate. This should be repeated until urine is aspirated.
- When urine is aspirated, leave the spinal needle in place.
- Using the suprapubic catheter and needle set, advance the catheter into the bladder, following the tract created by the spinal needle.
- In most sets, once the needle has been withdrawn it cannot be replaced in situ, and the entire catheter/needle apparatus must be reassembled outside of the patient.

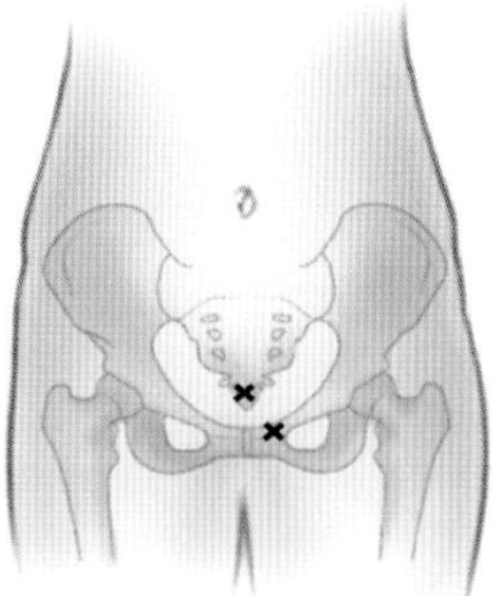

Fig. 29-3

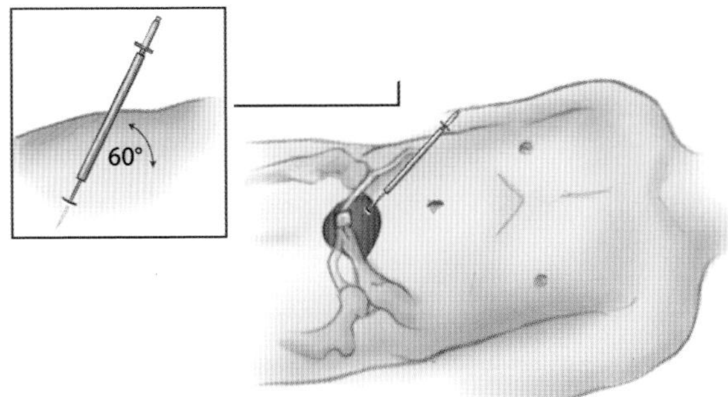

Fig. 29-4

- When urine is encountered, advance the catheter 2 cm farther.
- Disengage the needle obturator and catheter, stabilize the needle, and advance the catheter into the bladder.
- Aspirate from the catheter to confirm urine egress.
- Secure the catheter to the skin with 3-0 nylon suture.

PEARLS

- *At a minimum, patients should be given antibiotics that are effective against gram-positive organisms, and if a urinary tract infection is suspected, the coverage should be broadened.*
- *Ultrasound can help detect and view the distended bladder.*
- *As the spinal needle is passed into the skin, it may be possible to detect resistance points when penetrating the rectus sheath fascia and then the bladder wall.*

PITFALLS

- In patients with an inadequately distended bladder, there is a higher risk of bowel injury. If the bowel is entered, use a new spinal needle and attempt insertion into the bladder from different site. Begin broad-spectrum antibiotics and monitor for peritonitis.
- If bleeding is encountered during catheter insertion, it usually dissipates. If bleeding persists, consult urology.

✓ POSTPROCEDURE CHECK

- ❑ Ensure good urine output.
- ❑ Consult urology.

See Appendix E for additional helpful information.

30

Closed Reduction: Ankle Dislocation

A 27-year-old woman presents with a dislocated ankle.

INDICATIONS

- Dislocated ankle (Fig. 30-1)

CONTRAINDICATIONS

- Fracture of the tibia or fibula

SUPPLIES

- Conscious sedation
- Materials for soft cast

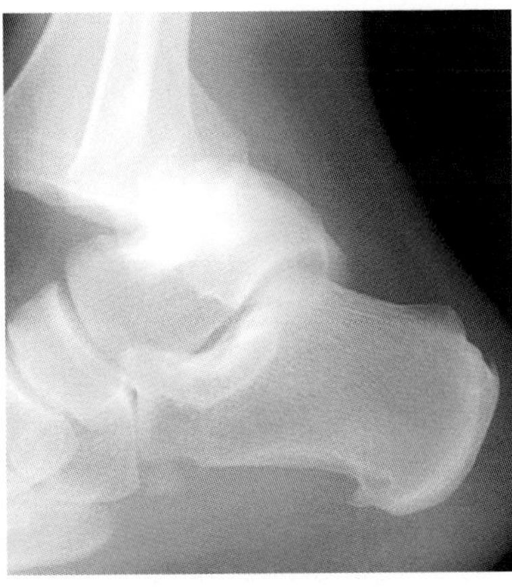

Fig. 30-1 Radiograph showing ankle dislocation.

POSITIONING

- Supine with legs hanging off the bottom of the bed

TECHNIQUE

- The assistant should grasp the patient's thigh to immobilize the upper leg.
- The clinician should grasp the heel of the foot in one hand and the forefoot in the other hand (Fig. 30-2).
- Twist the foot slightly toward the side on which it is located (same side as the talus).
- Twist the foot in the direction opposite the mechanism of injury, pulling the talus back into place underneath the tibia.

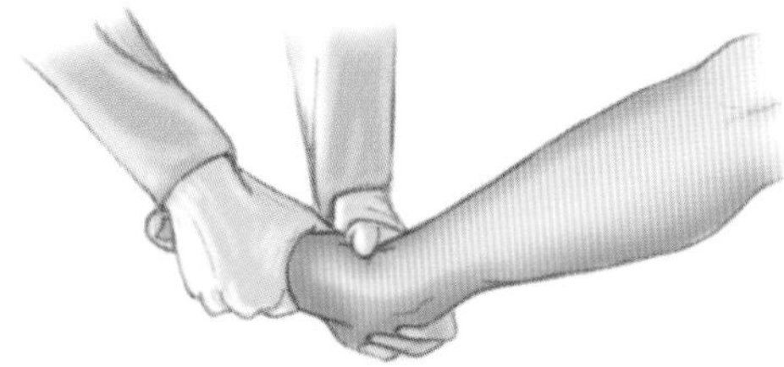

Fig. 30-2

PEARLS

- *Having the affected leg dangle off the bed allows gravity to assist in reducing the joint.*

PITFALLS

- Ankle dislocations can lead to damage of the neurovascular structures in the foot and need to be reduced urgently.
- Unreduced joints should lead to consultation with orthopedics.

See Appendix E for additional helpful information.

31

Closed Reduction: Hip Dislocation

A 67-year-old woman presents with a dislocated hip.

INDICATIONS

- Posterior dislocation of the hip (Fig. 31-1)

CONTRAINDICATIONS

- Any fracture of the femur

SUPPLIES

- Conscious sedation
- Sling

POSITIONING

- Supine

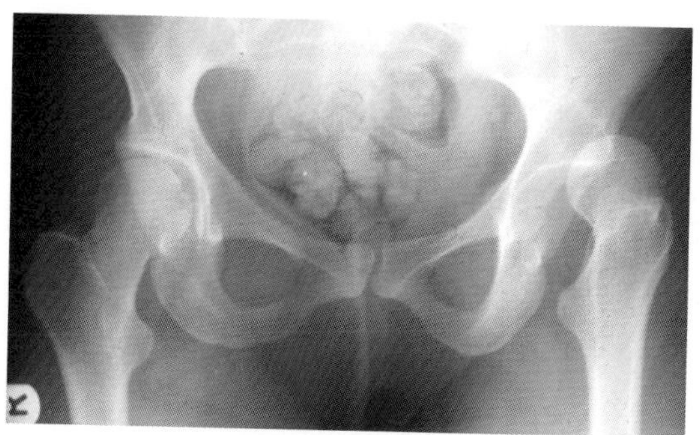

Fig. 31-1 Hip and pelvis radiograph showing left hip dislocation.

TECHNIQUE

- Assess the results of a neurologic examination of the sciatic nerve before and after closed reduction.
- An assistant stands on the side of the uninjured leg and stabilizes the patient's pelvis by grasping the anterior superior iliac spine.
- Flex the injured limb 90 degrees at both the hip and knee (Fig. 31-2).
- Grasp the calf and the back of the knee, and apply steady traction in line with the femur.
- Reduction is usually accompanied by a clicking sound.
- Place in a sling.
- Obtain radiographs.

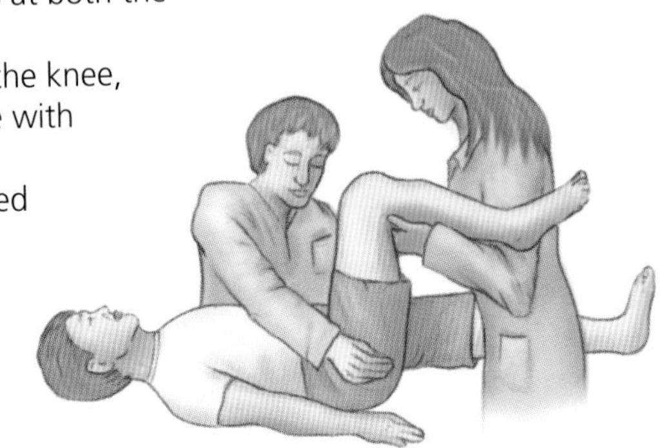

Fig. 31-2

PEARLS

- *Always apply steady constant traction; sudden traction can fracture the femoral neck.*

PITFALLS

- Unsuccessfully reduced dislocations should lead to orthopedic consultation.
- Injury to the sciatic nerve should lead to orthopedic consultation.

✓ POSTPROCEDURE CHECK

- ❑ Confirm reduction of the hip with radiographs.

See Appendix E for additional helpful information.

32

Closed Reduction: Radial Head Dislocation

A 12-year-old boy presents with a dislocated elbow.

INDICATIONS

- Dislocation of the radial head (Fig. 32-1)

CONTRAINDICATIONS

- Any fracture of the radius or elbow joint

SUPPLIES

- Conscious sedation
- Arm sling

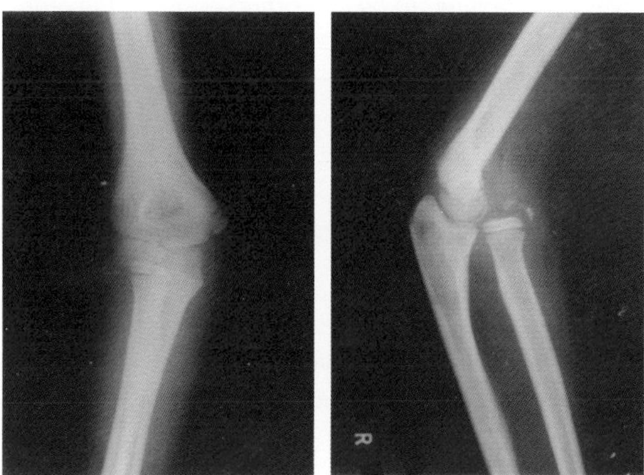

Fig. 32-1 Elbow radiographs revealing radial head dislocation.

POSITIONING

- Sitting

TECHNIQUE

- While the patient is sitting, grasp the hand of the injured arm.
- A handshake grasp is the most secure and allows the free hand to be placed on the patient's elbow (Fig. 32-2).
- With your free hand on the patient's elbow, use your thumb to apply pressure posteriorly.
- While applying pressure with your thumb, supinate the patient's forearm with your grasping hand.
- This may need to be repeated several times to achieve reduction of the radial head.
- Place the elbow in a sling.

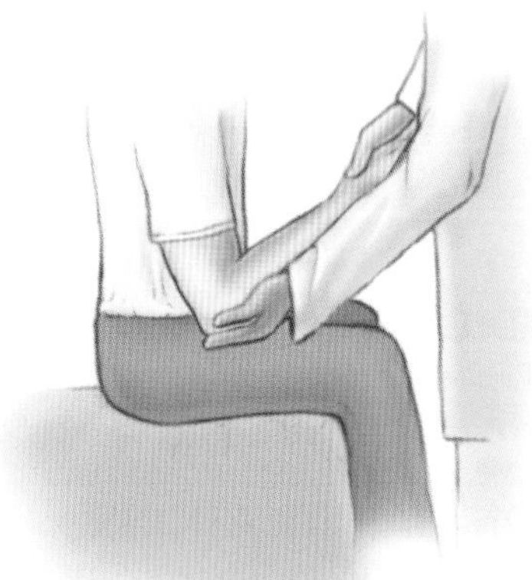

Fig. 32-2

PEARLS

- *If the patient is too sedated to be in a sitting position, the reduction can be safely attempted with the patient recumbent.*

PITFALLS

- Unsuccessfully reduced dislocations should lead to orthopedic consultation.

See Appendix E for additional helpful information.

33

Closed Reduction: Shoulder Joint Dislocation

A 22-year-old man presents with a dislocated shoulder.

INDICATIONS

- Anterior dislocation (Fig. 33-1)
- Posterior dislocation

CONTRAINDICATIONS

- Humeral shaft fracture

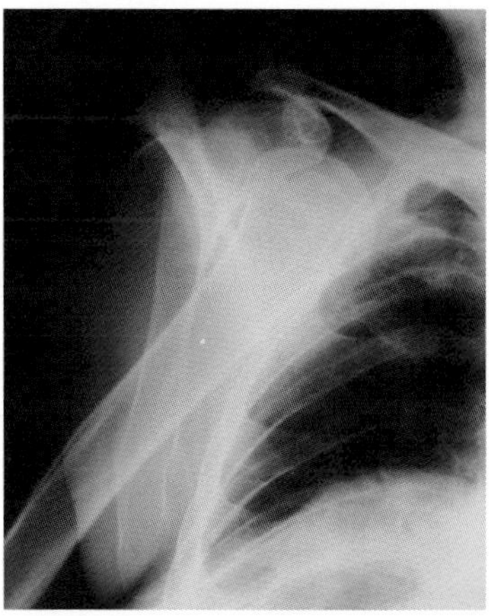

Fig. 33-1 Shoulder radiograph revealing right anterior shoulder dislocation.

SUPPLIES

- Conscious sedation
- Shoulder splint

POSITIONING

- Supine, with the head of the bed at 30 degrees, and the clinician standing next to the dislocated shoulder

TECHNIQUE

Anterior Dislocation

- Always assess axillary nerve function before and after closed reduction of the shoulder.
- Immobilize the patient in bed by wrapping a blanket around the thorax and tying it to the bed railing.
- Tie another sheet, folded into a narrow swath, around your waist, and drop a loop around the forearm of the patient's dislocated arm (Fig. 33-2).
- The arm should be flexed 90 degrees at the elbow and abducted 30 degrees at the shoulder.
- Traction is applied to the arm (the humerus) in this direction steadily for 5 to 10 minutes until the shoulder reduces into place (usually with a click).
- Confirm complete reduction by having the patient touch the contralateral shoulder with the injured arm.
- Immobilize the shoulder in internal rotation and adduction.
- Obtain AP and scapular Y radiographs.

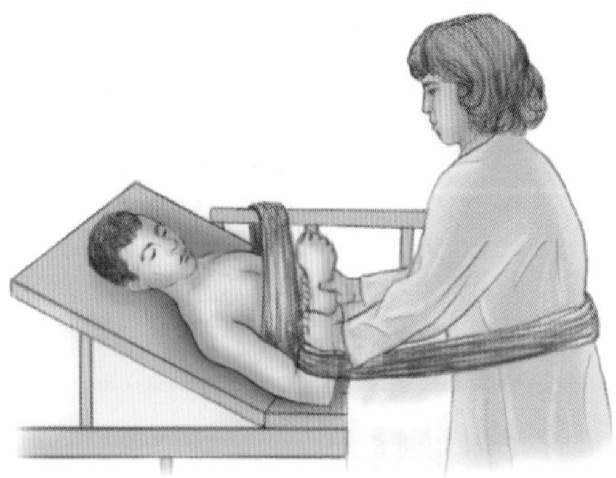

Fig. 33-2

Posterior Dislocation

- Always assess axillary nerve function before and after closed reduction of the shoulder.
- Use the same methods as for anterior dislocation.
- When applying traction on the arm, gentle internal rotation can help reduce the posteriorly dislocated shoulder.

PEARLS

- *Palpate the shoulder to help confirm the prominence of the deltoid muscle in a properly reduced shoulder.*
- *Posterior dislocations are more difficult to reduce, and excessive shoulder rotation should be avoided.*

PITFALLS

- Fractures and axillary nerve damage should lead to orthopedic consultation.
- Excessive external rotation during attempted reduction of a posteriorly dislocated fracture can fracture the humerus.

✓ POSTPROCEDURE CHECK

- ❑ Reduction of a dislocated shoulder should be confirmed by radiographs.

See Appendix E for additional helpful information.

34

Conscious Sedation

A 23-year-old man presents with a dislocated shoulder.

INDICATIONS

- Need for sedation for invasive or painful procedure

CONTRAINDICATIONS

- Unstable patient or patient for whom general anesthesia is indicated

SUPPLIES

- ACLS-certified clinician
- Cardiac monitoring
- Blood pressure monitoring
- Pulse oximetery
- Oxygen source and nasal cannula or face mask
- Bag mask resuscitator
- Emergency intubation equipment
- Intravenous access

POSITIONING

- Supine

DRUGS USED FOR SEDATION

Table 34-1 Analgesics

Drug Name	Initial Dose	Onset	Maximum Dose	Duration	Side Effects
Fentanyl	25-50 μg	60 sec	1-3 μg/kg	30-60 min	Respiratory depression, hypotension, bronchospasm
Morphine	2-4 mg	2 min	0.1 mg/kg	3-4 hr	Respiratory depression, hypotension, bronchospasm
Meperidine	25-50 mg	1-2 min	1-2 mg/kg	2-4 hr	Respiratory depression, seizures, contraindicated by monoamine oxidase inhibitors

Table 34-2 Sedatives (With Amnesic Properties)

Drug Name	Initial Dose	Onset	Maximum Dose	Duration	Side Effects
Midazolam	0.5-1.0 mg	60 sec	0.05-0.1 mg/kg	1-2 hr	Respiratory depression and hypotension
Diazepam	1-2 mg	2-5 min	0.1 mg/kg	1-4 hr	Respiratory depression and hypotension
Droperidol	1.0-2.5 mg	2-5 min	6.0 mg	2-4 hr	Respiratory depression and hypotension; sedative effects are synergistic with narcotics and other sedatives

Table 34-3 Reversal Drugs

Drug Name	Initial Dose	Onset	Maximum Dose	Duration	Side Effects
Naloxone (opioid antagonist)	0.1-0.2 mg	1-3 min	0.1 mg/kg	1 hr	Catecholamine surge
Flumazenil (benzodiazepine antagonist)	0.2 mg	30-60 sec	1.0 mg	30-90 min	Respiratory depression and hypotension

PEARLS

- *Morphine and fentanyl act similarly, but fentanyl may have a reduced incidence of bronchospasm (less histamine release).*

PITFALLS

- Meperidine cannot be used in patients taking monoamine oxidase inhibitors. Also, avoid using in patients with compromised renal function.

See Appendix E for additional helpful information.

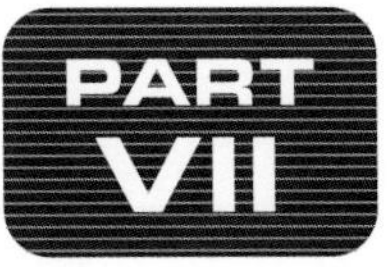

EMERGENCY MEDICAL MANAGEMENT

35

Advanced Cardiac Life Support (ACLS)

CARDIAC ARRHYTHMIAS

Normal Heart Rate and Rhythm

- A normal heart rate is between 60 and 100 beats/min.
- Heart rate is controlled by the heart's endogenous conduction system, which fires automatically to maintain a steady rate.
- Sympathetic and parasympathetic nervous systems can increase or decrease heart rate, respectively.
- Heart rhythm includes *how* the heart beats in addition to the heart rate, such as whether there is a consistent time interval between ventricular depolarization and atrial depolarization.
- Normal heart rhythm (sinus rhythm) is described by specific waves on an ECG. These waves depict the electrical activity of the heart responsible for its mechanical movement (such as contraction and relaxation).

Waves on a Normal ECG (Fig. 35-1)

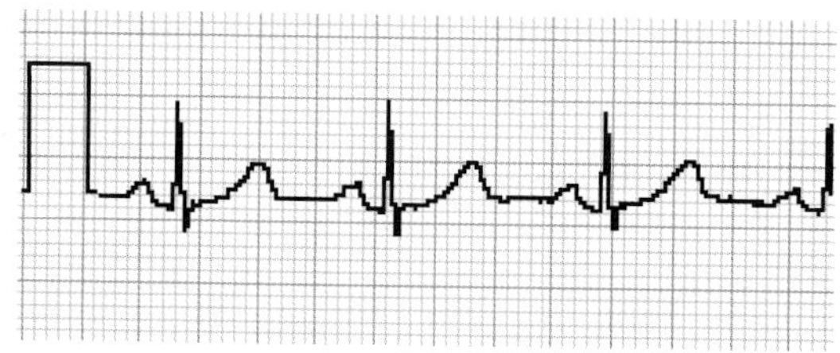

Fig. 35-1 Normal wave pattern from lead II of an ECG.

- Waves appear in the following order, and the time between waves is consistent within and between beats.
  - P wave: atrial depolarization
  - QRS complex: ventricular depolarization (normally <120 msec); masks atrial repolarization
  - T wave: ventricular repolarization

Interpretation of a Normal ECG

- PR interval: conduction delay through the atrioventricular (AV) node (normally <200 msec)
- QT interval: mechanical contraction of the ventricles

Abnormal Heart Rate and Rhythm (Arrhythmias)

- Bradycardia
- Tachycardia
- Cardiac arrest
- Asystole
- Pulseless electrical activity
- Ventricular fibrillation and pulseless ventricular tachycardia

PRIMARY SURVEY

The purpose of a primary survey is to detect and treat problems that pose an immediate threat to survival.

Airway

- Assess for responsiveness.
- Check whether the airway is patent.
- Open the airway if it is closed, and be careful of injuries to the cervical spine.

Breathing

- Assess breathing.
- Provide rescue breathing if necessary.
- Provide positive pressure ventilation when necessary and accessible.

Circulation

- Assess circulation (pulse and blood pressure).
- Check for bleeding that can be controlled.
- Administer CPR if necessary.

Disability

- Perform a neurologic examination and assess consciousness.
- Check for signs of severe central nervous system injury or penetrating injuries.

Defibrillate

- If ventricular fibrillation or pulseless ventricular tachycardia is present, defibrillation is needed.

SECONDARY SURVEY

The purpose of a secondary survey is to detect problems that do not pose an immediate threat to survival but need to be addressed to ensure patient recovery.

Airway

- Assess for possible flame or fire injury.
- Check for hoarseness or stridor.
- Position airway device as soon as possible.

Breathing

- Assess whether the patient is moving a sufficient amount of air.
- Secure the airway device and confirm its function by examination and testing.
- Ensure adequate oxygenation and ventilation.
- Consider bronchoscopy to check for airway damage and swelling.

Circulation

- Monitor blood pressure.
- Check for signs of perfusion (such as warm toes and sufficient urine outflow).
- Ensure IV access for resuscitating.
  - Peripheral lines are best if used early.
  - A central line is needed for drawing blood, monitoring hemodynamics, and aggressive fluid resuscitation.
- Identify and monitor rhythm.
- Treat rhythm abnormalities with appropriate drugs.

Disability

- Check the patient from head to toe and palpate bones.
- Treat traumatic injuries.

Differential Diagnosis

- Consider differential diagnosis and treat reversible causes.

BRADYCARDIA (Fig. 35-2)

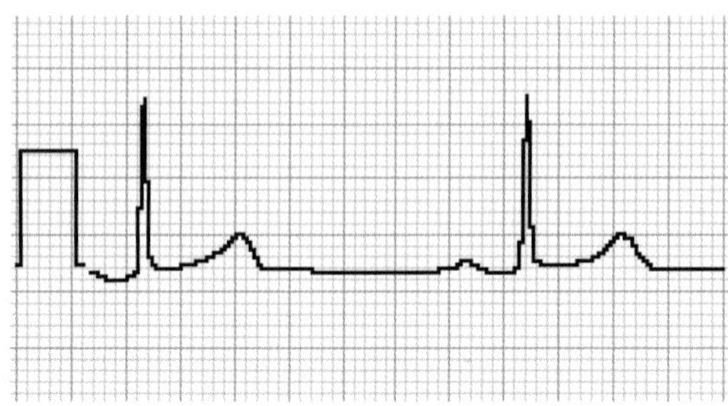

Fig. 35-2 Sinus bradycardia from lead II of an ECG.

Definition and Physiology

- Absolute bradycardia is a heart rate less than 60 beats/min.
- Relative bradycardia is a low heart rate (which can be more than 60 beats/min) that is inconsistent with a patient's underlying condition, such as a low heart rate in a patient with hypotension.
- A slow heart rate may be physiologically normal for some patients, but it can also present as an emergency medical situation when perfusion is compromised.

Signs and Symptoms

- Signs: low blood pressure, pulmonary congestion, congestive heart failure, and shock
- Symptoms: shortness of breath, chest pain, and decreased level of consciousness

Patient Evaluation

- The degree of bradycardia determines whether medical intervention is needed.
- Bradycardia may be present without symptoms, because the heart may be able to compensate for it.
- When bradycardia presents with the signs and symptoms given previously, poor perfusion is possible and medical intervention may be indicated.
- Methods of evaluation include the following:
  - Clinical history and physical examination
    - Precipitating factors associated with bradycardic episodes
    - Medications
  - Laboratory tests for underlying conditions (such as thyroid disease)
  - 12-lead ECG

Differential Diagnosis and/or Common Causes

- Myocardial infarction or ischemia
- Heart-related surgical trauma
- Infectious diseases (endocarditis, Chagas disease)
- Drugs
- Electrolyte disturbances

Workup

- See Primary Survey and Secondary Survey.

Treatment

- Asymptomatic bradycardia during a medical emergency requires monitoring for deterioration of perfusion.
- If a type II second-degree AV block or third-degree AV block is confirmed in an asymptomatic patient, transvenous pacing should be prepared. If the patient suddenly becomes symptomatic, administer transcutaneous pacing while transvenous pacing is being prepared.
- Symptomatic bradycardia should be treated with atropine, transcutaneous pacing, dopamine, and epinephrine.

TACHYCARDIA (Fig. 35-3)

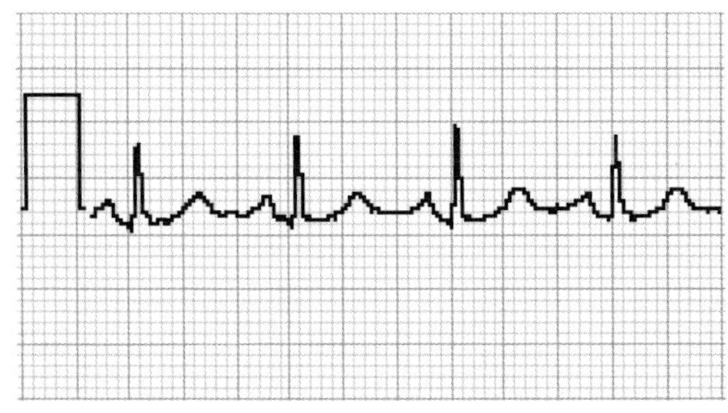

Fig. 35-3 Sinus tachycardia from lead II of an ECG.

Definition and Physiology

- Tachycardia is a heart rate greater than 100 beats/min.
- The increased rate can be in the upper or lower chambers of the heart.
- There are a variety of types and causes of tachycardia, described in the following sections.
- A fast heart rate can be asymptomatic, or it can cause serious problems, because the heart's ability to pump blood may be compromised.

Signs and Symptoms

- Dizziness
- Shortness of breath
- Lightheadedness
- Rapid pulse rate
- Palpitations
- Chest pain
- Fainting (syncope)

Patient Evaluation

- Tachycardia may be asymptomatic (stable) or symptomatic (unstable), indicating inadequate perfusion.
- Clinical history and physical examination
  - If patient is symptomatic, find out the number of episodes, duration, frequency, onset, and precipitating factors.
- 12-lead ECG
  - Is the rhythm regular (sinus) or irregular?
  - Is the QRS complex narrow or wide?

Differential Diagnosis and/or Common Causes

- Damage to heart tissue from heart disease
- Congenital abnormalities
- Abnormal electrical pathways in the heart
- Drugs or medications (such as cocaine)
- Overactive thyroid (hyperthyroid)

Workup

- See Primary Survey and Secondary Survey.
- Unstable patients should receive immediate electrical cardioversion.
- If the patient is stable, is the QRS narrow or wide?
  - For wide QRS (>120 msec), seek expert consultation (see Treatment).
  - For narrow QRS, check the regularity of the rhythm.
- Is the rhythm regular or irregular?
  - For irregular rhythm, atrial fibrillation or flutter is possible; seek expert consultation (see Treatment).
  - If the rhythm is regular, supraventricular tachycardia (SVT) is possible; see Treatment (Narrow QRS).
- If patient becomes unstable, perform immediate electrical cardioversion.

Treatment

Stable

Atrial fibrillation or flutter

- Treatment includes rate control and conversion to regular (sinus) rhythm, but the specific methods of treatment vary depending on the underlying cardiac function and pathology.
- Normal cardiac function (normal ejection fraction)
  - Rate control
    - Calcium channel blockers (diltiazem or verapamil) or beta-blockers
  - Conversion to sinus rhythm if duration less than 48 hours
    - Electrical cardioversion
    - Amiodarone, ibutilide, or other drugs
  - Conversion to sinus rhythm if duration more than 48 hours
    - No electrical cardioversion because of embolism risk (risk is reduced by more than 3 weeks of anticoagulation therapy)
    - Antiarrhythmics used with caution
    - Delayed cardioversion: after 3 weeks of anticoagulation therapy, administer electrical cardioversion followed by 4 more weeks of anticoagulation therapy
    - Early cardioversion: administer electrical cardioversion within 24 hours after administering IV heparin and excluding thrombi by transesophageal echocardiogram; followed by 4 weeks of anticoagulation therapy
- Impaired heart (ejection fraction <40% or CHF)
  - Rate control
    - Digoxin, diltiazem, or amiodarone
  - Conversion to sinus rhythm if duration less than 48 hours
    - Same as for normal cardiac function
  - Conversion to sinus rhythm if duration more than 48 hours
    - Same as for normal cardiac function
- Wolff-Parkinson-White Syndrome
  - Rate control
    - Do not attempt rate control.
    - Adenosine, beta-blockers, calcium channel blockers, and digoxin are all **harmful.**
    - If patient becomes unstable, or if duration is less than 48 hours, perform immediate electrical cardioversion.
  - Conversion to sinus rhythm if duration less than 48 hours
    - Electrical cardioversion
    - Primary antiarrhythmic treatment with only one of the following: amiodarone, flecainide, propafenone, or procainamide
  - Conversion to sinus rhythm if duration more than 48 hours
    - Anticoagulation therapy followed by early or delayed cardioversion (as described previously)

Stable ventricular tachycardia (Fig. 35-4)

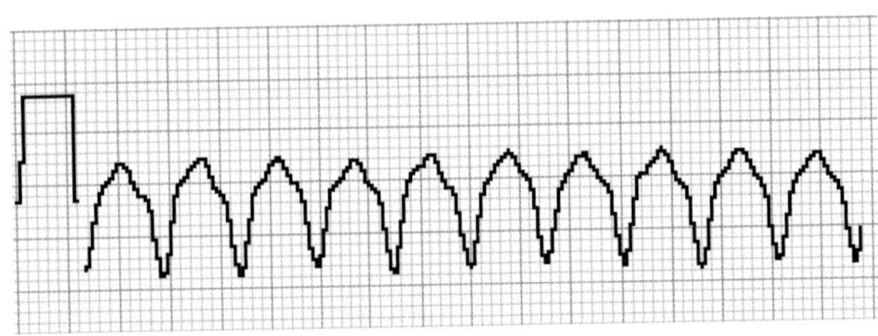

Fig. 35-4 Monomorphic sustained tachycardia from lead II of an ECG. Note that pulseless ventricular tachycardia is simply a ventricular tachycardia rhythm when there is no pulse.

- Is the rhythm monomorphic or polymorphic?
  - Monomorphic means that each beat on a given ECG lead is the same.
  - Polymorphic means that there is a beat-to-beat variation on the ECG.
- For monomorphic stable ventricular tachycardia, assess ventricular function.
  - For normal ventricular function, administer procainamide, sotalol, amiodarone, or lidocaine.
  - For impaired cardiac function, administer amiodarone or lidocaine, and then perform synchronized cardioversion.
- For polymorphic stable ventricular tachycardia, check baseline QT.
  - For normal baseline QT
    - Treat ischemia, correct electrolytes, and decrease beta-agonist.
    - Administer beta-blockers, lidocaine, amiodarone, procainamide, or sotalol.
  - For prolonged baseline QT
    - Correct electrolytes, including potassium, calcium, and magnesium.
    - Administer magnesium, overdrive pacing, isoproterenol (until pacing is available), phenytoin, or lidocaine.
  - For either monomorphic or polymorphic stable ventricular tachycardia, consider immediate electrical cardioversion.

Narrow QRS

- Diagnose specific rhythm.
- Obtain 12-lead ECG.
- Ascertain clinical information/history if possible.
- Perform vagal maneuvers, and administer adenosine.

- Supraventricular tachycardia is possible.
- If ventricular tachycardia is suspected, follow instructions under Stable Ventricular Tachycardia.

Stable wide QRS

- Diagnose specific rhythm.
- Obtain 12-lead ECG.
- Ascertain clinical information.
- Apply an esophageal lead.
- If wide QRS tachycardia of an unclear type is suspected, consider the following:
  - Electrical cardioversion
  - Amiodarone
  - Procainamide if ejection fraction is greater than 0.40 and no CHF
- If ventricular tachycardia is suspected, follow instructions under Stable Ventricular Tachycardia.
- Supraventricular tachycardia is possible.

Unstable

- Verify that rapid heart rate is the cause of patient's signs and symptoms.
- A heart rate of less than 150 beats/min is rarely a cause of instability.
- Immediate electrical cardioversion is indicated.

CARDIAC ARREST

Definition and Physiology

- Sudden loss of cardiac function, respiration, and consciousness
- Caused by an electrical disturbance in the heart (arrhythmia) that decreases the ability of the heart to pump and compromises circulation
- Varies from myocardial infarction in that MI is caused by decreased or blocked perfusion to the heart

Signs and Symptoms

- Sudden collapse
- No pulse
- No breathing
- Unconscious

Patient Evaluation (If Patient Is Successfully Resuscitated)

- Complete history
  - Look for underlying and correctible causes.
  - Inquire about new medications, illicit drugs (such as cocaine), and new diets.
- Physical examination
  - Check for findings of atherosclerosis (such as peripheral vascular disease, xanthomas, or xanthelasmas).
  - Cardiac examination may reveal murmurs (S_3 and S_4).
- Laboratory examinations
  - Cardiac enzymes
- ECG

Predisposing Factors/Differential Diagnosis

- Preexisting heart diseases can predispose a patient to lethal arrhythmia.
  - Coronary artery disease
  - Myocardial infarction
  - Enlarged heart
  - Valvular heart disease
  - Congenital heart disease (hypertrophic cardiomyopathy)
  - Primary heart rhythm abnormalities
- Triggers can cause lethal arrhythmia in a healthy heart.
  - Electric shock
  - Trauma to the chest
  - Drugs
- Some causes are reversible.
  - Hypovolemia
  - Hypoxia
  - H+ acidosis
  - Hyperkalemia
  - Hypothermia
  - Drug overdose
  - Tamponade
  - Tension pneumothorax
  - Thrombosis (coronary/pulmonary)

Treatment

- See Primary Survey.
- Assess rhythm and continue administering CPR if there is no pulse.
  - If ventricular fibrillation or ventricular tachycardia is present, then attempt defibrillation, followed by CPR for 1 minute.
  - If neither ventricular fibrillation nor ventricular tachycardia is present (the patient is in asystole or has pulseless electrical activity), then administer CPR for 3 minutes.
- See Secondary Survey.

ASYSTOLE (Fig. 35-5)

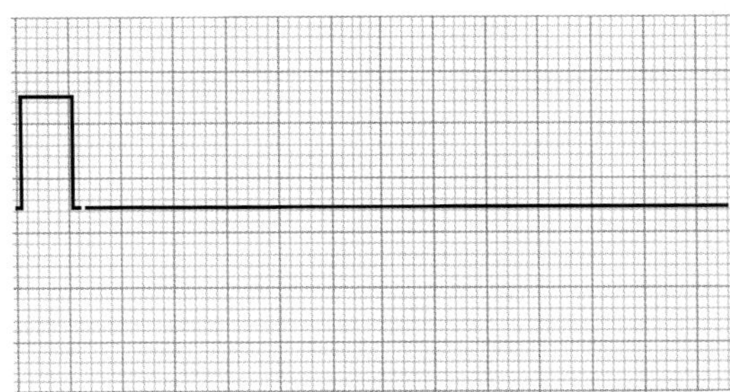

Fig. 35-5 Asystole.

Definition and Physiology

- Asystole is suspended cardiac function with no cardiac output and no ventricular depolarization.
- Asystole ultimately occurs in all dying patients.

Signs and Symptoms

- Unconscious
- Unresponsive
- Lack of heart sounds and peripheral pulses
- Possible presence of agonal breath sounds

Patient Evaluation

- ECG while administering resuscitation efforts

Differential Diagnosis and/or Common Causes

- Primary asystole is caused by an intrinsic defect in the heart's conduction system that results in a failure to generate ventricular depolarization.
  - May be a result of ischemia or degeneration of the sinoatrial or atrioventricular nodes
- Secondary asystole occurs when factors extrinsic to the heart create an inability to generate electrical depolarization.
  - Ultimately, tissue hypoxia and metabolic acidosis lead to asystole.

Treatment

- See Primary Survey and Secondary Survey.
- Transcutaneous pacing may be applied if it is considered an option; however, it is not usually considered, and it must be done early and in combination with medications.
- Vasopressin, epinephrine, and atropine may be helpful in reviving patients.
- Consider terminating resuscitation efforts if asystole persists.
  - Consider the quality of resuscitation efforts and how they can be improved.
  - Check for atypical clinical features, including hypothermia, drowning, and reversible therapeutic or illicit drug overdose.
  - Ensure support for termination of resuscitation efforts.

PULSELESS ELECTRICAL ACTIVITY

Definition and Physiology

- Presence of electrical activity in the heart combined with a lack of palpable pulse and unresponsiveness
- Can be caused by extreme cardiac insults that result in decreased preload, increased afterload, or decreased contractility

Signs and Symptoms

- Pulselessness
- Apnea
- Electrical activity present on ECG
- No heart tones heard on auscultation

Patient Evaluation

- ECG

Differential Diagnosis and/or Common Causes

- Caused by inability of the heart to generate a forceful contraction following electrical depolarization
- May be caused by profound respiratory, cardiovascular, or metabolic insult
- Often caused by hypoxia from respiratory failure

Treatment

- See Primary Survey and Secondary Survey.
- Check for frequent causes:
  - Hypovolemia
  - Hypoxia
  - Acidosis
  - Hyperkalemia
  - Hypothermia
  - Drug overdose
  - Tamponade
  - Tension pneumothorax
  - Thrombosis (coronary)
  - Pulmonary thromboembolism
- Vasopressin followed by epinephrine
- Atropine

VENTRICULAR FIBRILLATION AND PULSELESS VENTRICULAR TACHYCARDIA (Fig. 35-6)

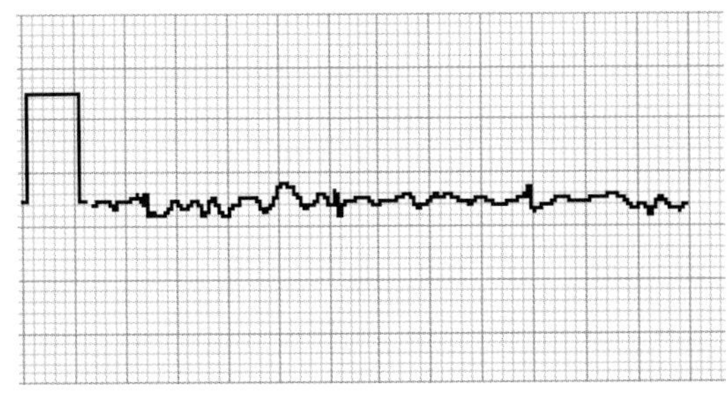

Fig. 35-6 Ventricular fibrillation from lead II of an ECG.

Definition and Physiology

- Ventricular fibrillation is uncontrolled twitching of the lower chambers of the heart; blood is not pumped from the ventricles.
- Pulseless ventricular tachycardia is a fast heart rate originating in the ventricles; this form of ventricular tachycardia has no effective cardiac output or pulse and is best treated in the same way as ventricular fibrillation.
- Both of these conditions lead to compromised blood circulation, cardiac arrest, and death.

Signs and Symptoms

- No pulse
- No respiration
- Unconscious
- Wide and chaotic QRS complexes on ECG
- Before ventricular fibrillation there may be the following:
  - Chest pain
  - Dyspnea
  - Easy fatigue
  - Palpitations or syncope

Differential Diagnosis and/or Common Causes

- Ventricular fibrillation
  - The most common cause of ventricular fibrillation is myocardial infarction.
  - Predisposing factors include congenital heart disease, electrocution, heart injury, cardiomyopathy, heart surgery, ischemia, and sudden cardiac death.
- Pulseless ventricular tachycardia
  - See causes of Ventricular Tachycardia in Tachycardia section.

Treatment

- See Primary Survey (Defibrillate) and Secondary Survey.
- Administer vasopressin followed by epinephrine.
- Resume defibrillation attempts.
- Administer antiarrhythmics: amiodarone, lidocaine, magnesium, procainamide, bicarbonate.
- Resume defibrillation attempts.

Suggested Readings

Cummins RO, ed. ACLS: Principles and Practice. Dallas: American Heart Association, 2004.

Delacrétaz E. Supraventricular tachycardia. N Engl J Med 354:1039-1051, 2006.

Desbeins NA. Simplifying the diagnosis and management of pulseless electrical activity in adults: a qualitative review. Crit Care Med 36:391-396, 2008.

Jalife J. Ventricular fibrillation: mechanism of initiation and maintenance. Annu Rev Physiol 62:25-50, 2000.

Mangrum JM, DiMarco JP. The evaluation and management of bradycardia. N Engl J Med 342:703-709, 2000.

Roth JJ, Hughes WB. The Essential Burn Unit Handbook. St Louis: Quality Medical Publishing, 2004.

36

ANAPHYLAXIS

Table 36-1 Managing Anaphylaxis

Airway	Administer 100% O_2 and consider early intubation for airway edema
Cardiac	Apply cardiac monitor and pulse oximeter; assess vital signs frequently
Skin	Remove stinger; apply ice; epinephrine (0.1-0.3 mg of 1:1000) subcutaneously local to site if not an end organ (i.e., finger, toe, or nose)
Gastrointestinal	Consider charcoal, 50 g by mouth, for an ingested allergen

Drug	**Dose**	**Route**	**Indications**
Epinephrine*	0.01 g/kg	Subcutaneous or intramuscular IV	Mild/moderate symptoms • Airway compromise • Severe hypotension Use with extreme caution and only in severe, life-threatening situations
Normal saline solution	20 ml/kg	IV	Hypotension
Methylpred-nisolone	2 mg/kg	IV	Moderate/severe symptoms
Diphenhydramine	1 mg/kg	IV/intramuscular	Moderate/severe symptoms (maximum 50 mg)
Cimetidine	5 mg/kg	IV/intramuscular	If no wheezing (bronchoconstricts)
Glucagon	2-5 mg	IV	If patient is taking a beta-blocker
Albuterol	2.5 mg	Nebulized	Bronchospasm
Racemic epinephrine	0.2-0.4 ml	Nebulized	Stridor (2.25% solution)

*Use with extreme caution, because severe, life-threatening complications can occur.

37

Status Epilepticus

DEFINITION

- Persistent seizure or repeated seizures without full recovery between episodes; operationally defined as a seizure lasting longer than 5 minutes or two seizures between which there is incomplete recovery of consciousness

ETIOLOGIC FACTORS

- Acute structural injury: trauma, tumor, stroke, hemorrhage, or anoxia
- Remote structural injury: head trauma, previous stroke or neurosurgery, or arteriovenous malformation (AVM)
- Central nervous system (CNS) infection: encephalitis or meningitis
- Toxin: penicillins, imipenem, fluoroquinolones, metronidazole, isoniazid, cyclic antidepressants, lithium, antipsychotics, lidocaine, meperidine, theophylline, cyclosporine, or cocaine (often dose-related or in patients with renal or hepatic insufficiency)
- Drug withdrawal: ethanol, opiates, barbiturates, or benzodiazepines (flumazenil)
- Metabolic: hypoglycemia or hyperglycemia, electrolytes (↓Na^+, ↓Ca^{++}, ↓Mg^{++}), hyperosmolar state, hypoxia, or uremia
- New-onset or inadequately controlled chronic epilepsy: change in anticonvulsant drug levels (drug interactions, noncompliance, and altered absorption); intercurrent infection or metabolic abnormality; ethanol excess, or withdrawal

COMPLICATIONS

- Neuronal death after 30 to 60 minutes of continuous seizure activity (even with little or no motor activity; for example, paralyzed for airway management)
- Mortality rate is as much as 35%, depending on underlying etiologic factors
- Other: rhabdomyolysis, aspiration, metabolic/lactic acidosis, respiratory failure, or neurogenic pulmonary edema

MANAGEMENT

Table 37-1 Suggested Management Algorithm[1]

Time	Intervention
0-5 minutes	• Assess ABCs; cardiac monitor • Give O_2; intubate if necessary • Obtain the patient's medical history and perform a physical examination, including a neurologic examination • Start an IV and draw blood for electrolytes (including Mg^{++}/Ca^{++}), glucose, complete blood count, renal/liver function, toxicology screen, and anticonvulsant drug levels • Check fingerstick glucose; give thiamine, 100 mg IV, before dextrose • Treat hyperthermia promptly with antipyretics or cooling blankets • Lorazepam, 0.1 mg/kg IV, at 2 mg/min • Call for EEG monitoring
5-25 minutes	If seizures continue • Phenytoin, 20 mg/kg IV, at 50 mg/min ***or*** • Fosphenytoin, 20 mg/kg PE* IV, at 150 mg/min • Monitor ECG and vital signs
25-30 minutes	If seizures continue • Phenytoin, additional 5-10 mg/kg IV, at 50 mg/min ***or*** • Fosphenytoin, additional 5-10 mg/kg PE* IV at 150 mg/min
30-50 minutes	If seizures continue • Phenobarbital, 20 mg/kg IV, at 50-75 mg/min ***or*** • Consider proceeding directly to anesthesia with midazolam or propofol (see the section for >60 minutes) if (1) patient is already in the ICU, (2) there is a severe systemic disturbance (e.g., hyperthermia), or (3) seizures have continued for >60-90 minutes
50-60 minutes	If seizures continue • Phenobarbital, additional 5-10 mg/kg IV at 50-75 mg/min
>60 minutes	If seizures continue, begin anesthesia in the ICU with • Midazolam, 0.2 mg/kg IV, followed by 75-100 μg/kg/hr or propofol, 1-2 mg/kg IV, followed by 2-10 mg/kg/hr • Adjust dosage to EEG response • Therapeutic levels may require intubation and pressor support

*Fosphenytoin dispensed in phenytoin equivalents (PEs).

INITIAL DRUG THERAPY

- Benzodiazepines are often given first because of their rapid onset and ease of delivery; their effectiveness is limited by sedation/respiratory depression.
- Lorazepam and diazepam have similar onsets (3 minutes versus 2 minutes), but diazepam has a shorter half-life because it is redistributed out of the CNS; diazepam may also be given per rectum (PR).
- Benzodiazepines and phenytoin are incompatible if given through the same IV.
- Fosphenytoin (a water-soluble product of phenytoin) may be given more rapidly than phenytoin, although the time to onset of clinical effect is similar.

Reference

1. Working Group on Status Epilepticus. Treatment of convulsive status epilepticus. JAMA 270:854-859, 1993.

38

Adult Trauma Life Support (ATLS)

Table 38-1 Initial Approach to Trauma Assessment and Management

Primary Survey	
Assess **Airway** (immobilize C-spine)	• If poor or no air movement, perform jaw thrust or insert oral or nasal airway • Intubate if Glasgow Coma Scale (GCS) $\leq$8, response to above is poor, or there is severe shock, flail chest, or a need to hyperventilate • Perform cricothyrotomy or apply a laryngeal mask airway if unsuccessful
Assess **Breathing**	• Examine neck and thorax for deviated trachea, flail chest, sucking chest wound, and breath sounds • Needle chest for tension pneumothorax; apply occlusive dressing to three sides of sucking chest wound; reposition ET tube or insert chest tubes (36-38 Fr) if needed • Administer O_2, apply pulse oximeter; measure ET CO_2
Assess **Circulation**	• Apply pressure to external bleeding sites; establish two large peripheral IV lines; obtain blood for basic labs and type and crossmatch; administer 2 liters NS IV as needed • Check pulses; listen for heart sounds; observe neck veins; assess cardiac rhythm; treat cardiac tamponade • Apply cardiac monitor; obtain BP and HR (pulse quality)
Assess **Disability** (neurologic status)	• Measure Glasgow Coma Scale, or • Assess whether alert or responsive to verbal cues or pain, or unresponsive to pain • Pupil assessment—size and reactivity
Patient **Exposure**	• Completely undress patient (but keep warm)

Continued

Table 38-1 Initial Approach to Trauma Assessment and Management—cont'd

Resuscitation (perform simultaneously during primary survey)	
Reassess ABCs	• Reassess ABCs if patient deteriorates; address abnormality as identified; place chest tube if needed • Emergent thoracotomy if >1.2-1.5 L of blood is obtained from initial chest tube, if there is >100-200 ml/hr after first hour, or if there is persistent low BP • Administer second 2 L NS bolus, then blood as needed • Place NG tube and Foley catheter (unless contraindicated)
Secondary Survey	
History	• Obtain AMPLE history (**A**llergies, **M**edications, **P**ast history, **L**ast meal, and **E**vents leading up to injury)
Physical examination	• Perform head-to-toe examination (including rectal/back).
Radiographs	• Obtain cervical spine, chest, and pelvic radiographs, plus CT scans and any other needed images
Address injuries	• Reduce/splint fractures; call consultants as soon as needed; administer analgesics, tetanus shot, and/or antibiotics as needed
Disposition	• Initiate transfer; admit or readmit to OR; document all findings, radiographs, laboratory values, and consultants; and talk to family

Table 38-2 Trauma Score*

Respiratory Rate	Systolic BP	Glasgow Coma Scale	Respiratory Effort	Capillary Refill
2 = ≥36/min	4 = ≥90 mmHg	5 = GCS 14-15	1 = Normal	2 = Normal
3 = 25-35/min	3 = 70-89 mm Hg	4 = GCS 11-13	0 = Shallow	1 = Delayed
4 = 10-24/min	2 = 50-69 mm Hg	3 = GCS 8-10	0 = Retractive	0 = None
1 = 0-9/min	1 = 0-49 mm Hg	2 = GCS 5-7		
0 = None	0 = No pulse	1 = GCS 3-4		

*A score ≤12 needs trauma center; a score >14 has <1% mortality; 13-14, 1%-2% risk; 11-12, 2-5% risk; ≤10, >10% risk.

Table 38-3 Glasgow Coma Scale*

Eye Opening	Best Verbal	Best Motor
4 = Spontaneous	5 = Oriented, converses	6 = Obeys commands
3 = Eyes open to verbal commands	4 = Disoriented, converses	5 = Localizes pain
2 = Eyes open to pain	3 = Inappropriate words	4 = Withdraws from pain
1 = No response	2 = Incomprehensible	3 = Abnormal flexion/ decorticate posture
	1 = No response	2 = Extension/decerebrate
		1 = No response

*Total score indicates mild (13-15), moderate (9-12), or severe (≤8) head injury.

Table 38-4 American College of Surgeons Classification of Shock

Class	Blood Volume Lost	Signs or Symptoms
I	<15% (<750 ml if 70 kg)	Normal HR, normal vital signs, few symptoms
II	15%-30% (750-1500 ml)	HR >100, low pulse pressure, anxiety, urine output 20-30 ml/hr, capillary refill >2 sec, RR 20-30
III	30%-40% (1500-2000 ml)	HR >120, low BP, RR 30-40, confused, urine output 5-15 ml/hr, capillary refill >2 sec
IV	>40% (>2000 ml)	HR >140, low BP, RR >35, confused/ lethargic, urine output negligible, capillary refill >3-4 sec

Table 38-5 High-Yield Criteria for Cranial CT Scan in Trauma Patients With a GCS of 13-15

Major Risk Factors

- Failure to reach GCS of 15 in 2 hr
- Suspected open skull fracture
- Any sign of basal skull fracture
- Vomiting, >1 episode
- Age >64 years

Minor Risk Factors

- Amnesia before impact >30 min
- Dangerous mechanism (pedestrian struck, assault by blunt object, fell >3 feet or down >5 stairs, heavy object fell on head, vehicle ejection)

Utility of Major Criteria in Predicting Need for Neurologic Intervention*

Sensitivity	100% (92%-100%)†
Specificity	68.7% (67%-70%)

Utility of Major and Minor Criteria in Predicting Clinically Important CNS Injury‡

Sensitivity	98.4% (96%-99%)
Specificity	49.6% (48%-51%)

From Stiell IG, Wells GA, Vandemheen K, et al. The Canadian CT Head Rule for patients with minor head injury. Lancet 357:1391-1396, 2001.

*Death ≤7 days, craniotomy, elevation of skull fracture, ICP monitor, intubate for head injury.

†Numbers in parentheses are 95% confidence intervals.

‡Any finding from a CT scan that requires admission and neurologic follow-up.

SEVERE HEAD INJURY MANAGEMENT

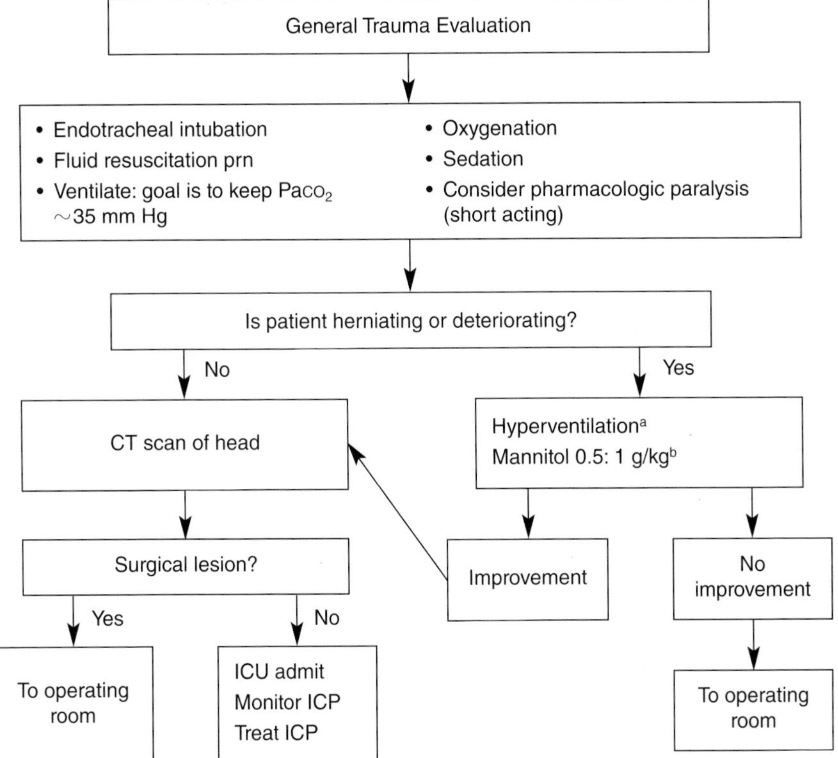

Fig. 38-1 Management of severe head injury (Glasgow Coma Scale ≤8). *a,* Hyperventilation should only be instituted for brief periods if there is acute neurologic deterioration. $Paco_2$ ≤35 mm Hg will cause decreased cerebral perfusion and can worsen the outcome. *b,* Mannitol is only indicated before ICP monitoring if signs of herniation or progressive neurologic deterioration occur. Bolus therapy is most effective. Keep serum Osm <320. (From the American Association of Neurological Surgeons/Brain Trauma Foundation. Guidelines for the Management of Severe Head Injury. Copyright © 2000 Brain Trauma Foundation.)

CERVICAL, THORACIC, AND LUMBAR SPINE INJURIES

NEXUS Cervical Spine Radiograph Criteria

- Neck tenderness—midline
- Motor or sensory deficit
- Altered mental status
- Intoxication with drugs or alcohol
- Distracting painful injury

These criteria were 99% sensitive, with a 99.9% negative predictive value for detecting clinically significant cervical spine fractures (if these features are absent there is only a 0.1% probability of fracture).[1]

Canadian C-Spine Rule (CCR)

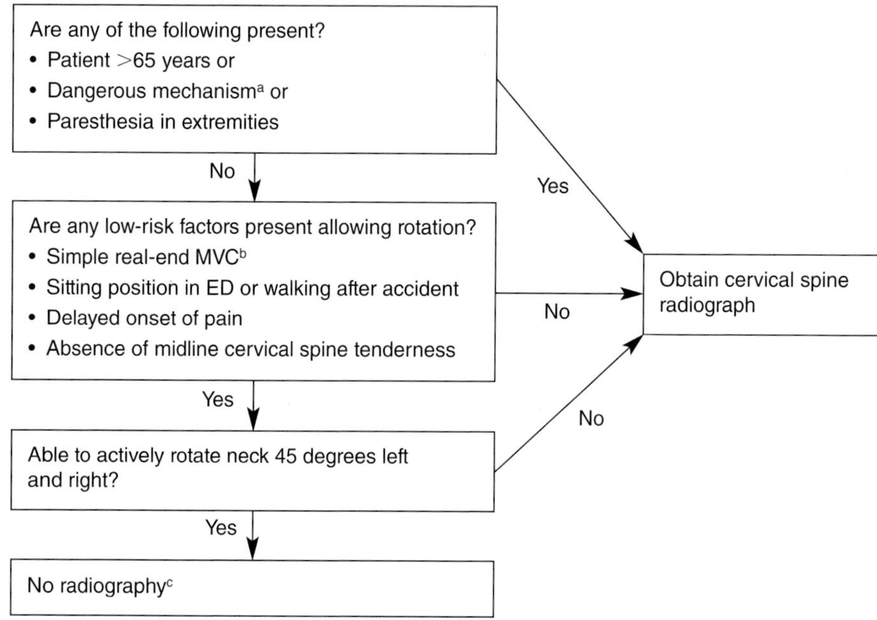

Fig. 38-2 *a,* Fall ≥3 feet/5 stairs, axial load to head (e.g., diving), high-speed MVC (>100 km [65 miles]/hr), rollover, ejection, motorized recreational vehicle crash, bicycle crash. *b,* Pushed into oncoming traffic, hit by bus/truck, rollover, hit at high speed. *c,* These criteria are 100% sensitive (98% to 100%, 95% confidence interval) in detecting clinically important C-spine fractures. A prospective study found the CCR to be more sensitive than the NEXUS rule for identifying C-spine injuries in stable alert patients in Canada. (From Stiell IG, Wells GA, Vandemheen KL, et al. The Canadian C-spine rule for radiography in alert and stable trauma patients. JAMA 286:1841-1848, 2001.)

Indications for Thoracolumbar Spine Radiographs in Blunt Trauma

- Back pain or tenderness
- Neurologic deficit
- Glasgow Coma Scale ≤14
- Drug or alcohol intoxication
- Fall ≥10 feet
- Ejection from motorcycle/vehicle
- Motor vehicle crash (MVC) ≥50 miles per hour
- Major distracting injury
- Pelvic or long bone fracture
- Intrathoracic or abdominal injury

Criteria were 100% sensitive in detecting thoracolumbar fractures in all five studies cited.

The mechanism (e.g., fall, MVC, or ejection) did not add to 100% sensitivity in several studies.[2-6]

TRAUMA—NECK INJURIES, PENETRATING

Wounds through platysma muscle are a major concern. Some experts believe that zone I and zone III injuries generally require angiography to identify major vascular injury, whereas zone II injuries generally do not (Fig. 38-3). Other experts manage penetrating injuries using the algorithm outlined in Fig. 38-4.

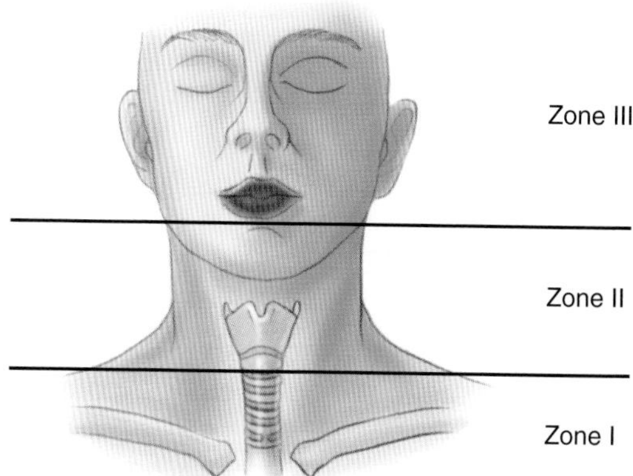

Fig. 38-3 Zone I, II, and III injuries.

Initial Management of Patient With Penetrating Neck Injury

- Airway: note that expanding hematomas, stridor, or other indicators of impending airway compromise mandate endotracheal intubation
- Breathing: obtain a chest radiograph to exclude pneumothorax; insert chest tube as needed
- Circulation: control bleeding by direct compression; give NS or blood
- Other evaluation: contact consultants early and exclude cervical, neurologic, vascular, airway, lung, and gastrointestinal injuries clinically, using chest radiographs or exploration

Neck Injury Management Based on Clinical Examination

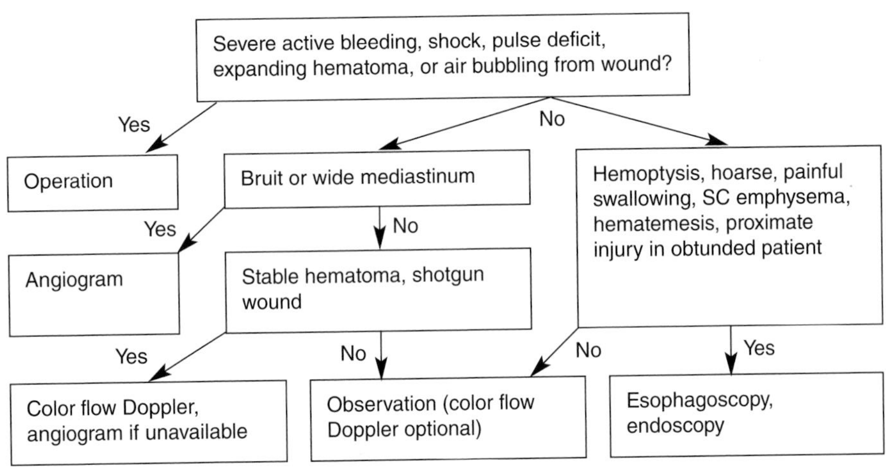

Fig. 38-4 (From Kendall JL, Anglin D, Demetriades D. Penetrating neck trauma. Emerg Med Clin North Am 16:85-105, 1998.)

TRAUMA: CHEST INJURIES

Myocardial Contusion

Overview and Emergency Room Diagnosis

- The most common injuries are to the right ventricle, anterior septum, and anterior apical left ventricle
- Diagnosis: chest radiograph, ECG, and O_2 saturation
  - Chest radiograph: pulmonary contusion, first or second rib fractures, clavicle or sternal fractures, congestive heart failure (CHF)
  - ECG findings may take 24 hours to develop
  - Cardiac markers are not useful diagnostically

Features

- Anginal pain (1 to 3 days after trauma) that is not relieved by nitroglycerin
- External thoracic trauma (73%)
- Tachycardia (70%)
- Friction rub
- Beck's triad (cardiac tamponade): decreased BP, jugular venous distention, and increased heart rate (present in <50%)

Radiologic Studies

- Echocardiogram: right ventricle (RV) wall dyskinesia with or without chamber dilation; echocardiography identifies most problems that require treatment
- Radionuclide angiography: assesses ejection fraction (EF); left and right ventricular EF are abnormal at <50% or <40%, respectively
- Single Photon Emission Computed Tomography (SPECT): can detect contusions and ischemia

ECG

- Sinus tachycardia: 70%
- Nonspecific ST-T changes: 60%
- Repolarization disturbances: 61%
- Atrial arrhythmia or conduction defects: 12%
- Ventricular arrhythmia: 22%
- Normal ECG: 12%
- Myocardial infarction: 2%

Management

Consider admission for monitoring if the ECG changes, or if the patient has cardiac disease, coexisting trauma, or is older than 45 to 55 years of age. Consider echocardiography or other tests (radionuclide angiography or SPECT). Additional studies should be performed only if there are problems or complications (e.g., arrhythmia, hemodynamic instability). If the patient is younger than 45 years and has a normal ECG, and if the tachycardia resolves, discharge after 4 hours of observation and cardiac monitoring.

Traumatic Thoracic Aortic Rupture

Only 10% to 20% of patients with traumatic thoracic aortic rupture survive to reach the emergency room. Rupture most frequently occurs at the fixed immobile ligamentum arteriosum as a result of a rapid deceleration injury.

Clinical Features

- Retrosternal or intrascapular pain
- Dyspnea, stridor, hoarseness, dysphagia
- Increase or decrease in BP (mean BP 152/98 mm Hg)
- Depressed lower extremity BP
- Systolic intrascapular/precordial murmur, swelling at base of neck
- Sternal, scapular, or multiple rib fractures (especially the first or second rib)
- Chest tube with initial output >750 ml

Chest Radiograph

- Increased mediastinal width* (52% to 90%)
- Obscured aortic knob
- Opacified aorticopulmonary window
- NG tube >2 cm to the right of T4
- Tracheal strip >5 mm from the right lung
- Left main-stem bronchus 40 degrees below horizontal
- Left hemothorax/apical pleural cap
- Normal chest radiograph (up to 15%)

Diagnosis

- Spiral CT scan: >97% to 100% sensitive for aortic rupture
- Transesophageal echocardiogram: very accurate—best reserved for unstable patients
- Intraarterial digital subtraction angiography (IA-DSA): 100% sensitive in one series

Management of Suspected Thoracic Aortic Rupture

- Manage ABCs as for all trauma patients

NOTE: Some experts state that repairing life-threatening hemoperitoneum and brainstem herniation takes precedence over aortic rupture.

- Maintain systolic BP ≤120 mm Hg by controlling fluids, sedation, and pain; consider short-acting IV agents, beta-blockade (esmolol with nitroprusside [Nipride])
- Contact thoracic surgeon and prepare for surgery

---

*A mediastinal width on an erect PA chest radiograph of >6 cm, a mediastinal width on a supine AP radiograph of >8 cm and >7.5 cm at the aortic knob, or the mediastinal width at the aortic knob ÷ chest width >0.25 all correlate with thoracic aortic rupture.

BLUNT ABDOMINAL TRAUMA

Management

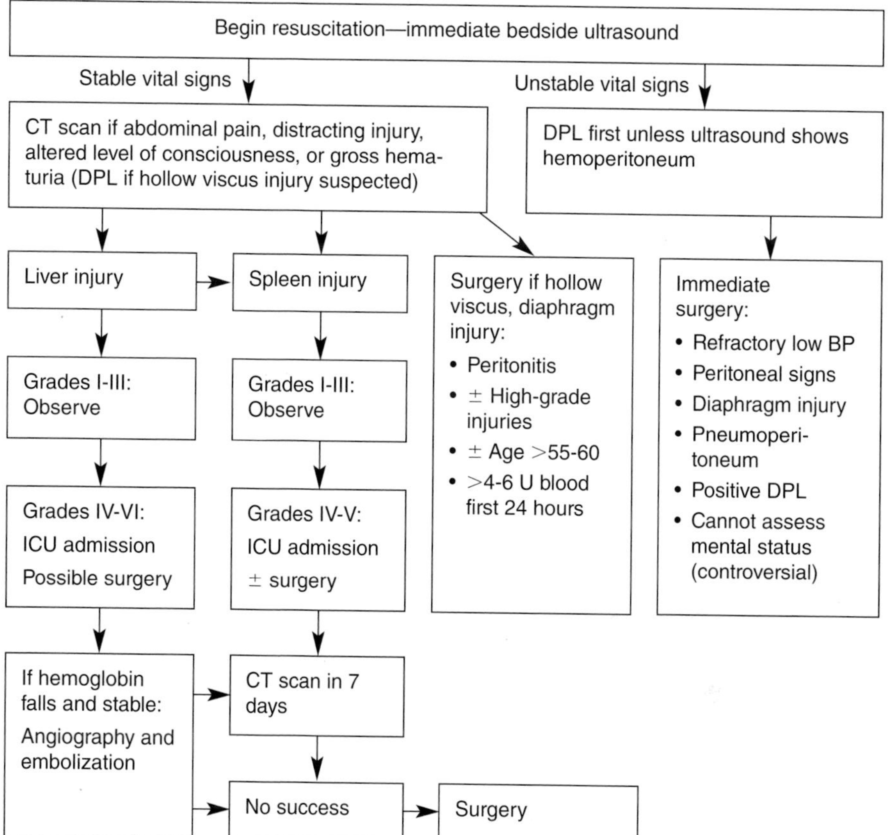

Fig. 38-5 Management of adults with blunt abdominal trauma. (Compiled from Pachter HL, Feliciano DV. Complex hepatic injuries. Surg Clin North Am 76:763-782, 1996; Brasel KJ, DeLisle CM, Olson CJ, et al. Splenic injury: trends in evaluation and management. J Trauma 44:283-286, 1998.)

Diagnostic Adjuncts for Blunt Abdominal Trauma

- Physical examination: 20% of patients with left lower rib fractures have an injured spleen, and 10% with right lower rib fractures have an injured liver. Nonspecific indicators of liver damage include AST or ALT >130 IU/L and laparotomy; need = base deficit ≤−6
- Diagnostic tests
  1. CT scans may miss hollow viscus, pancreatic, mesenteric, and diaphragm injuries. It requires hemodynamic stability. Oral contrast aids in detecting less than 1% of additional pathology in CT scans, increases aspiration, and adds time.[7]
  2. Diagnostic peritoneal lavage (DPL) is more sensitive than CT scans for identifying a need for laparotomy. DPL has more false positive results and leads to unnecessary laparotomies in many cases.
  3. Ultrasound is less sensitive than DPL for detecting peritoneal blood (80% to 90% versus 98% for DPL), although ultrasound detects hemoperitoneum in most cases that require surgery.

Positive Diagnostic Peritoneal Lavage

- Aspiration of ≥10 ml of gross blood
- Blunt or penetrating trauma, abdomen
  - ≥100,000 red blood cells/μl
  - 20,000-100,000 red blood cells/μl equivocal
- Penetrating trauma, lower chest
  - ≥5000 red blood cells/μl
- ≥500 white blood cells/ml (4-hour lag)
- Amylase lavage, ≥20 IU/L
- Alkaline phosphatase lavage, ≥3 IU/L
- Bile, food, or vegetable matter

PENETRATING ABDOMINAL TRAUMA

Indications for Laparotomy

- Unstable vital signs
- Peritoneal signs
- Evidence of diaphragm injury
- Significant gastrointestinal bleeding
- Bowel protrusion or evisceration
- Impaled or weapon embedded
- Gunshot wound to abdomen*
- Positive DPL (see previous section)

*Debate exists whether laparotomy is needed for stab wounds entering the peritoneum.

PELVIC TRAUMA

Criteria for Pelvic Radiography After Blunt Trauma*

- Glasgow Coma Scale <14
- Intoxication with drugs or alcohol
- Hypotension or gross hematuria
- Lower extremity neurologic deficit
- Femur fracture or painful or tender pelvis, symphysis pubis, or iliac spine
- Pain, swelling, and/or bruise to medial thigh, groin, genitals, suprapubic area, back
- Instability of pelvis with anteroposterior or lateral-medial pressure
- Pain with abduction, adduction, rotation, or flexion of either hip

Management of Pelvic Fractures

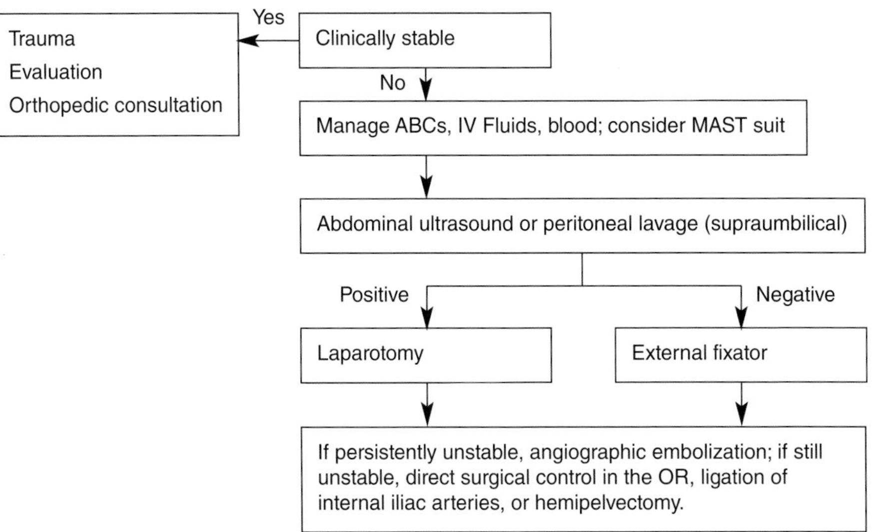

Fig. 38-6 Initial management of pelvic fractures. (From Coppola PT, Coppola M. Emergency department evaluation and treatment of pelvic fractures. Emerg Med Clin North Am 18:1-27, 2000.)

*These criteria are 100% sensitive.[8,9]

MANAGEMENT OF PENETRATING FLANK OR BACK INJURIES

- Immediate laparotomy if patient is in shock or has obvious intraperitoneal or vascular injury
- CT scan with triple contrast (oral, IV, and rectal) if there are no signs or symptoms of significant injury or gross hematuria alone in a hemodynamically stable patient
- Angiography should be considered if patient has significant retroperitoneal hematoma or bleeding

GENITOURINARY TRAUMA

Urethral Trauma

Overview

Pelvic fractures cause most proximal urethral injuries, whereas falls or straddle injuries usually cause anterior urethral injuries. Perform abdominal, perineal, and rectal examination, and obtain a urethrogram if injury is suspected.

Management

If there is partial urethral disruption, a urologist may attempt to gently place a 14 to 16 Fr catheter. If unsuccessful, or if complete urethral disruption is found, a suprapubic catheter needs to be placed.

*Retrograde Urethrogram Indication**

- Penile, scrotal, or perineal trauma
- Blood at urethral meatus
- High-riding prostate on examination
- Suspected pelvis fracture (controversial)
- Unable to easily place a Foley catheter

*Retrograde Urethrogram Technique**

- Obtain a preinjection kidney, ureter, and bladder (KUB) film
- Place a Cooke adapter on a 60 ml syringe (do not use a Foley catheter)
- Inject 10 to 15 ml of contrast medium in 60 seconds
- Obtain oblique radiographs during the last 10 seconds

---

*Use diatrizoate sodium (Hypaque) 50%, diatrizoate meglumine (Renografin-60; Cystografin) 40, or nonionic dye (Omnipaque or Isovue) diluted to ≤10% solution with NS.

Bladder Trauma

Overview

- All patients with bladder trauma have pelvic fractures, abdominal trauma requiring CT scan, or gross hematuria (98%); if gross hematuria is present, obtain a cystogram
- Abdominal CT scans can miss this injury; obtain a CT scan of the abdomen before a cystogram so that the dye does not obscure the CT scan

Management

- Intraperitoneal rupture releases dye into the abdomen; exploration of the abdomen plus repair are often required
- Extraperitoneal rupture releases dye into perivesical tissues, whereas washout may show dye behind the bladder. Treat with catheter alone (Foley if small; suprapubic if large)

Cystogram Indications

- Penetrating injury to the lower abdomen/pelvis
- Blunt abdominal or perineal trauma with gross hematuria, blood at the urethral meatus, pelvic fracture, abnormal retrograde urethrogram, or inability to void or little or no urine from Foley catheter

Cystogram Technique

- After urethrogram, insert Foley catheter
- Obtain baseline KUB film, instill dye* by gravity until 400 ml is instilled or there is bladder contraction
- Clamp the Foley catheter, obtain both anteroposterior and oblique radiographs, and empty the bladder with or without washing it out using saline solution
- Obtain final KUB film with oblique film

---

*Use diatrizoate sodium (Hypaque) 50%, diatrizoate meglumine (Renografin-60; Cystografin), or nonionic dye (Omnipaque or Isovue) diluted to ≤10% solution with NS.

RENAL TRAUMA

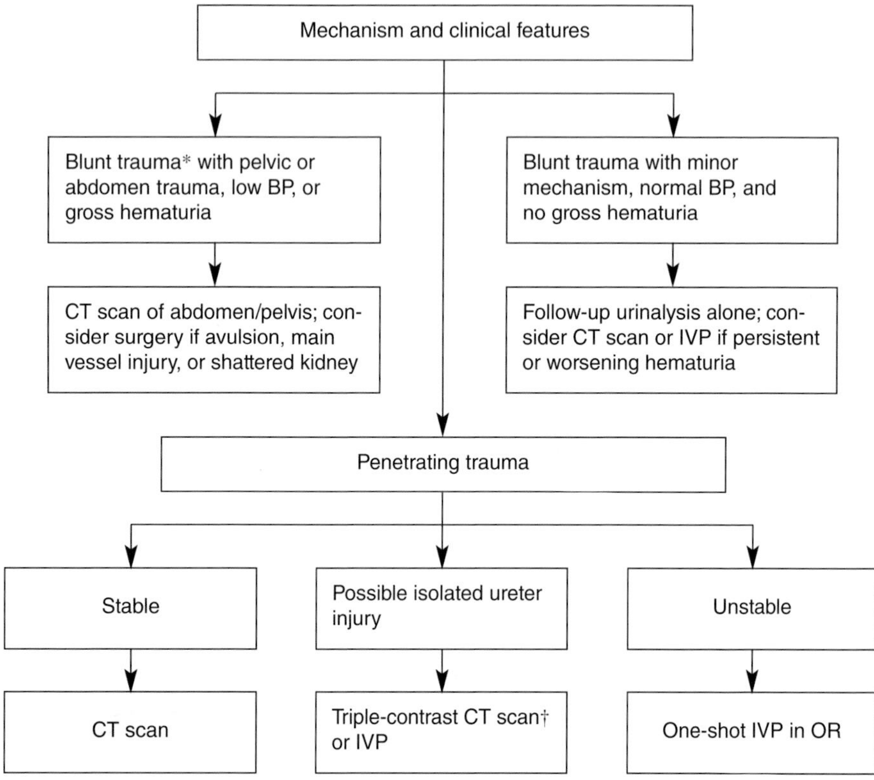

*Regardless of level of hematuria.
†Use triple contrast (IV, oral, and rectal).

Fig. 38-7 Diagnostic evaluation of suspected renal trauma. (From Ahn JH, Morey AF, McAninch JW. Workup and management of traumatic hematuria. Emerg Med Clin North Am 16:145-164, 1998.)

References

1. Hoffman JR, Mower WR, Wolfson AB, et al. Validity of a set of clinical criteria to rule out injury to the cervical spine in patients with blunt trauma. National Emergency X-Radiography Utilization Study Group. N Engl J Med 343:94-99, 2000.
2. Holmes JF, Panacek EA, Miller PQ, et al. Prospective evaluation of criteria for obtaining thoracolumbar radiographs in trauma patients. J Emerg Med 24:1-7, 2003.
3. Durham RM, Luchtefeld WB, Wibbenmeyer L, et al. Evaluation of the thoracic and lumbar spine after blunt trauma. Am J Surg 170:681-684, 1995.
4. Samuels LE, Kerstein MD. 'Routine' radiologic evaluation of the thoracolumbar spine in blunt trauma patients: a reappraisal. J Trauma 34:85-89, 1993.
5. Frankel HL, Rozycki GS, Ochsner MG, et al. Indications for obtaining surveillance thoracic and lumbar spine radiographs. J Trauma 37:673-676,1994.
6. Meldon SW, Moettus LN. Thoracolumbar spine fractures: clinical presentation and the effect of altered sensorium and major injury. J Trauma 39:1110-1114, 1995.
7. Tsang BD, Panacek EA, Brant WE, et al. Effect of oral contrast administration for abdominal computed tomography in the evaluation of acute blunt trauma. Ann Emerg Med 30:7-13, 1997.
8. Civil ID, Ross SE, Botehlo G, et al. Routine pelvic radiography in severe blunt trauma: is it necessary? Ann Emerg Med 17:488-490, 1988.
9. Koury HI, Peschiera JL, Welling RE. Selective use of pelvic roentgenograms in blunt trauma patients. J Trauma 34:236-237, 1993.

39

STROKE CODE

INITIAL ASSESSMENT

- Assess airway, breathing, circulation (ABCs), and vital signs.
- Provide O_2; protect airway.
- Establish the onset of symptoms: 3-hour window for thrombolytic therapy (best results if given within 90 minutes; up to 6 hours for intraarterial therapy).
- Obtain IV access and ECG. Order initial studies (complete blood count [CBC], platelets, electrolytes, PT/PTT, glucose, liver/kidney function, blood type, and screen for blood transfusion). Consider toxicology screen and hypercoagulable workup in young patients without apparent risk factors.
- Complete C-spine radiography if trauma or comatose.
- Check glucose level and treat if indicated.
- Perform focused general physical and neurologic examinations; also assess level of consciousness (see Table 38-3 on p. 177) and stroke severity.
- Assess for coexisting acute cardiovascular disease (such as myocardial infarction [MI] or aortic dissection) or unusual cause of stroke.
- Obtain urgent noncontrast head CT scan or diffusion-weighted MRI to determine whether the stroke is ischemic or hemorrhagic—the goal is completion within 25 minutes of arrival and interpretation within 45 minutes.
- CT scans are generally preferred because of availability and rapid diagnosis of intracranial bleeding.
- CT scans are 50% sensitive for ischemic changes within 6 hours of stroke.
- Diffusion-weighted MRI is >90% sensitive for ischemic changes and reveals positive results earlier than CT scans.
- Perform CT angiogram (if available) to assess for large-vessel thrombosis.

Table 39-1 American Heart Association Recommended Studies for Patients With Suspected Acute Ischemic Stroke

All patients		***If clinically suspected alternate disease***	
CT (or MRI)	Renal function	Liver function	O_2 saturation
ECG	CBC/platelets	Toxicology screen	Chest radiograph
Glucose	PT/INR	Blood alcohol level	Lumbar puncture
Electrolytes	PTT	Pregnancy test	EEG

From Guidelines 2000 for Cardiopulmonary Resuscitation and Emergency Cardiovascular Care. Part 7: the era of reperfusion: section 2: acute stroke. The American Heart Association in collaboration with the International Liaison Committee on Resuscitation. Circulation 102(Suppl 8):204S-216S, 2000.
INR, International normalized ratio.

GENERAL TREATMENT

Do not treat hypertension unless BP is >220/120 mm Hg or patient has intracranial bleeding, acute MI, or aortic dissection. If SBP is >220 or DBP is 120 to 140, aim for a 10% to 15% reduction with labetalol or nicardipine; consider nitroprusside if DBP is >140. If considering thrombolysis, lower SBP to ≤185 and DBP to ≤110 with labetalol (10 mg IV, may repeat once) or nitroglycerin paste, 1 to 2 units.

- Replenish fluid deficit (this may improve cerebral perfusion), but avoid hypotonic fluids.
- Treat seizures with lorazepam (0.1 mg/kg IV at 2 mg/min) or with phenytoin (20 mg/kg IV at ≤50 mg/min). Infuse slowly to avoid drug-induced hypotension (for status epilepticus, see Chapter 37).
- If patient is febrile, assess for infection/meningitis. Sterile fever (fever with negative results on the infectious workup) may be found. Maintaining normothermia with antipyretics or cooling blankets may improve outcome after stroke.
- Manage elevated ICP in deteriorating patient, regardless of cause.
  - Elevate the head of bed 30 degrees.
  - Induce a hyperosmolar intravascular state while maintaining euvolemia. Give mannitol IV, 1 g/kg (50 to 100 g), followed by 0.25 g/kg (15 to 25 g) every 6 hours. Check Na^+ and osmolarity every 6 hours and hold if Na is >152 mEq/L and/or osmolarity is >305 mOsm/L. If the patient is fluid overloaded (or if there is risk of CHF), give furosemide IV every 6 hours or as needed.
  - Intubate and hyperventilate until Pco_2 is 25 to 30 mm Hg. Decreasing Pco_2 by 5 to 10 mm Hg will lower the ICP by 20 to 30 mm Hg; however, this is useful only as a temporary measure, because the pH equilibrates in several hours.

  - Steroids (e.g., dexamethasone, 10 mg IV followed by 6 mg IV every 6 hours) work only for vasogenic edema (e.g., tumors) and not for cytotoxic edema (e.g., strokes).

TREATMENT OF ACUTE ISCHEMIC STROKE[1]

- Intravenous thrombolytic therapy (tissue plasminogen activator [tPA]) should be considered for patients with ischemic stroke (i.e., CT scan without evidence of hemorrhage), those for whom the duration of symptoms is ≤3 hours, and those with no contraindications.
- Angiographic intraarterial thrombolytic therapy appears to be beneficial if given within 6 hours, particularly with documented occlusion of middle cerebral or basilar artery.
- Aspirin is not a contraindication to thrombolytics, but all antiplatelet and anticoagulant agents should be withheld for 24 hours after thrombolysis.
- Patients not receiving thrombolysis should receive aspirin.

TREATMENT OF BLEEDING COMPLICATIONS FROM THROMBOLYTIC THERAPY

- There is a 6% average rate (3% to 16% range) of symptomatic intracerebral hemorrhage in clinical trials; a higher rate occurs when thrombolytic therapy is used in patients who fall outside current guidelines.
- Clinical deterioration after thrombolysis should be presumed to represent intracerebral bleeding until proven otherwise—stop tPA infusion immediately (and heparin, if used), and obtain a noncontrast CT scan of the head immediately.
- Check CBC, PT, PTT, platelets, and fibrinogen.
- Give 6 to 8 units of cryoprecipitate and/or fresh-frozen plasma (FFP) plus 10 units of single-donor platelets to reverse the thrombolytic effect.
- Consult with neurosurgery for early decompression.

ACUTE SUBARACHNOID HEMORRHAGE[2]

- Diagnosis:
  - CT scans are 92% sensitive if performed within 24 hours of event.
  - Perform lumbar puncture if the history suggests a risk or if a head CT scan is revealing, or if the patient presents more than 72 hours after the event.
  - Xanthochromia does not appear until 4 hours after the event and reaches a maximum level at 1 week.

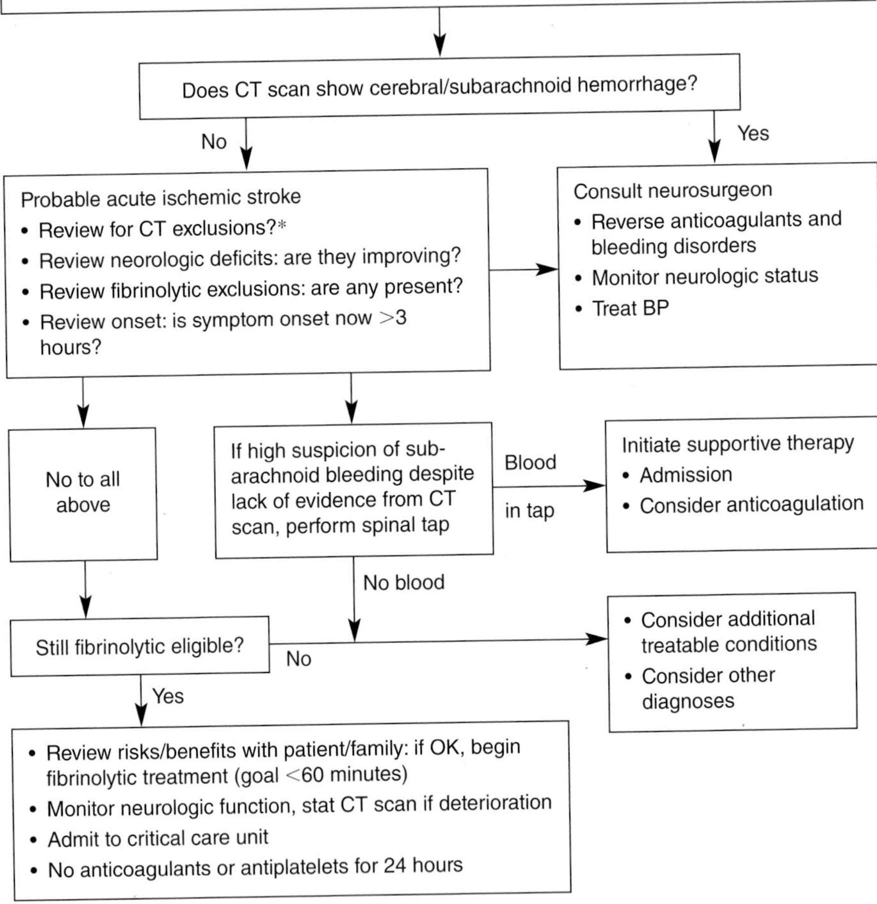

IMMEDIATE GENERAL ASSESSMENT
(<10 minutes from ED arrival)
• Assess ABCs, vital signs, O_2 blood sugar
• IV, CBC, electrolytes, PT/PTT (INR)
• 12-lead ECG, cardiac monitor
• General neurologic screening
• Alert neurologist, radiologist, CT
IMMEDIATE NEUROLOGIC ASSESSMENT
(goal <25 minutes from ED arrival)
• Review history (establish onset <3 hr)
• Glasgow Coma Scale, NIH Stroke Scale, or Hunt and Hess scale
• Stat noncontrast CT scan, rapid review
• C-spine series if possible trauma
Does CT scan show cerebral/subarachnoid hemorrhage?
No
Yes
Probable acute ischemic stroke
• Review for CT exclusions?*
• Review neorologic deficits: are they improving?
• Review fibrinolytic exclusions: are any present?
• Review onset: is symptom onset now >3 hours?
Consult neurosurgeon
• Reverse anticoagulants and bleeding disorders
• Monitor neurologic status
• Treat BP
No to all above
If high suspicion of subarachnoid bleeding despite lack of evidence from CT scan, perform spinal tap
Blood in tap
Initiate supportive therapy
• Admission
• Consider anticoagulation
No blood
Still fibrinolytic eligible?
No
Yes
• Consider additional treatable conditions
• Consider other diagnoses
• Review risks/benefits with patient/family: if OK, begin fibrinolytic treatment (goal <60 minutes)
• Monitor neurologic function, stat CT scan if deterioration
• Admit to critical care unit
• No anticoagulants or antiplatelets for 24 hours
*Edema, sulcal effacement, mass effect, or possible hemorrhage.

Fig. 39-1 American Heart Association (AHA) Suspected Stroke Algorithm. (From Guidelines 2000 for Cardiopulmonary Resuscitation and Emergency Cardiovascular Care. Part 7: the era of reperfusion: section 2: acute stroke. The American Heart Association in collaboration with the International Liaison Committee on Resuscitation. Circulation 102[Suppl 8]: 204S-216S, 2000.)

- Consult a neurosurgeon.
- Treatment of hypertension is generally avoided unless the patient is alert (in which case lowering the blood pressure may reduce the risk of rebleeding).
- Nimodipine, 60 mg by mouth every 6 hours, reduces vasospasm and improves outcomes.
- Prescribe analgesics and sedatives as needed; consider empiric anticonvulsants.
- Complete an urgent angiography and consider surgery (there is a 4% chance of recurrent bleeding within 24 hours and a cumulative 20% risk of rebleeding at 2 weeks).

ACUTE HYPERTENSIVE INTRACEREBRAL HEMORRHAGE

- Type and cross-match 4 units of packed red blood cells (PRBCs), 4 to 6 units of cryoprecipitate or FFP, and 1 unit of single-donor platelets for emergency use.
- Use labetalol or nitroprusside to lower SBP to 140 to 160 mm Hg (or blood pressure before stroke).
- Neurosurgical decompression may be indicated for large cerebellar or intracerebral hemorrhage, especially if there is associated hydrocephalus or a deteriorating level of consciousness.
- Ventriculostomy is indicated for basal ganglia hemorrhage associated with hydrocephalus.

References

1. Meschia JF, Miller DA, Brott TG. Thrombolytic treatment of acute ischemic stroke. Mayo Clin Proc 77:542-551, 2002.
2. Stieg PE, Kase CS. Intracranial hemorrhage: diagnosis and emergency treatment. Neurol Clin North Am 16:373-389, 1998.

Appendixes

Appendix

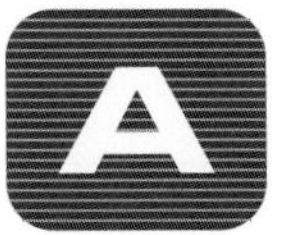

GASTROINTESTINAL

A

GASTROINTESTINAL BLEEDING

Upper GI Bleeding

Diagnostic Evaluation

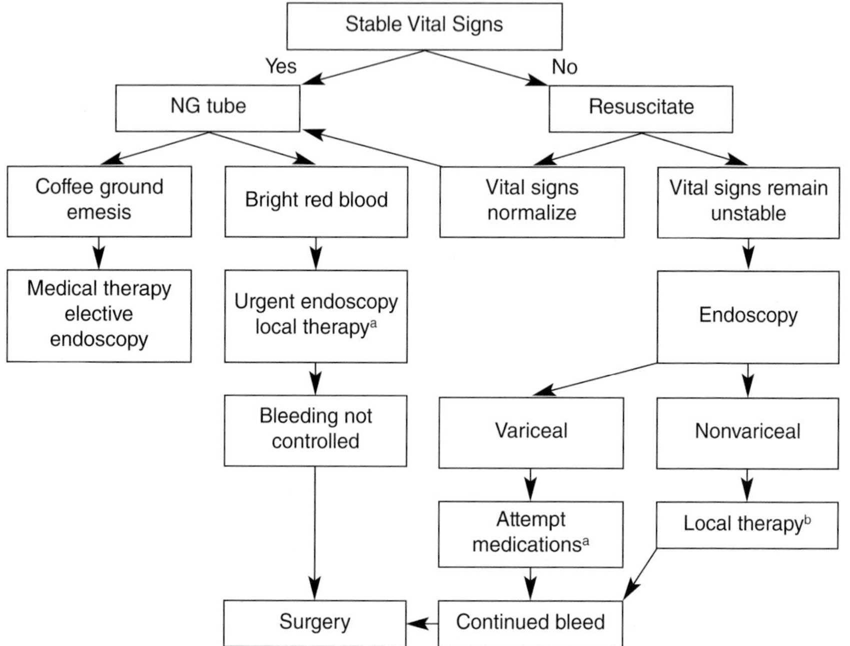

Fig. A-1 *a,* Medications include (1) octreotide or somatostatin (to lower portal venous pressure by splanchnic vasoconstriction). *Octreotide dose:* 50 μg bolus, then 50 μg/hour IV. *Somatostatin dose:* 250 μg IV, then 250 μg/hour **or** (2) vasopressin: Start with 0.4 units/minute, gradually increase to a maximum of 0.9 units/minute IV. Side effects are decreased BP, bowel ischemia, myocardial ischemia, and skin necrosis. Nitroglycerin IV (40-400 μg/minute) can limit these effects. *b,* Bipolar electrocoagulation controls 90% to 95% of acute ulcer bleeding. Injection and sclerotherapy are effective against ulcers and variceal bleeding. Results differ depending on the site and the magnitude of bleeding. (From Talbot-Stern JK. Gastrointestinal bleeding. Emerg Med Clin North Am 14:173-184, 1996.)

Causes and Management

Box A-1

Resuscitation With Upper GI Bleeding	Causes of Upper GI Bleeding—Admitted	
O_2, cardiac monitor, insert NG tube, NS 2 L IV. Consider transfusion, FFP if unknown coagulopathy or if PT or PTT >1.5 times normal	Duodenal ulcer	36%
	Gastric ulcer	24%
	Varices and gastritis	6% (each)
Type and cross 4 to 6 units packed RBCs; obtain CBC, platelets, electrolytes,* LFTs, and PT/PTT. Obtain chest radiograph and ECG	Esophagitis	4% (each)
	Gastroduodenitis	3%
	Other, or source not found	17%
Administer platelets if level is <50,000/ml		

From Longstreth GF. Epidemiology of hospitalization for acute upper gastrointestinal hemorrhage: a population-based study. Am J Gastroenterol 90:206-210, 1995.
*BUN/Cr ratio ≥36 indicates a greater than 95% likelihood that the source of bleeding is in the upper GI tract.

Indications for ICU Admission and Surgery Consultation

Box A-2

Indications for *ICU Admission* With Upper GI Bleeding*	Indications for *Surgery Consultation* With Upper GI Bleeding*
Hypotension or orthostasis	Variceal bleeding
Hematochezia or hematemesis	Peptic ulcer with >4 units transfused
Active GI bleeding	Endoscopy: ulcer larger than 2 cm
Two or more comorbidities	Endoscopy: recent bleeding
Significant coronary artery disease	Vascular malformation bleeding
Endoscopy: recent bleeding, visible vessels	Aortoenteric fistula known or suspected
Onset or recurrence of bleeding in hospital	Bowel perforation known or suspected
Multiple units of blood transfused	
Variceal bleeding	

Compiled from McGuirk TD, Coyle WJ. Upper gastrointestinal tract bleeding. Emerg Med Clin North Am 14:523-545, 1996; and Peter DJ, Dougherty JM. Evaluation of the patient with gastrointestinal bleeding: an evidence based approach. Emerg Med Clin North Am 17:239-261, 1999.
*These are not absolute indications, and clinical judgment must be used.

Lower GI Bleeding

Sources

- The most common source of massive lower GI bleeding is an upper GI site; therefore all patients need an NG tube. 80% to 90% of lower bleeding will stop without therapy.
- *Diverticulosis:* 75% of bleeds are from the right colon. Bleeding is arterial and often massive. Pain is mild and crampy. 50% of patients bleed again, and 20% require surgery.
- *Angiodysplasia:* Angiodysplasia is an acquired disorder of unknown cause. Lesions are usually in the cecum and ascending colon. Barium studies and colonoscopy may not show these lesions. Selective mesenteric angiography is accurate (Table A-1).

Table A-1 Most Common Sources of Lower GI Bleeding*

Cause	Incidence in Patients With Lower GI Bleeding
Diverticulosis	35%
Angiodysplasia	30%
Cancer polyps	10%
Rectal disease	7%
Other causes	3%
Undiagnosed	15%

*Excludes upper GI tract.

A

Assessment and Management

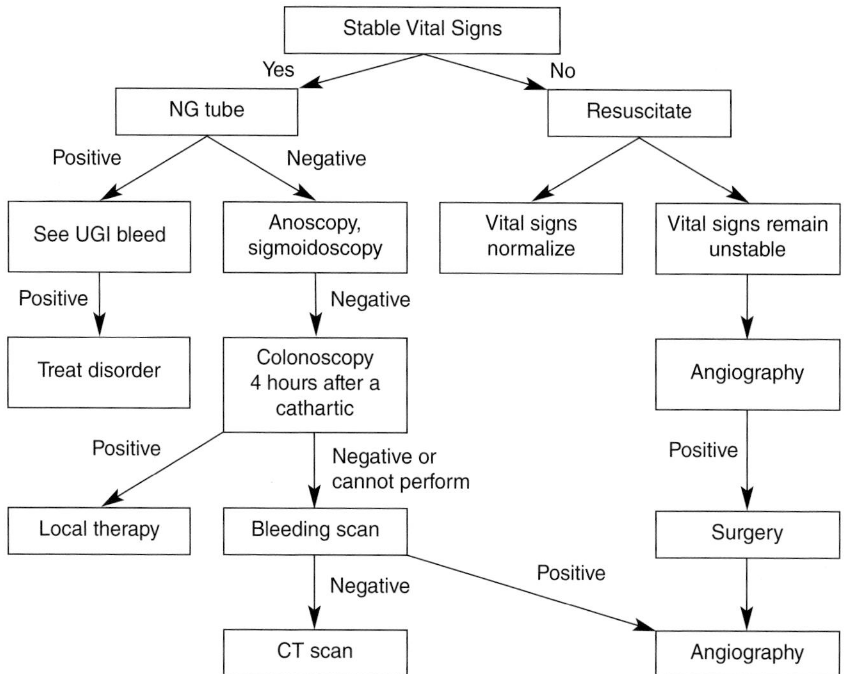

Fig. A-2 (Compiled from Talbot-Stern JK. Gastrointestinal bleeding. Emerg Med Clin North Am 14:173-184, 1996; and Peter DJ, Dougherty JM. Evaluation of the patient with gastrointestinal bleeding: an evidence based approach. Emerg Med Clin North Am 17:239-261, 1999.)

LIVER DISEASE

Liver Function Tests

Table A-2*

Condition	AST	ALT	Alkaline Phosphatase	Bilirubin	Albumin
Abscess	1-4 × ↑	1-4 × ↑	1-3 × ↑	1-4 × ↑	Normal
Acetaminophen	50-100 × ↑	50-100 × ↑	1-2 × ↑	1-5 × ↑	Normal
Alcohol hepatitis	AST >ALT by 2:1 (2-5 × ↑)		10 × ↑	1-5 × ↑	Chronically low
Biliary cirrhosis	1-2 × ↑	1-2 × ↑	1-4 × ↑	1-2 × ↑	Low
Chronic hepatitis	1-20 × ↑	1-20 × ↑	1-3 × ↑	1-3 × ↑	Low
Viral hepatitis	5-50 × ↑	5-50 × ↑	1-3 × ↑	1-3 × ↑	Normal

*Levels for different diseases can vary, and numbers given here are not absolute. Numbers indicate the magnitude of test results above normal (10 × ↑) = 10-fold increase above normal.

Ascitic-Peritoneal Fluid Analysis

Table A-3

Condition	SAAG*	WBCs (per μl)	PMNs (per μl)	Ascitic RBCs	Protein (g/dl)	Glucose (mg/dl)	LDH (IU/L)
Cardiac	>1.1	~500	<250	Few	~4.0	~150	~100
Cirrhosis	>1.1	<500	<250	Few	~2.0	~130	½ serum
Liver cancer†	>1.1	Varies	Varies	Few	~2.0	~130	~150
Liver metastasis	>1.1	~2000	~500	Few	~2.0	~100	~200
Pancreas	<1.1	~4000	~3000	Few	~3.0	~200	~2000
Perforation of bowel	Varies	>1000	>250	Varies	~2.5	<50	~1000
Renal	<1.1	<500	<250	Few	~0.5	~100	½ serum
Spontaneous bacterial peritonitis	>1.1	>1000	>250	Few	~1.0	~130	~200
Tuberculosis	Varies	~500	~1000	High	~4.0	<100	~300

*Ratio of serum to ascetic fluid albumin concentration.

†Hepatocellular carcinoma.

Serum-Ascites Albumin Gradient[1]

- SAAG = Serum albumin − Ascetic fluid albumin
- SAAG ≥1.1 mg/dl suggests the presence of *portal hypertension*
- 97% accuracy for classifying the cause (superior to the exudate-transudate concept)

Box A-3

SAAG ≥1.1 mg/dl (Portal Hypertension Present)	SAAG <1.1 mg/dl (Portal Hypertension Absent)
Cirrhosis (with or without infection or cancer)	Peritoneal carcinomatosis
Cardiac ascites (CHF, tricuspid regurgitation, constrictive pericarditis, or tamponade)	Peritonitis in absence of cirrhosis (bacterial, tuberculous)
Massive liver metastases	Nephrotic syndrome
Portal vein thrombosis	Pancreatic or biliary ascites
Budd-Chiari syndrome	Malignant chylous ascites
Fulminant hepatic failure	Bowel infarction or obstruction
Hepatocellular carcinoma	Hypothyroidism
Acute hepatitis (viral or alcoholic) superimposed on cirrhosis	

Jaundice[2]

Skin pigment change is generally seen if serum bilirubin >2.5 mg/dl.

Table A-4

Major Laboratory Abnormality	Cause	Examples	Evaluation
None	Pseudojaundice	• Carotenemia • Normal pigmentation	• Assess vegetable intake
Isolated increase in indirect (unconjugated) bilirubin	Increased bilirubin load or production, or decreased bilirubin conjugation	• Hemolysis • Transfusion • Hematoma resorption • Gilbert syndrome	• Transfusion load* • Blood smear • Haptoglobin • Direct Coombs test • CT scan of abdomen and pelvis for hematoma
Increase in transaminases and direct (conjugated) bilirubin	Hepatocellular injury	• Drug injury • Hypotension • Hypoxemia • Acute hepatitis (viral, ethanol, or autoimmune) • Wilson's disease • Nonalcoholic steatohepatitis • Venoocclusive disease • Budd-Chiari syndrome • Worsening of preexisting liver disease	• Rule out drug injury • Assess tissue perfusion (Doppler ultrasound) • Hepatitis serologies • Liver biopsy

Compiled from Pasha TM, Lindor KD. Diagnosis and therapy of cholestatic liver disease. Med Clin North Am 80:995-1019, 1996; and Hawker F. Liver dysfunction in critical illness. Anaesth Intensive Care 19: 165-181, 1991.

*Each unit of PRBCs contains ~250 mg bilirubin.

Table A-4—cont'd

Major Laboratory Abnormality	Cause	Examples	Evaluation
Increase in alkaline phosphatase with or without direct (conjugated) bilirubin	Cholestatic injury	• Drug injury • Benign postoperative effect† • Sepsis • TPN	• Rule out drug injury • Amylase, lipase • Ultrasound or CT scan • ERCP or MRCP if ducts are dilated • Liver biopsy
	Biliary obstruction (intrahepatic or extrahepatic)	• Choledocholithiasis • Pancreatitis • Biliary stricture (benign or malignant) • Hepatic metastasis • Sarcoidosis‡ • AIDS cholangiopathy	

Compiled from Pasha TM, Lindor KD. Diagnosis and therapy of cholestatic liver disease. Med Clin North Am 80:995-1019, 1996; and Hawker F. Liver dysfunction in critical illness. Anaesth Intensive Care 19: 165-181, 1991.

†Mild elevations in bilirubin (2 to 4 mg/dl) are seen in 25% of postsurgical patients.[2]

‡Injury is often at the level of portal triad; radiographic evidence of obstruction is often absent.

Risks of Surgery in Patients With Liver Disease

Modified Child-Pugh Score

Table A-5

Modified Child-Pugh Score		1 Point	2 Points	3 Points
Encephalopathy*		None	Grades I-II	Grades III-IV
Ascites		Absent	Slight	Moderate
Bilirubin (mg/dl)	Noncholestatic Cholestatic†	<2 <4	2-3 4-10	>3 >10
Albumin (g/dl)		>3.5	2.8-3.5	<2.8
INR		<1.7	1.7-2.3	>2.3

Modified from Pugh RN, Murray-Lyon IM, Dawson JL, et al. Transection of the oesophagus for bleeding oesophageal varices. Br J Surg 60:646-649, 1973.

*Grade I: mild confusion or slowing, no asterixis; Grade II: drowsy, asterixis present; Grade III: marked confusion, somnolence, asterixis present; Grade IV: unresponsive or responsive only to painful stimuli, no asterixis.

†Primary biliary cirrhosis, for example.

Modified Child-Pugh Class

Table A-6

Class	Child-Pugh Score	Perioperative Mortality[3]	Description	Survival 1 year	Survival 2 year
A	5-6	10%	Near-normal response to all operations; normal regenerative ability; increased risk of complications if portal hypertension present	100%	85%
B	7-9	31%	Moderate liver impairment; tolerates noncardiac surgery with preoperative preparation; limited regeneration; sizable resections contraindicated	80%	60%
C	≥10	76%	Poor response to all operations regardless of preparatory efforts; liver resection contraindicated regardless of size	45%	35%

Contraindications to Elective Surgery

- Acute alcoholic or viral hepatitis
- Fulminant hepatic failure
- Severe chronic hepatitis
- Child-Pugh class C
- PT prolongation >3 seconds despite vitamin K
- Platelet count <50,000 ml
- Coexisting renal failure, cardiomyopathy, or hypoxemia

Optimizing Medical Therapy

- Adequate nutrition
- Correct PT (≤3 seconds of normal) with vitamin K, FFP, or recombinant human factor VIIa
- Maintain platelet count >50,000 ml
- Treat prolonged bleeding time with DDAVP
- Prophylactic beta-blocker for varices

- Correct hypokalemia and metabolic alkalosis
- For encephalopathy: use lactulose with a target of 3 to 4 bowel movements per day; avoid narcotics and sedatives
- For ascites: salt restriction and potassium-sparing with or without loop diuretic

A

PANCREATITIS[4]

Diagnosis

Amylase and Lipase

- A value >3 times normal supports clinical diagnosis
- A value <3 times normal is nonspecific (differential diagnosis includes perforated ulcer, mesenteric ischemia, and renal failure)
- Lipase is probably the better test; no need to measure both
- Absolute values do not correlate with disease severity or prognosis
- Serial measurements do not predict clinical response or prognosis

Alanine Aminotransferase

- >80 units/ml is highly specific for gallstone pancreatitis

Abdominal Ultrasound

- Indicated to assess for gallstones or bile duct dilation

Dynamic Contrast CT Scan

- Perform at 72 hours in severe pancreatitis to assess for presence and degree of necrosis

Prognosis

Organ Failure

- Most important indicator of severity
- Defined by any of the following:
  - SBP <90
  - $Pa{O_2}$ <60 mm Hg
  - Creatinine >2 mg/dl
  - GI bleeding >500 ml/24 hours

Hemoconcentration

- Hct >44% predicts pancreatic necrosis

APACHE-II Score

- Most sensitive and specific for severity

Ranson Criteria[5]

Box A-4

On Arrival	48 Hours After Admission
Age >55 years	Hct <30%, or falls >10%
WBC >16,000 cells/μl	Serum calcium <8 mg/dl
Blood glucose >200 mg/dl	BUN increases >5 mg/dl
Serum LDH >2× normal	Pa_{O_2} <60 mm Hg
Serum AST >6× normal	Base deficit >4 mEq/L
	Estimated fluid sequestration >6 L
	Massive volume resuscitation

Ranson Factors

Table A-7

Ranson Factors	Mortality	Dead, or More Than 7 Days in ICU
0-2	0.9%	3.7%
3-4	16%	40%
5-6	40%	93%
7-8	100%	100%

Treatment

Supportive Care

- Fluid resuscitation
- Pain control
- Nutritional support if NPO >1 week

Urgent ERCP

- Indicated in severe gallstone pancreatitis
- Sphincterotomy should be performed if stones are detected[6]

Prophylactic Broad-Spectrum Antibiotics

- Indicated in necrotizing pancreatitis associated with organ failure[7]

Percutaneous Aspiration

- Indicated to exclude superinfection in patients with necrotizing pancreatitis who fail to show clinical improvement

Surgical Intervention

- Gallstones (cholecystectomy should be performed after resolution of episode; increased mortality if performed within the first 48 hours)
- Abscess or superinfected necrosis
- Sterile necrosis with prolonged organ failure (4 to 6 weeks)
- Symptomatic pseudocyst that survives conservative treatment and cannot be drained endoscopically or percutaneously

BILIARY TRACT DISEASE (BILIARY COLIC)

Clinical Features

- Pain duration <6 to 8 hours
- Absence of fever
- WBC count <11,000 cells/μl in most
- Normal liver function test results in 98%
- Ultrasound is >98% sensitive for gallstones

Management

- Treat pain
- Anticholinergics (such as dicyclomine or atropine) are no more effective than placebos for pain relief
- Surgery follow-up

ACUTE CHOLECYSTITIS[8,9]

Clinical Features

- Pain duration >6 to 8 hours: >90%
- Temperature ≥100.4° F: 25%
- Murphy's sign: >95%
- WBC >11,000 cells/μl: 65%
- Elevated liver function tests: 55%
- Ultrasound sensitivity: 85%

Management

- Use ultrasound or CT scan to exclude complications (such as choledocholithiasis, acute pancreatitis in 15%, or gallstone ileus)
- Treat pain
- Administer antibiotics
- IV NS and NPO

COMPLICATED INTRAABDOMINAL INFECTIONS

Complicated infections are those extending beyond the hollow viscus into the peritoneum, with or without abscess.

Table A-8

Severity	Antimicrobial Agents
Mild to Moderate	• **Single agent regimen:** Ampicillin and sulbactam (Unasyn)* 1.5-3.0 g IV q6 hours **or** ticarcillin and clavulanate potassium (Timentin) 3.1 g IV q4-6 hours **or** ertapenem (Invanz) 1 g IM or IV q24 hours • **Combination regimen:** Metronidazole (Flagyl) 15 mg/kg (1 g maximum) IV + 7.5 mg/kg (500 mg maximum) IV q6 hours, plus any one of the following: cefazolin (Ancef, Kefzol) 1-1.5 g IV q6 hours **or** cefuroxime (Ceftin) 1.5 g IV q6-8 hours **or** ciprofloxacin (Cipro) 400 mg IV q12 hours **or** (levofloxacin [Levaquin] 500 mg, moxifloxacin [Avelox] 400 mg, or gatifloxacin [Tequin] 400 mg IV q24 hours)
Severe	• **Single agent regimen:** Piperacillin and tazobactam (Zosyn) 3.375-4.5 g IV q8 hours **or** imipenem and cilastatin (Primaxin) 0.5-1.0 g IV q6-8 hours **or** meropenem (Merrem) 1 g IV q8 hours • **Combination regimen:** Metronidazole (Flagyl) 15 mg/kg (1g maximum) IV + 7.5 mg/kg (500 mg maximum) IV q6 hours, plus any one of the following: ciprofloxacin (Cipro) 400 mg IV q12 hours **or** aztreonam (Azactam) 2 g IV q8 hours **or** ceftriaxone (Rocephin) 1-2 g IV q24 hours **or** ceftazidime 2 g IV q8 hours **or** cefepime (Maxipime) 2 g IV q12 hours

Modified from Solomkin JS, Mazuski JE, Baron EJ, et al. Guidelines for the selection of anti-infective agents for complicated intra-abdominal infections. Clin Infect Dis 37:997-1005, 2003.

*Avoid ampicillin in areas that have increasing *E. coli* resistance.

A

MESENTERIC ISCHEMIA

Causes
- Arterial embolus: 25% to 50% (especially to superior mesenteric artery)
- Arterial thrombosis: 12% to 25%
- Venous thrombosis (especially coagulopathy) with low cardiac output

Risk Factors
- Age
- Vascular/valvular disease
- Arrhythmias
- CHF
- Recent MI
- Hypovolemia
- Diuretics
- Beta-blockers
- Splanchnic vasoconstrictors (such as digoxin)

Clinical Features[10]

Table A-9

Signs and Symptoms	Incidence
Abdominal pain	80%-90%
Sudden-onset pain	60%
Vomiting	75%
Diarrhea (often heme positive)	40%
Gross GI bleeding	25%
Early: Increased pain with minimal abdominal tenderness	Variable
Late: Shock, fever, confusion, distension, rebound, and rigidity	Variable

Diagnostic Studies

Table A-10

Values in Mesenteric Ischemia	Incidence
Elevated lactate	70%-90%
WBC >15,000 cells/μl	60%-75%
Elevated LDH	70%
Elevated creatine kinase	63%
Elevated phosphate	30%-65%
Plain radiograph: obstruction	60%
Plain radiograph: thumbprinting portal gas, or free air	<20%
CT scan, ultrasound sensitivity	<50%-70%
Angiography sensitivity	>95%

Management[10]

- Fluid and blood resuscitation
- Broad-spectrum antibiotics
- Surgical consultation and emergency laparotomy (especially if there is bowel necrosis or perforation)
- Mesenteric arteriography reveals thrombosis, emboli, and mesenteric vasoconstriction and allows for selective papaverine administration until symptoms are gone or surgery is performed
- Avoid digoxin and vasopressors because of vasoconstriction

NUTRITION SUPPORT[11,12]

Nutritional Requirements

Calories (Kcal/kg/day, up to 2500/day maximum)

- Mild stress: 20-25
- Typical ICU patient: 25-30
- Severe stress or BMI <20: 30-40
- BMI >30: 15-220

Protein (g/kg/day, up to 150 g/day maximum)

- Normal: 0.8
- Illness or injury: 1.0-1.5
- Uremia (not dialyzed): 0.8-1.0
- Dialysis: 1.2-1.5
- Hepatic encephalopathy: 0.5

Fluid

- Typically 30 ml/kg/day

Nitrogen Balance

- Protein intake (g) / 6.25 – (urine urea nitrogen + 4)
- (6.25 because protein ≈16% N; 4 represents N loss in skin/stool)
- Goal is 0; 0-5: moderate stress; >5: severe stress

Timing to Initiate Feeding

Table A-11

	Enteral	Parenteral
Well nourished, nonhypercatabolic	7-10 days	14-21 days
Malnourished *or* hypercatabolic	1-5 days	1-10 days
Malnourished *and* hypercatabolic	1-3 days	1-7 days

Parenteral Nutrition Components

Table A-12

Component	Typical Values	Comments
Volume	2 L/day	1.5 L/day if weight <60 kg
Rate	Start 1 L/day (42 ml/hour); can increase to goal on day 2 if stable	To prevent hypoglycemia, do not stop abruptly (hang D10 if needed, or cut rate in half during surgery/procedures)
Dextrose	10%-30% solution (D10-D30)	D25 is typical using a dedicated central line. Maximum in other lines as follows: femoral, D15; nondedicated central, D10; peripheral line, D5. 3.4 Kcal/g (340 Kcal/L D10)
Protein	30-70 g/L (3%-7% amino acid solution)	4 Kcal/g (200 Kcal in 1 L 5% solution)
Lipids	200 g/L (20% solution); may be given separately	9 Kcal/g—20% lipid solution (contains glycerol and phospholipids) provides 2 Kcal/ml. Total dose is 20% to 30% of total Kcal. Decrease dose if triglycerides increase, or if increased phosphates
Electrolytes	K^+ 30 mEq/L, Na^+ 30 mEq/L, Mg^{++} 4 mEq/L, Ca^{++} 4 mg/L, phosphates 15 mmol/L	Add acetate (HCO_3) if hyperchloremic acidosis; additional phosphate for severe malnourishment
Vitamins	Standard multivitamin (10 ml MVI-12 or MVI-13) plus trace minerals (Zn, Cu, Mn, Se, and Cr)	
Optional	H2 blocker, vitamin K, insulin	

Enteral Feeding Commercial Products

Table A-13

Type	Example Products	Kcal/ml	Protein (g/L)	mOsm/L
Standard polymeric*	Osmolite HN Plus	1.2	45-55	360-450
Standard polymeric with fiber	Jevity 1.2 CAL, Fibersource HN	1.2	45-55	360-450
Polymeric reduced protein	Jevity, Osmolite, Isocal HN, Ultracal	1.06	35-42	300
High protein and calories	Ensure Plus HN, Boost Plus	1.5	63	650
Fluid restricted	TwoCal HN, Magnacal, Nutren 2.0	2.0	84	690-720
Elemental†	Criticare HN, Vital HN, Vivonex TEN	1.0	38-42	500-650
Liver disease	NutriHep	1.5	40	690
Renal	Nepro	2.0	70	635
Pulmonary	Pulmocare, Respalor	1.5	60-75	475-580

*Appropriate for most patients.
†For patients with malabsorption (e.g., short bowel syndrome or IBD).

Gastric Feeding
- Start with full strength at 30 ml/hour, advance 20 ml q8 hours to goal
- Check residual volume q4 hours, continue if <150 ml, hold 1 hour if >150 ml

Jejunostomy Feeding
- Start with full strength at 20 ml/hour, advance 20 ml q8 hours to goal
- Follow clinical examination to assess tolerance (do not check residuals)
- Do not bolus feed using a jejunostomy tube

Intermittent/Bolus Feeding
- Start with full strength at 120 ml q4 hours
- Advance 60 ml q2-3 boluses to goal

General

- Elevate head of bed 30 degrees
- Consider jejunostomy feeding if patient develops recurrent aspiration with gastric feeding
- If patient develops diarrhea, consider the following:
  1. Decrease the rate, then titrate upward at slower pace
  2. Evaluate for *Clostridium difficile* or bacterial overgrowth
  3. Eliminate GI irritants, including magnesium and sorbitol (found in elixir medications)
  4. Use a low-fat, peptide-containing formula
  5. Add fiber or kaolin-pectin
- Avoid using blue food dye[13]

HEPATIC ENCEPHALOPATHY

Grades

- Grade 1: Irritable, slurring, and asterixis
- Grade 2: Lethargy and confusion
- Grade 3: Somnolence and reacts to pain
- Grade 4: Coma (decreased ICP)

Common Precipitants

- Azotemia: 26%
- Drugs: 24%
- GI bleed: 20%
- Protein use: 7%
- Alkalosis: 7%
- Infection: 5%
- Constipation: 5%
- Other: 6%

Management

- Exclude precipitant/complication; check glucose; manage ABCs
- Admit to ICU if grade 2 encephalopathy; intubate if grade 3
- Lactulose 30-45 ml po tid/qid or 300 ml using a retention enema, low protein diet
- Neomycin 1-2 g/day po (or substitute vancomycin, or Flagyl because of toxicity)
- Determine eligibility for liver transplant

References

1. Runyon BA, Montano AA, Akriviadis EA, et al. The serum-ascites albumin gradient is superior to the exudate-transudate concept in the differential diagnosis of ascites. Ann Intern Med 117:215-220, 1992.
2. Becker SD, Lamont JT. Postoperative jaundice. Semin Liver Dis 8:183-190, 1988.
3. Garrison RN, Cryer HM, Howard DA, et al. Clarification of risk factors for abdominal operations in patients with hepatic cirrhosis. Ann Surg 199:648-655, 1984.
4. Banks P. Practice guidelines in acute pancreatitis. Am J Gastroenterol 92:377-386, 1997.
5. Ranson JH, Rifkind KM, Roses DF, et al. Prognostic signs and the role of operative management in acute pancreatitis. Surg Gynecol Obstet 139:69-81, 1974.
6. Fan ST, Lai EC, Mok FP, et al. Early treatment of acute biliary pancreatitis by endoscopic papillotomy. N Engl J Med 328:228-232, 1993.
7. Sainio V, Kemppainen E, Puolakkainen P, et al. Early antibiotic treatment in acute necrotising pancreatitis. Lancet 346:663-667, 1995.
8. Gruber PJ, Silverman RA, Gottesfeld S, et al. Presence of fever and leukocytosis in acute cholecystitis. Ann Emerg Med 28:273-277, 1996.
9. Sarasin FP, Louis-Simonet M, Gaspoz JM, et al. Detecting acute thoracic aortic dissection in the emergency department: time constraints and choice of the optimal diagnostic test. Ann Emerg Med 28:278-288, 1996.
10. Walker JS, Dire DJ. Vascular abdominal emergencies. Emerg Med Clin North Am 14:571-592, 1996.
11. Kirby DF, Delegge MH, Fleming CR. American Gastroenterological Association technical review on tube feeding for enteral nutrition. Gastroenterology 108:1282-1301, 1995.
12. Koretz RL, Lipman TO, Klein S. AGA technical review on parenteral nutrition. Gastroenterology 121:970-1001, 2001.
13. Maloney JP, Halbower AC, Fouty BF, et al. Systemic absorption of food dye in patients with sepsis. N Engl J Med 343:1047-1048, 2000.

APPENDIX

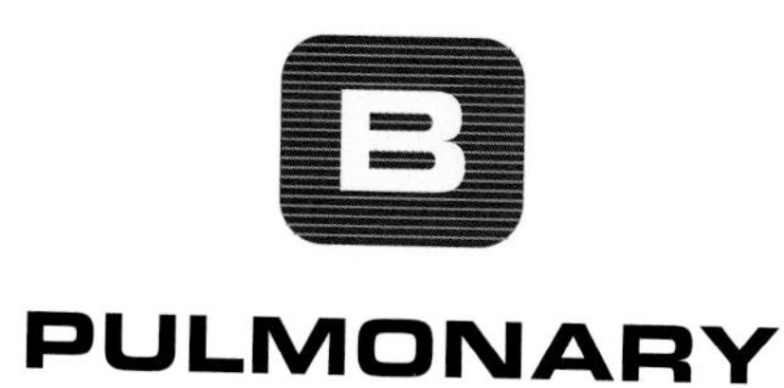

PULMONARY

B

PULMONARY EQUATIONS

Tidal volume: $V_T = (V_{dead\ space} + V_{alveolar\ space}) = V_D + V_A$

Minute ventilation: $V_E = \dfrac{0.863 \times V_{CO_2}\ ml/min}{Paco_2 \times (1 - V_D/V_T)}$ (Normal 4 to 6 L/min)

Bohr dead space: $\dfrac{V_D}{V_T} = \dfrac{PAco_2 - P_{expired\ CO_2}}{PAco_2}$ (Normal 0.2 to 0.3)

Physiologic dead space: $\dfrac{V_D}{V_T} = \dfrac{Paco_2 - P_{expired\ CO_2}}{Paco_2}$

Static compliance $= \dfrac{V_T}{P_{plateau} - P_{end\ expiration}}$ (Normal >60 ml/cm H_2O)

LaPlace law of surface tension: Pressure $= \dfrac{2 \times \text{Tension}}{\text{Radius}}$

Alveolar O_2 estimate: $Pao_2 = Fio_2\ (p_{atmospheric} - p_{H_2O}) - \dfrac{pco_2}{\text{Resp quotient}} =$

$Fio_2\ (760 - 47\ \text{mm Hg}) - \dfrac{pco_2}{0.8}$

Alveolar − Arterial O_2 gradient $= PAo_2 - Pao_2 \approx 2.5 + 0.21 \times$ Age (years) upright

Pao_2 upright $\approx 104.2 - 0.27 \times$ Age (years)

$$Pa_{O_2} \text{ supine} \approx 103.5 - 0.42 \times \text{Age (years)}$$

$$Pa_{CO_2} = K \times \frac{CO_2 \text{ production}}{\text{Alveolar ventilation}} = 0.863 \times \frac{V_{CO_2}}{V_A}$$

$$\text{Shunt fraction: } \frac{Q_S}{Q_T} = \frac{0.0031(A - aDO_2)}{0.0031(A - aDO_2) + Ca_{O_2} - Cv_{O_2}}$$

Ca_{O_2} = Arterial O_2 content

Cv_{O_2} = Mixed venous O_2 content (from PA catheter)

$Cx_{O_2} = ([1.39 \times \text{Hb (g/d)}] \times [O_2\text{sat}]) + (0.0031 \times Px_{O_2})$

$A - aDO_2$ = Alveolar − Arterial oxygen difference (mm Hg)

B

PULMONARY FUNCTION TESTING[1]

Abbreviations

- ERV, Expiratory reserve volume
- $FEF_{25\% \text{ to } 75\%}$, Forced expiratory flow from 25% to 75% VC
- FET, Forced expiratory time
- FEV_1, Forced expiratory volume in 1 second
- FRC, Functional residual capacity
- FVC, Forced vital capacity
- IC, Inspiratory capacity
- RV, Residual volume
- TLC, Total lung capacity
- VC, Vital capacity

Spirometry Patterns

- Normal: FVC, FEV_1, PEFR, and $FEF_{25\% \text{ to } 75\%}$ >80% predicted; FEV_1/FVC >95% predicted
  - Can be seen with intermittent disease (such as asthma), pulmonary emboli, and pulmonary vascular disease
- Obstructive: Obstruction to airflow prolongs expiration
  - FEV_1 /FVC <95% predicted and increased airway resistance
  - Differential diagnosis: Asthma, COPD, bronchiectasis, cystic fibrosis, bronchiolitis, or proximal airway obstruction
- Restrictive: Reduced volumes without changes in airway resistance
  - Decreased VC and TLC, FEV_1 and FVC decreased proportionately (FEV_1/FVC ratio >95% predicted)
  - Must confirm lung volumes by helium dilution or plethysmography (reduced FVC on spirometry not specific for restrictive disease, although normal FVC predicts normal TLC)
  - Differential diagnosis: Interstitial disease, CHF, pleural disease, pneumonia, neuromuscular disease, chest wall abnormalities, obesity, and lung resection
- Bronchodilator response: Positive if FVC or FEV_1 increase 12% and ≥200 ml
- Poor effort: Most reliably diagnosed by technician performing test rather than from spirometric values. FET <6 seconds suggests inadequate expiration

PLEURAL FLUID ANALYSIS[2]

Light's Criteria

Any of the following is 98% sensitive and 83% specific for exudative effusion (*excludes* transudates) (Box B-1):

1. Pleural/serum LDH >0.6
2. Pleural LDH >two thirds of upper limit for serum LDH
3. Pleural/serum protein >0.5
4. Serum albumin − pleural albumin <1.2 g/dl: More specific for exudates (92%),[3] but should not be used as the only criterion

Appearance

- Bloody
  - Fluid hematocrit <1% is not significant
  - Hematocrit 1% to 20% suggests cancer, PE, or trauma
  - Fluid hematocrit >50% of serum hematocrit suggests hemothorax
- Turbidity despite centrifugation suggests chylothorax or pseudochylothorax
- Putridity suggests empyema
- Viscosity suggests mesothelioma
- "Anchovy paste" or "chocolate sauce" consistency suggests amebiasis

Box B-1 **Pleural Fluid Analysis**

ALWAYS TRANSUDATIVE

CHF

Cirrhosis with ascites

Hypoalbuminemia

Nephrotic syndrome

SOMETIMES TRANSUDATIVE

PE (35%)

Malignancy (10%)

Sarcoidosis

SOMETIMES EXUDATIVE

Diuretic-treated CHF

Additional Useful Tests for Exudative Effusions

Leukocytes

- Total WBC count is rarely helpful
- Neutrophil predominance suggests pneumonia, PE, pancreatitis, or abdominal abscess
- Lymphocyte predominance suggests tumor, TB, or resolving acute process
- Eosinophilia (>10% suggests blood or air in pleural space, asbestos, drug reaction, or paragonimiasis; uncommon in TB and malignancy)

Cytology (Cell Block and Smears)

- 70% yield for metastatic adenocarcinoma, lower for other cancers
- Mesothelial cells are nonspecific, but >2% or 3% makes tuberculosis unlikely
- Send flow cytometry if lymphoma is suspected

Glucose

Glucose <60 mg/dl:

- Complicated parapneumonic effusion (<40 mg/dl → chest tube)
- Neoplasm
- TB
- Hemothorax
- Churg-Strauss syndrome
- Rheumatoid arthritis or SLE
- Paragonimiasis

Amylase

Elevated in:

- Esophageal perforation
- Pancreatic disease
- Malignancy

Triglycerides

Elevated in:

- Chylous effusions
- >110 mg/dl is 100% specific; <50 mg/dl excludes

LDH

- Nonspecific indicator of inflammation

pH

- <7.0: Complicated parapneumonic effusion (empyema)
- <7.20: Empyema, systemic acidosis, esophageal rupture, rheumatoid arthritis, TB, neoplasm, hemothorax, or paragonimiasis

Useful Tests for Tuberculous Pleuritis

- Adenosine deaminase >40 units/L
- Interferon gamma >140 pg/ml
- Positive PCR

Useful Tests for Effusion of Unknown Cause

- Pulmonary embolism evaluation
- Serial LDH measurement (reassuring if decreasing)
- Thoracoscopy

VENTILATION

NPPV

Box B-2

Disease States Amenable to NPPV	**Relative Contraindications for NPPV**
Acute respiratory failure (such as from ARDS, pneumonia, asthma/COPD, pulmonary edema, or neuromuscular disease)	Failure of previous NPPV attempts
Chronic respiratory failure	Hemodynamic instability/GI bleed
Acute pulmonary edema	Life-threatening arrhythmias
Chronic congestive heart failure with breathing-related sleep disorder	High risk of aspiration
	Airway obstruction
Clinical Criteria for NPPV Use	Impaired mental status
Moderate to severe respiratory distress • Increased dyspnea • RR >24 • Accessory muscles • Paradoxical breathing	Inability to use nasal or face mask
$Paco_2$ >45 mm Hg and pH <7.35	Life-threatening refractory hypoxemia
Pao_2/Fio_2 <200	Pao_2 <60 mm Hg with $Fio_2 = 1.0$
	pH <7.20

Modified from Hillberg RE, Johnson DC. Noninvasive ventilation. N Engl J Med 337:1746-1752, 1997; and Spiro SG, Jett JR, Albert RK, eds. Comprehensive Respiratory Medicine. Philadelphia: Mosby–Year Book, 1999.

NPPV Modes and Parameters

Table B-1

Mode	Parameter
Volume mechanical	• Breaths of 250 to 500 ml (4 to 8 ml/kg), pressures vary
Pressure mechanical	• Pressure support or pressure control at 8 to 20 cm H_2O • End-expiratory pressure of 0 to 6 cm H_2O, volumes vary
BiPAP	• Inspiratory pressure of 8 cm H_2O (range 6 to 14 cm H_2O) • End expiratory pressure of 4 cm H_2O (range 3 to 5 cm H_2O), volumes vary, initial RR = 8 breaths/min
CPAP	• 5 to 13 cm H_2O, volumes vary
Weaning parameters for all NPPV modes	• Clinically stable for 4 to 6 hours • RR $<$24 breaths/min, heart rate $<$110 beats/min • Compensated pH $>$7.35 • Sao_2 $>$90% to 92% on $\leq$3 L face mask O_2

From Hillberg RE, Johnson DC. Noninvasive ventilation. N Engl J Med 337:1746-1752, 1997.

Drugs for Rapid Sequence Intubation

Table B-2

Agent	Dose IV (mg/kg)	Onset (min)	Key Properties
Defasciculating Drugs			**Defasciculation (Optional)**
Rocuronium*	0.06	2	Tachycardia, mild histamine release
Succinylcholine	0.1	<1	Increased ICP, GI, and eye pressures
Vecuronium	0.01	2.5 to 5	Minimal tachycardia
Sedation Drugs			
Etomidate*	0.3 to 0.4	1	Minimal BP decrease
Fentanyl	2 to 10 μg/kg	1	Increased ICP, chest wall rigidity
Ketamine	1 to 2	<1	Increased BP, ICP, GI, and eye pressures
Midazolam	0.1 to 0.3	2	Hypotension
Propofol	1 to 2.5	<1	Hypotension
Thiopental	3 to 5	<1	Hypotension, bronchospasm
Paralyzing Drugs			
Succinylcholine*	1 to 2	<1	Increased ICP, K^+, GI, and eye pressures
Rocuronium	0.6 to 1.2	2	Tachycardia, mild histamine release
Vecuronium	0.15 to 0.25	2.5 to 5	Prolonged action

*Rocuronium → etomidate → succinylcholine: Standard drug sequence if no contraindications exist.

B

After Intubation

1. Check tube placement (CO_2 detector and esophageal detector device). Other methods, including examination, can be inaccurate
2. Inflate cuff, then release cricoid pressure
3. Reassess patient's BP, pulse, and pulse oximetry
4. Obtain chest radiograph to verify correct ET tube depth (should be between T2 and T4)
5. Sedate and consider long-acting paralytics

Modes of Mechanical Ventilation

Table B-3

Mode	Advantages	Disadvantages
AC	• Full TV regardless of respiratory effort or drive • Can preset minute volume	• Tachypnea may lead to respiratory alkalosis • Poor synchrony between patient and ventilator may lead to "breath-stacking" and auto-PEEP
IMV	• Patient determines TV for spontaneous breath • Potentially less respiratory alkalosis • May facilitate weaning or respiratory conditioning	• May increase work of breathing and respiratory muscle fatigue • Must overcome resistance of respiratory circuit for spontaneous breath (unless pressure support is added)
PSV	• Patient determines own volumes, rate, and flow (more physiologic) • Potentially reduces PIPs	• Requires careful monitoring to ensure adequate TV and minute ventilation • Requires consistent respiratory effort
PCV	• Can more easily control inspiratory time and peak airway pressures • May be used with AC or IMV modes	• Requires careful monitoring to ensure adequate TV and minute ventilation • May increase risk of auto-PEEP
NPPV	• Allows ventilation without intubation • Easily taken on and off	• Requires careful patient selection and trained respiratory therapists • No airway control

Ventilator Parameters and Settings

Table B-4

Parameter	Suggested Initial Settings or Normal Range	Comments
FiO_2	100%	• May taper rapidly to level adequate to maintain PaO_2/O_2sat • Ideally, keep <60% to prevent oxygen toxicity and lung injury
RR	8 to12 breaths/min	• Titrate to pH • Consider 18 to 24 breaths/min for therapeutic hyperventilation (decreases respiratory effort in shock) • Rate of >20 breaths/min may increase auto-PEEP
Mode	IMV or AC	• Consider PSV in neuromuscular disease if respiratory effort is enough to trigger cycle
TV	6 ml/kg of ideal body weight	• Higher volumes may increase risk of alveolar overdistention (barotrauma) and worsen ventilator-associated lung injury
IFR	60 L/min	• Set only on volume-cycled ventilators • IFR set too low may increase auto-PEEP by allowing insufficient exhalation time • IFR set too high may increase PIPs
I/E ratio	1:3	• Determined by IFR and RR during volume-cycled ventilation • Can be specifically adjusted during PCV • Increased I/E ratio (such as 1:4) may be useful in severe obstruction (↑ expiratory phase) • Inverse ratio (2:1) may be used to increase PaO_2 in severe hypoxemia
Plateau pressure	<35 cm H_2O	• A noninvasive measure of transpulmonary pressure • Ideally kept low to decrease risk of barotrauma
PIP	<45 cm H_2O	• Ideally kept low, but may not be achievable (less important than plateau pressure)

Continued

B

Table B-4—cont'd

Parameter	Suggested Initial Settings or Normal Range	Comments
PEEP	5 cm H_2O (considered physiologic)	• Improves oxygenation by preventing alveolar collapse and V/Q mismatch • Titrate PEEP by 5 cm H_2O increments until Fio_2 requirement ≤ 0.6 **or** plateau pressure >35 cm H_2O **or** compliance decreases • Increases airway pressures and risk of barotrauma • Decreases venous return and cardiac output
Compliance	70 to 100 ml/cm H_2O	• Δvolume/Δpressure = TV/(plateau pressure − PEEP) • Decreased in CHF, pneumothorax, ARDS, effusions, pneumonia, and chest wall disorders
Resistance	<5 to 10 cm H_2O/L/sec	• Δpressure/flow rate = (PIP − plateau) ÷ IFR • Increased in bronchoconstriction and mucous plugging

Weaning from Mechanical Ventilation

Optimize Before Extubation

- Withdraw sedative drugs
- Ensure adequate rest and nutrition
- Prepare patient psychologically
- Diurese to minimize pulmonary edema
- Treat bronchospasm
- Minimize secretions
- Normalize electrolytes affecting muscle function (such as PO_4, Mg^{++}, and Ca^{++})
- Suppress fever with antipyretics
- Treat systemic illness (such as infections)
- Institute effective antianginal therapy
- Exclude drug-induced neuromuscular blockade (such as with aminoglycosides)

Criteria for Starting Weaning[4]

- Cause of respiratory failure improved
- Adequate oxygenation: $Pao_2 \geq 60$ mm Hg or $Fio_2 \leq 0.4$ (Pao_2/Fio_2 = 150 to 300) with positive PEEP ≤ 5 cm H_2O

- Hemodynamic stability: No myocardial ischemia or hypotension
- Temperature <38° C
- Hemoglobin ≥8 to 10 g/dl
- Patient awake or easily roused

Predicting Successful Extubation[5]

- RR/TV <105 during T-piece trial best predicts successful weaning[6]
- Higher values may be compatible with weaning in certain populations (such as small, elderly women[7]) or if clinical judgment predicts success

Trial of Spontaneous Breathing

- Give 30-minute trial of T-tube or pressure support ventilation of 7 ± 3 cm H_2O
- Consider adding CPAP (5 cm H_2O) for patients with obstruction (such as those with asthma or COPD)
- Successful trial:
  - O_2sat >90% or $Pa{O_2}$ >60 mm Hg or $Fi{O_2}$ <0.4 to 0.5
  - Increase in $Pa{CO_2}$ <10 mm Hg or decrease in pH to <0.10
  - RR <35
  - RR/TV <100 to 105
  - HR <140 or increased <20% from baseline
  - SBP 80 to 160 mm Hg or changes <20% from baseline
  - No signs of increased work of breathing (such as paradoxical breathing or accessory muscle use) or other signs of distress (such as diaphoresis or agitation)
- If successful, proceed with extubation
- If unsuccessful, repeat trial daily and gradually withdraw ventilator support (pressure support and T-piece weaning equally effective and superior to IMV weaning)[8,9]

Ventilator Emergencies

High Pressure

- If O_2 saturation ≤80% or if patient is hemodynamically unstable, disconnect from ventilator and bag at $Fi{O_2}$ 100%; check for causes
- If oxygenation and hemodynamics are stable, check ventilator peak and plateau pressures (Table B-5)
  - PIP: Maximum pressure is registered with each volume-cycled breath
  - Plateau: Pressure at end-inspiration (may use 0.5 sec hold to measure)

B

Table B-5 Ventilator Peak and Plateau Pressures

Increased Resistance	Decreased Compliance
Peak pressure elevated (>35 cm H_2O) Plateau pressure normal (≤35 cm H_2O)	Peak and plateau pressures elevated (>35 cm H_2O)
Causes	
Endotracheal tube mucus or plugs Biting the endotracheal tube Tracheal obstruction Bronchospasm	Tube in mainstem bronchus Asynchronous breathing Auto-PEEP Atelectasis, pneumonia, or CHF Pneumothorax
Interventions	
Check ventilator circuit Suction Bronchodilators Reposition tube Consider bronchoscopy	Stat chest radiograph to determine underlying cause Decrease auto-PEEP by decreasing TV/RR ratio or temporarily disconnecting from ventilator circuit

Low Pressure

- If O_2 saturation ≤80% or if patient is hemodynamically unstable, disconnect from ventilator and bag at FiO_2 100%
- Causes:
  - Endotracheal tube has slipped out of trachea → reintubate
  - Cuff leak → instill more air into cuff or reintubate
  - Tracheoesophageal fistula → attempt to reposition tube
  - Leak within mechanical ventilator circuit

ASTHMA AND COPD

Management of Acute Asthma

Box B-3

General

Administer O_2 and apply cardiac monitor and pulse oximeter

Inhaled Beta-2 Agonist

Administer using a nebulizer, continuous or q30 minutes if moderate to severe **or** with MDI, 2 to 4 puffs q4 hours if mild asthma

Albuterol (Ventolin) 2.5 to 5 mg **or** levalbuterol (Xopenex) 0.63 to 1.25 mg

Anticholinergic Agent

Ipratropium bromide (Atrovent) 0.5 mg in 2.5 ml NS using a nebulizer **or** 4 to 8 puffs q6 hours (18 μg/puff)

Steroids

Methylprednisolone (Solu-Medrol) 1 to 2 mg/kg IV (if cannot take po) **or** prednisone 1 to 2 mg/kg po; continue for 5 to 7 days (do not taper)

Inhaled steroids (triamcinolone [Azmacort], flunisolide [AeroBid], beclomethasone [Beclovent, Vanceril], or fluticasone [Flovent]) after stopping oral steroids, if frequent oral steroids or severe asthma

Other Options

Magnesium sulfate ($MgSO_4$) 2 g IV over 15 minutes if severe asthma and no renal failure

Epinephrine 0.3 mg SC **or** terbutaline 0.25 mg SC q20 minutes $\times$ 2

Prophylaxis (not acute treatment) with oral zafirlukast (Accolate), montelukast (Singulair), or zileuton (Zyflo)

ED Management of Asthma

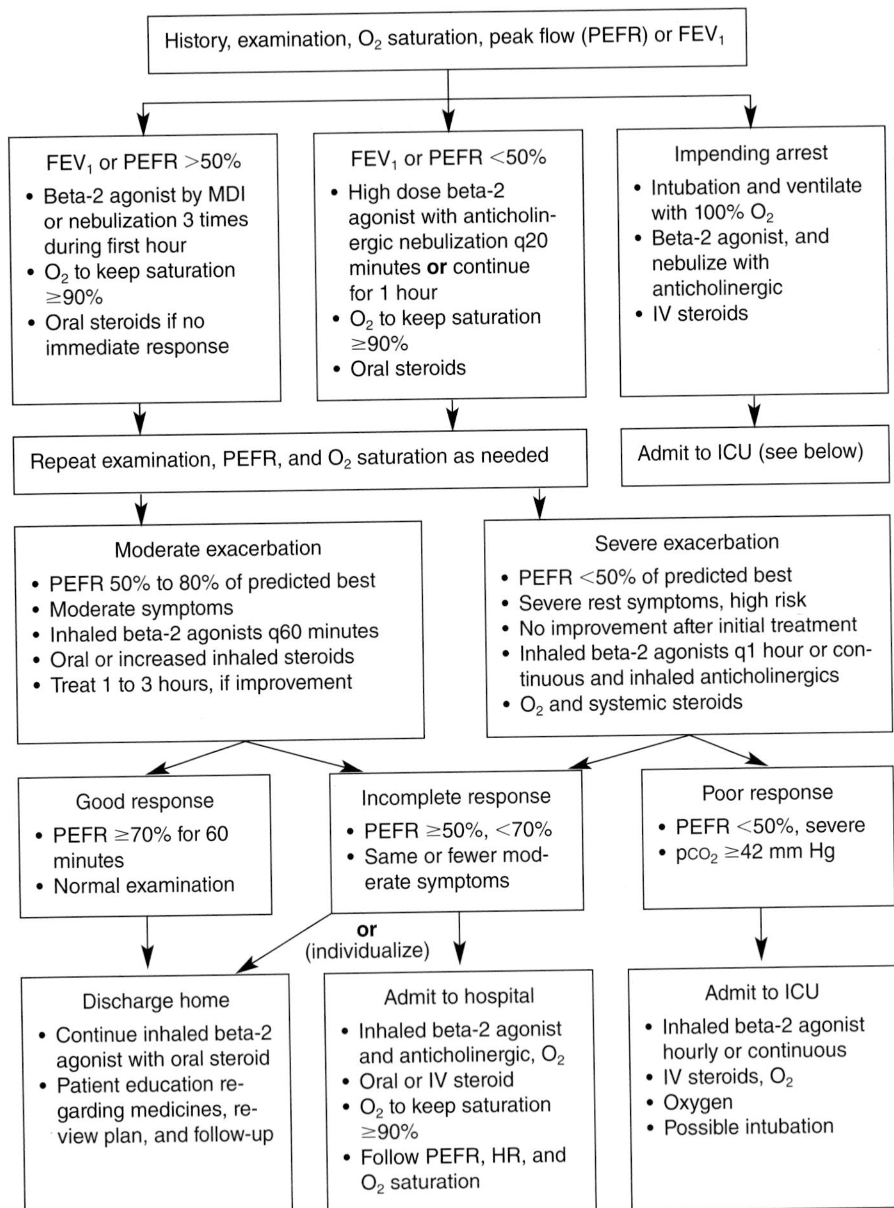

Fig. B-1 NIH Guidelines for Emergency Department Management of Asthma. (From Emond SD, Camargo CA Jr, Nowak RM. 1997 National Asthma Education and Prevention Program guidelines: a practical summary for emergency physicians. Ann Emerg Med 31:579-589, 1998.)

American Thoracic Society COPD Guidelines

COPD Severity

Table B-6 COPD American Thoracic Society Disease Severity Scale

Individual Features	Disease Severity
Worsening dyspnea	Mild if one feature plus additional finding*
Increased sputum purulence	Moderate if two features
Increased sputum volume	Severe if three features

*Upper respiratory infection in the past 5 days, fever, increased wheezing or cough, increased HR or RR by ≥20%.

COPD Exacerbation

Box B-4 American Thoracic Society Recommendations for Managing COPD Exacerbation

Useful Treatments/Procedures	Not Useful Treatments/Procedures
Beta-agonists/anticholinergics (inhaled)	Spirometry for severity assessment
Steroids up to 2 weeks	Mucolytics
Oxygen cautiously if there is hypoxemia	Chest physiotherapy
BiPAP or CPAP	Methylxanthines
Narrow-spectrum antibiotic agents (amoxicillin [Amoxil], sulfamethoxazole with trimethoprim [Septra], or tetracycline) if outpatient, no pneumonia present	Any risk stratification methods for predicting relapse or inpatient mortality

Compiled from Snow V, Lascher S, Mottur-Pilson C, et al. Joint Expert Panel on Chronic Obstructive Pulmonary Disease of the American College of Chest Physicians and the American College of Physicians-American Society of Internal Medicine. Evidence base for management of acute exacerbations of chronic obstructive pulmonary disease. Ann Intern Med 134:595-599, 2001.

B

THROMBOEMBOLISM, PULMONARY EMBOLISM, AND DEEP VEIN THROMBOSIS

PE Risk Factors

- Immobility, venous damage
- Hypercoagulability (such as cancer, a previous clot, nephritic syndrome, inflammatory disease, or a recent pregnancy [<3 months]), estrogens, sepsis, or lupus
- No risk factors in 15% overall
- No risk factors in 28% <40 years old

Diagnostic Studies

- Chest radiograph: Abnormal in 60% to 84%
- Arterial blood gas: 92% ↑ A-a gradient*
- Ventilation perfusions scan V/Q
- D-dimer: 85% to 95% sensitive
- Angiography: >98% sensitive/specific
- Echocardiography: Detects 90% of cardiac movement defects causing ↓ BP
- CT: ~90% sensitive for central PE
- MRI: >90% sensitive for PE

Clinical Features

- Chest pain (pleuritic 75%): 80% to 90%
- Dyspnea: 73% to 84%
- Cough (wheeze 9%): 37% to 53%
- Hemoptysis: 13% to 30%
- Respirations ≥16 breaths/min (≥20 breaths/min): 92 (70%)
- Fever >100° F with tachycardia: 43 (40%)
- Calf swelling: 30%

ECG Findings

- Nonspecific ST-T changes: 50%
- T-wave inversion: 42%
- New right bundle branch: 15%
- S in 1, Q in 3, T in 3: 12%
- Right axis deviation: 7%
- Shift in transition to V5: 7%
- Right ventricle hypertrophy: 6%
- P pulmonale: 6%

---

*A-a gradient: 150 − (pao_2 + pco_2/0.8); normal = (age/4) + 4.

Charlotte Rule for Excluding Pulmonary Embolism

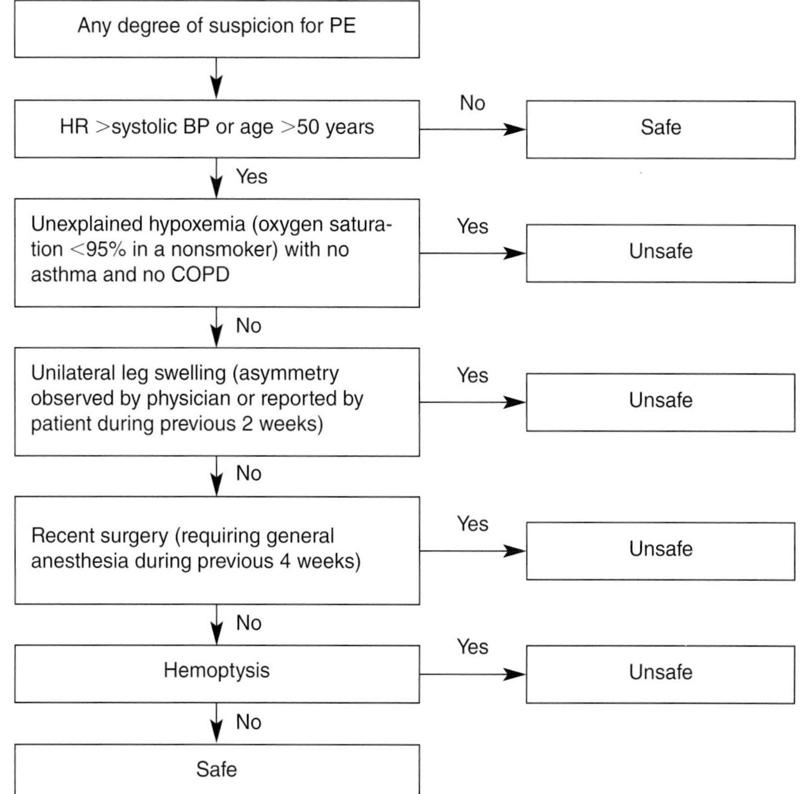

Charlotte Rule Application

- Patients designated as safe have a 13.3% probability of having a PE. In the cited studies, safe patients with either (1) a negative whole blood D-dimer (SimpliRED or SimpliFY) plus a normal dead space (<20%, modified dead space = 100[$Paco_2$ − $Petco_2$]/$Paco_2$) or (2) a quantitative D-dimer assay <500 ng/ml were judged to have a low enough probability of PE that no further evaluation was necessary. If any of these tests are abnormal (any abnormal D-dimer or dead space ≥20%), then radiologic imaging (CT, V/Q, or angiogram) is required.
- Patients designated as unsafe have a 42% probability of having a PE. These patients require radiologic imaging (CT, V/Q, or angiogram) to exclude PE.

Fig. B-2 (Application modified from Kline JA, Nelson RD, Jackson RE, et al. Criteria for the safe use of D-dimer testing in emergency department patients with suspected pulmonary embolism: a multicenter US study. Ann Emerg Med 39:144-152, 2002; algorithm from Kline JA, Wells PS. Methodology for a rapid protocol to rule out pulmonary embolism in the emergency department. Ann Emerg Med 42:266-275, 2003.)

Management Options for Pulmonary Embolism

Box B-5

Heparin	**Vena Cava Filter**
Load 80 U/kg, drip 18 U/kg/hour IV **Thrombolytics** Indications (controversial): Shock, significant respiratory distress, or significant hypoxia Dose: tPA 100 mg IV over 2 hours **or** streptokinase 250,000 U IV over 30 minutes, then 100,000 U/hour for 24 hours (administer infusion over 72 hours if concurrent DVT is suspected) May be used up to 1 to 2 weeks after symptom onset	Indications: Strong contraindication to anti-coagulation **or** clot develops during adequate anticoagulation **Embolectomy** Indication: If patient is not an anticoagulation candidate and is acutely unstable

References

1. American Thoracic Society. Lung function testing: selection of reference values and interpretive strategies. Am Rev Respir Dis 144:1202-1218, 1991.
2. Light RW. Pleural effusion. N Engl J Med 346:1971-1977, 2002.
3. Roth BJ, O'Meara TF, Cragun WH. The serum-effusion albumin gradient in the evaluation of pleural effusions. Chest 98:546-549, 1990.
4. Frutos-Vivar F, Esteban A. When to wean from a ventilator. An evidence-based strategy. Cleve Clin J Med 70:389, 392-393, 2003.
5. Alia I, Esteban A. Weaning from mechanical ventilation. Crit Care 4:72-80, 2000.
6. Yang KL, Tobin MJ. A prospective trial of indexes predicting the outcome of trials of weaning from mechanical ventilation. N Engl J Med 324:1445-1450, 1991.
7. Krieger B, Isber J, Breitenbucher A, et al. Serial measurements of the rapid shallow breathing index as a predictor of outcome in elderly medical patients. Chest 112:1029-1034, 1997.
8. Esteban A, Frutos F, Tobin MJ, et al. A comparison of four methods of weaning patients from mechanical ventilation. Spanish Lung Failure Collaborative Group. N Engl J Med 332:345-350, 1995.
9. Esteban A, Alía I, Gordo F, et al. Extubation outcome after spontaneous breathing trials with T-tube or pressure support ventilation. Spanish Lung Failure Collaborative Group. Am J Respir Crit Care Med 156:459-465, 1997.

Appendix

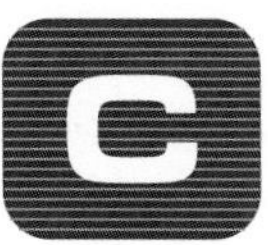

CARDIOVASCULAR

C

HEMODYNAMIC VALUES

Table C-1

Pressure Parameter	Normal (mm Hg)	Parameter	Normal
Right atrium		Cardiac output	4.0 to 6.0 L/min
• Mean	0 to 8	Cardiac index	2.6 to 4.2 L/min/m^2
• a-wave	2 to 10	Systemic vascular resistance	1130 ± 178 dynes/sec/cm^{-5}
• v-wave	2 to 10	Pulmonary vascular resistance	67 ± 23 dynes/sec/cm^{-5}
Right ventricle		O_2 consumption	110 to 150 ml/min/m^2
• Systolic	15 to 30	Arterial-venous O_2 difference	3.0 to 4.5 ml/dl
• Diastolic	0 to 8		
Pulmonary artery			
• Mean	9 to 16		
• Diastolic	3 to 12		
• Systolic	15 to 30		
Pulmonary artery wedge			
• Mean	1 to 10		
• a-wave	3 to 15		
• v-wave	3 to 12		

Modified from Lambert CR, Pepine CJ, Nichols WW. Pressure measurement and determination of vascular resistance. In Pepine CJ, Hill JA, Lambert CR, et al, eds. Diagnostic and Therapeutic Cardiac Catheterization, 3rd ed. Baltimore: Lippincott Williams & Wilkins, 1998.

CARDIAC PARAMETERS AND FORMULAS

Table C-2

Parameters and Formulas	Normal Values
CO = HR × SV	4 to 8 L/min
CI = CO / BSA	2.8 to 4.23 L/min/m^2
MAP = ([SBP − DBP] / 3) + DBP	80 to 100 mm Hg
SVR = (80 [MAP − CVP]) / CO	800 to 1200 dynes/sec/cm^2
PVR = (80[PAM − PCWP]) / CO	45 to 120 dynes/sec/cm^2
CVP	5 to 12 cm H_2O
Pulmonary artery systolic pressure	20 to 30 mm Hg
Pulmonary artery diastolic pressure	10 to 15 mm Hg
Pulmonary artery mean pressure	15 to 20 mm Hg
PCWP	8 to 12 mm Hg

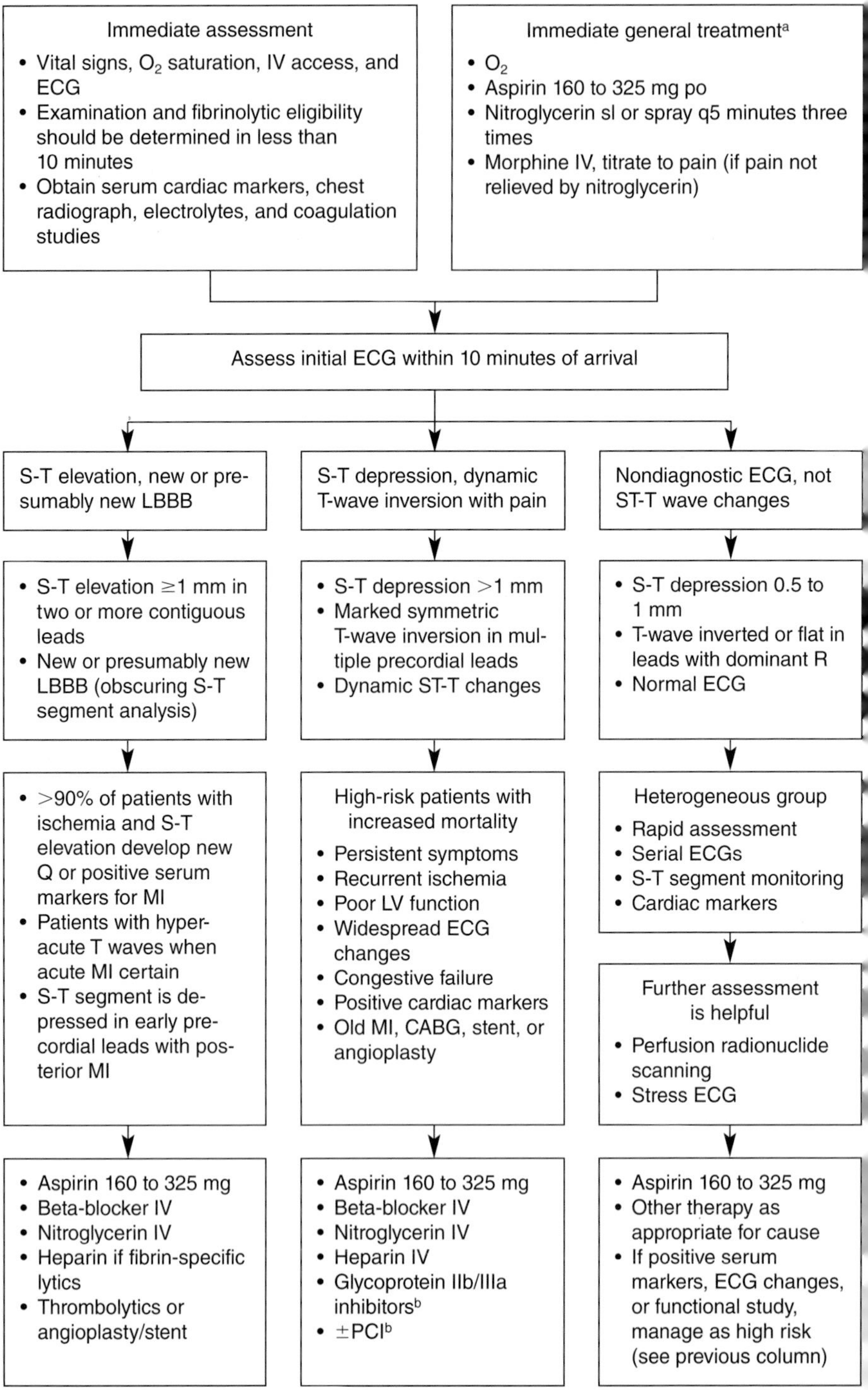

Immediate assessment

- Vital signs, O_2 saturation, IV access, and ECG
- Examination and fibrinolytic eligibility should be determined in less than 10 minutes
- Obtain serum cardiac markers, chest radiograph, electrolytes, and coagulation studies

Immediate general treatment[a]

- O_2
- Aspirin 160 to 325 mg po
- Nitroglycerin sl or spray q5 minutes three times
- Morphine IV, titrate to pain (if pain not relieved by nitroglycerin)

↓

Assess initial ECG within 10 minutes of arrival

↓

S-T elevation, new or presumably new LBBB

- S-T elevation ≥1 mm in two or more contiguous leads
- New or presumably new LBBB (obscuring S-T segment analysis)

↓

- >90% of patients with ischemia and S-T elevation develop new Q or positive serum markers for MI
- Patients with hyperacute T waves when acute MI certain
- S-T segment is depressed in early precordial leads with posterior MI

↓

- Aspirin 160 to 325 mg
- Beta-blocker IV
- Nitroglycerin IV
- Heparin if fibrin-specific lytics
- Thrombolytics or angioplasty/stent

S-T depression, dynamic T-wave inversion with pain

- S-T depression >1 mm
- Marked symmetric T-wave inversion in multiple precordial leads
- Dynamic ST-T changes

↓

High-risk patients with increased mortality

- Persistent symptoms
- Recurrent ischemia
- Poor LV function
- Widespread ECG changes
- Congestive failure
- Positive cardiac markers
- Old MI, CABG, stent, or angioplasty

↓

- Aspirin 160 to 325 mg
- Beta-blocker IV
- Nitroglycerin IV
- Heparin IV
- Glycoprotein IIb/IIIa inhibitors[b]
- ±PCI[b]

Nondiagnostic ECG, not ST-T wave changes

- S-T depression 0.5 to 1 mm
- T-wave inverted or flat in leads with dominant R
- Normal ECG

↓

Heterogeneous group

- Rapid assessment
- Serial ECGs
- S-T segment monitoring
- Cardiac markers

↓

Further assessment is helpful

- Perfusion radionuclide scanning
- Stress ECG

↓

- Aspirin 160 to 325 mg
- Other therapy as appropriate for cause
- If positive serum markers, ECG changes, or functional study, manage as high risk (see previous column)

Fig. C-1 Acute chest pain/coronary syndrome algorithm. *a,* Substitute clopidogrel if unable to take aspirin (withhold for 5 to 7 days before CABG). *b,* Abciximab (ReoPro), eptifibatide (Integrilin), or tirofiban (Aggrastat). (Compiled from Kinsara AJ. 2000 Guidelines for Cardiopulmonary Resuscitation Emergency Cardiovascular Care. Circulation 104:E45, 2001. ACC/AHA guideline update for the management of patients with unstable angina and non–ST-segment elevation myocardial infarction—2002: summary article. A report of the American College of Cardiology/American Heart Association Task Force on Practice Guidelines [Committee on the Management of Patients With Unstable Angina]. Circulation 106:1893-1900, 2002.)

ECG DIAGNOSIS OF ARRHYTHMIA, BLOCKS, AND MEDICAL DISORDERS

Normal Adult ECG (small box: 1 mm = 0.04 seconds; large box: 5 mm = 0.20 seconds)

- P wave
  - <0.10 second ↑ in I and II, ↓ in aVR
  - P-R interval 0.12 to 0.20 seconds
- QRS complex
  - 0.05 to 0.10 seconds
  - Normally ↑ in I, II, V5, and V6
  - ↓ in aVR and V1
  - Transition zone in V3
  - ↑ or ↓ in aVL, aVF, and III
  - Left chest lead's height is <27 mm
- Q wave
  - Normally <0.04 seconds and <25% height of following R
- Q-T interval
  - 0.34 to 0.42 seconds or 40% of R-R interval

$$\text{QTc (corrected Q-T interval)} = \frac{\text{Q-T interval}}{\sqrt{\text{R-R}}} \text{ (Normal} < 0.47 \text{ seconds)}$$

- T wave
  - ↑ in I and V6 and ↓ in aVR
  - Normal ↓ T waves may be found in III, aVF, aVL, and V
  - Abnormal ↓ T waves may signify LVH (especially V6), LBBB, ischemia, and MI
- Axis
  - Normal is −30 degrees to +100 degrees
  - LAD: −30 to −90 degrees
  - RAD: +100 to +180 or −90 to −180 degrees

Conduction Blocks

- First-degree AV block
  - P-R interval >0.2 seconds
  - P precedes each QRS
- Second-degree AV block
  - Type 1 (Wenckebach): increasing P-R interval until QRS is dropped
  - Type 2: QRS is dropped without increasing P-R interval

- Third-degree AV block
  - P and QRS are independent
  - Fixed P-P intervals
- RBBB
  - QRS ≥0.12 seconds (±0.1 to 0.12 seconds)
  - R-R′/R-S-R′ in V1/V2
  - ST-T opposite to terminal QRS
  - S in I, aVL, V5, or V6
- LBBB
  - QRS ≥0.12 seconds
  - R or R-R′ in I, aVL, or V6
  - Negative wave (RS or QS) in V1
  - ST-T waves directed opposite to the terminal 0.04 seconds QRS
- Anterior hemiblock
  - LAD >45
  - QRS 0.10 to 0.12 seconds
  - Small Q in I or aVL
  - R in II, III, and aVF
  - Terminal R in aVR
- Posterior hemiblock
  - RAD
  - QRS 0.10 to 0.12 seconds
  - S in I
  - Q in II, III, or aVF

Hypertrophy

- RAH
  - P >2.5 mm in II or large diphasic P in V1 (tall initial phase)
- Left atrial
  - Diphasic P in V1 with large terminal downward phase
- RVH
  - R >S in V1
  - R >5 mm in V1
  - Decreasing R in V1 to V4
  - S-T depression with flipped Ts in V1 to V3, with or without RAH
- LVH
  - Romhilt and Estes criteria, Cornell criteria

ECG Findings in Pericarditis

- S-T segment elevation is typically diffuse, involving ↑ in I, II, and III or at least two bipolar limb leads and precordial leads V1 through V6 or V2 through V6
- S-T depression is common in aVR and may occur in II and V1
  - S-T segment ↑ is typically concave upward and ≤5 mm high
  - Pathologic Q waves are rare, unless associated with MI
  - P-R segment depression is common
- Sequence of ST-T changes
  1. Initial S-T ↑
  2. S-T returns to baseline before T waves flip (↓)
  3. T wave ↓ is usually ≤5 mm
  4. T waves normalize
- Low voltage QRS or electrical alternans suggests pericardial fluid
- Positive or negative height of S-T segment/T wave >0.25 mm in V5, V6, or I

ECG Findings in Medical Disorders

Table C-3

Disorder	Class ECG Findings (Not Necessarily Most Common)
CNS bleed	Diffuse deep T inversion Prominent U wave Q-T interval >60% normal
COPD	RAD (negative lead) Overall low voltage RAH ± RBBB
Pulmonary emboli	ST-T wave changes RAD RBBB Large S in I, Q in III, T in III
Hyperkalemia	Peaked Ts Wide and flat Ps Wide QRS and Q-T interval Sine wave
Hypokalemia	Flat T waves U waves U waves >T waves S-T depression
Calcium	High calcium → short Q-T interval Low calcium → long Q-T interval
Pericarditis	Flat or concave S-T ↑ P-R ↓ ↓ voltage
Digoxin effect	Downward curve of S-T segment Flat/inverted Ts Shorter Q-T interval
Digoxin toxicity	PVCs (60%) AV block (20%) Ectopic SVT (25%) V tachycardia
Hypothyroidism	Sinus bradycardia Low voltage S-T ↓ Flat or inverted T waves
Hyperthyroidism	Sinus tachycardia

Typical ECG Findings in Acute MI

- Marked increase in R-wave voltage may occur early
- Prominent (hyperacute) T waves with normal direction occur early (especially >5 mm); T waves are peaked and symmetric (church steeple–shaped) (± wider than ↑ K)
- S-T segment elevation that is flat or convex (Table C-4)
- Q waves >0.04 seconds, other than leads aVR + V1, and T-wave flattening/inversion

Table C-4 Predictive Values of Initial ECG in Acute MI

Predictive Value	Sensitivity	Specificity
New Q waves or S-T segment elevation	40%	>90%
The above or S-T segment depression	75%	80%
Any of the above or previous ischemia/infarction changes	85%	76%
Any of the above or nonspecific ST-T changes	90%	65%

From Gibler WB, Lewis LM, Erb RE, et al. Early detection of acute myocardial infarction in patients presenting with chest pain and nondiagnostic ECGs: serial CK-MB sampling in the emergency department. Ann Emerg Med 19:1359-1366, 1990.

Myocardial Injury and Ischemia

Table C-5

Location	ECG ST Elevation or Q Waves	Coronary Arteries Involved
Anterior	V2 to V4	Left anterior descending
Anteroseptal	V1 to V4	Left anterior descending
Anterolateral	V1 to V6, I, aVL	Left anterior descending, diagonal
Inferior	II, II, aVF	Right coronary, circumflex
Lateral	I, aVL, V5, V6	Circumflex, diagonal
Posterior	Large R in V1, V2, and V3; reciprocal S-T segment ↓	Right coronary artery
Posterolateral	V6 to V9	Right coronary artery

S-T↑ ≥1 mm = injury/infarction in two contiguous leads; Q >0.04 seconds = infarction.

Arrhythmia Identification

- Multifocal atrial tachycardia
  - Three or more different P waves; normal QRS complex
  - Associated with COPD, hypoxia, digoxin or theophylline toxicity, or ASCVD
- Paroxysmal atrial tachycardia
  - P waves occur before each QRS complex; rate 150 to 250 beats/min
- Paroxysmal supraventricular tachycardia
  - Rate 120 to 250 beats/min
  - Narrow or wide QRS (if there is a bundle branch block or preexcitation)
  - P waves are visible or hidden in QRS
- Atrial flutter
  - Atrial rate 200 to 400 beats/min
  - Sawtooth pattern (especially leads II and III)
  - Common ventricular rate of 150/min as a result of a 2:1 block (with atrial rate of 300 beats/min)
- Atrial fibrillation
  - Highly irregular rhythm
  - No discernible P waves
  - Ventricular rate may be rapid or slow, depending on conduction
- Ventricular tachycardia
  - Three or more premature ventricular beats in a row
  - Broad QRS rhythm at 100 to 250 beats/min
  - Fusion beats
  - AV dissociation
  - Precordial concordance
- Ventricular fibrillation
  - Irregular chaotic baseline, no beats, no BP
- Torsades de pointes
  - Twisting QRS, prolonged Q-T interval, may progress to ventricular fibrillation

INDICATIONS FOR TRANSCUTANEOUS PATCHES/PACING FOR PATIENTS WITH ACUTE MI

- Hemodynamically unstable bradycardia (<50 beats/min)
- Mobitz type II second-degree AV block, or third-degree heart block
- Bilateral BBB, alternating BBB, or RBBB and alternating LBBB
- Left anterior fascicular block or newly acquired or age-determinate LBBB
- RBBB or LBBB and first-degree AV block

THROMBOLYTICS

Contraindications to Thrombolytic Agents

Absolute Contraindications

- Previous CNS bleed or CNS neoplasm
- Active internal bleeding (not menses)
- Stroke/TIA in the past year
- Suspicion of aortic dissection or pericarditis

Relative Contraindications

- BP >180/110 (arrival or during treatment)
- Anticoagulation (INR ≥2) or bleed diathesis
- Ready, high-volume cardiac catheterization laboratory
- Previous stroke or known CNS pathology not already listed
- Pregnancy or active peptic ulcer
- Noncompressible vascular puncture
- Internal bleeding in the previous 2 to 4 weeks
- Streptokinase use (in the past 1 to 2 years)—tPA is OK
- Trauma during the previous 4 weeks (head/spine trauma, CPR >10 min, or major surgery)
- History of chronic severe hypertension

Thrombolytic Dose and Choice of Agent

Table C-6

Agent	Dose	Criteria
rPA	• 10 U IV over 2 minutes, repeat dose in 30 minutes • Administer heparin as detailed for tPA	• See tPA
TNKase	• Single IV bolus over 5 seconds; if <60 kg, then 30 mg; 60 to 69 kg, 35 mg; 70 to 79 kg, 40 mg; 80 to 89 kg, 45 mg; ≥90 kg, 50 mg	• See tPA
tPA	• 15 mg bolus + 0.75 mg/kg (maximum 50 mg) over 30 minutes + 0.50 mg/kg (maximum 35 mg) over 60 minutes + heparin 60 U/kg bolus + 12 U/kg/hour. PTT goal is 1.5× to 2.0× control.	• ≤75 years old • Anterior wall or possibly large infero-lateral MI derive most benefit
SK	• 1.5 million U IV over 1 hour	• All others (unless previously given SK)

From Ryan TJ, Anderson JL, Antman EM, et al. ACC/AHA guidelines for the management of patients with acute myocardial infarction. A report of the American College of Cardiology/American Heart Association Task Force on Practice Guidelines (Committee on Management of Acute Myocardial Infarction). J Am Coll Cardiol 28:1328-1428, 1996.

rPA, reteplase (Retavase); *SK,* streptokinase (Streptase); *TNKase,* tenecteplase; *tPA,* tissue plasminogen activator or alteplase (Activase).

C

HYPERTENSION

Hypertensive Emergencies

- Definition: An elevated BP with end-organ damage or dysfunction
  - Treatment goal is to reduce MAP by 20% to 25% in 30 to 60 minutes

MAP = DBP + ([SBP − DBP] / 3)

- Catecholamine-induced hypertension
  - Acute increase in catecholamines with acute sympathetic overactivity and hypertension resulting from pheochromocytomas, monoamine oxidase inhibitors, sympathomimetics, clonidine, or withdrawal of beta-blockers
  - Treat with labetalol or alpha-blockers (for example, phentolamine)

Drugs for Hypertensive Emergencies

Table C-7

Drug	Dose and Route	Mechanism
Enalapril (Vasotec)	1.25 to 5 mg IV over 5 minutes, q6 hours	ACE inhibitor
Esmolol (Brevibloc)	500 μg/kg IV over the first minute, then titrate 50 to 200 μg/kg/min	Beta-blockade
Fenoldopam (Corlopam)	0.1 to 1.6 μg/kg/min IV	Dopamine-1 receptor agonist
Hydralazine (Apresoline)	5 to 10 mg IV q30 to 60 minutes or 10 to 50 mg IM	Arteriolar dilator
Labetalol (Normodyne)	0.25 mg/kg IV, double q15 minutes prn (maximum is lesser of 300 mg or 2 mg/kg)	Alpha- and beta-blockade in 1:7 ratio
Nicardipine (Cardene)	Start at 2 to 4 mg/hour IV, then ↑ 1 to 2 mg/hour q15 minutes; maximum 15 mg/hour	Calcium channel blocker
Nitroglycerin	5 to 200 μg/min SL	Vasodilator
Propranolol (Inderal)	1 mg IV over 1 minute q5 minutes up to maximum of 5 to 8 mg	Beta-blockade
Phentolamine (Regitine)	2 to 10 mg IV q5 to 15 minutes	Alpha-blocker
Sodium nitroprusside (Nipride)	0.5 to 8 μg/kg/min IV	Arterial and venous dilator

- Left ventricular failure and coronary insufficiency
  - Increased afterload can lead to pulmonary edema and myocardial ischemia
  - Nitroglycerin IV is the drug of choice
- Hypertensive encephalopathy
  - Headache, vomiting, and confusion resulting from cerebral hyperperfusion, with loss of cerebral blood flow autoregulation
  - Late: Cerebral vasodilation, decreased blood flow, cerebral edema, papilledema, or exudates
  - Treat with sodium nitroprusside or labetalol (Normodyne); lower MAP to normalize CNS flow within 30 to 60 minutes; do not lower MAP to <120 mm Hg
- Pregnancy-induced hypertension or preeclampsia
- Renal failure
  - Decreased renal function resulting from increased BP
  - Proteinuria and elevated BUN/creatinine occur
  - Red cells and red cell casts found in urine
- Thoracic dissection
  - Treat with labetalol or with nitroprusside and esmolol

Onset	Duration	Features
15 minutes	6 hours	Avoid in renal artery stenosis, useful if ↑ rennin (scleroderma)
Seconds	9 minute half-life	Worsens bronchospasm, heart blocks, and CHF
4 minutes	10 minutes	↑ Renal flow and Na^+ excretion; especially useful if ↓ renal function
<30 minutes	4 to 12 hours	Causes tachycardia, headache
Seconds	4 to 8 hours	Worsens bronchospasm, heart blocks, and CHF
1 to 5 minutes	20 minutes	Rarely precipitates angina; ↑ HR and ↑ ICP
2 to 5 minutes	5 to 10 minutes	May ↑ HR and ↓ BP
Seconds	Up to 8 hours	Worsens bronchospasm, heart blocks, and CHF
1 to 2 minutes	30 to 60 minutes	Tachycardia in pheochromocytoma
Seconds	1 to 3 minutes	No ↓ CO; possible cyanide toxicity and ↑ ICP

C

SHOCK

Classification

Table C-8

Causes	PCWP	CO	SVR	Comments
CARDIOGENIC				
Myocardial dysfunction	↑	↓	↑	Hemodynamic goals: PCWP = 15 to 18 mm Hg; MAP ≥70 mm Hg; CI ≥2.2 L/min/m^2; SVR = 1000 to 1200 dynes/sec/cm^2
Acute regurgitation	↑	$\downarrow_{\text{(forward)}}$	↑	
Acute VSD	↑	↓	↑	CO_{RV} >CO_{LV} O_2 step-up RV
RV infarction	↔/↓	↓	↑	RA pressure >> PCWP
Tamponade	↑	↓	↑	RAP = RVEDP = PAD = PCWP pulsus paradoxus increased
DISTRIBUTIVE				
Sepsis (early)	↔/↓	Usually ↑	↓	CO may ↓ as a result of sepsis-mediated LV dysfunction, especially in later phases (mixed cardiogenic-septic physiology)
Anaphylaxis, liver disease, spinal shock, or adrenal insufficiency	↔/↓	↑	↓	Epinephrine for anaphylaxis after treating underlying cause; pure alpha-agonists in spinal shock
HYPOVOLEMIC				
Hemorrhage or dehydration	↓	↓	↑	Invasive monitoring needed only if there is a coexisting LV dysfunction

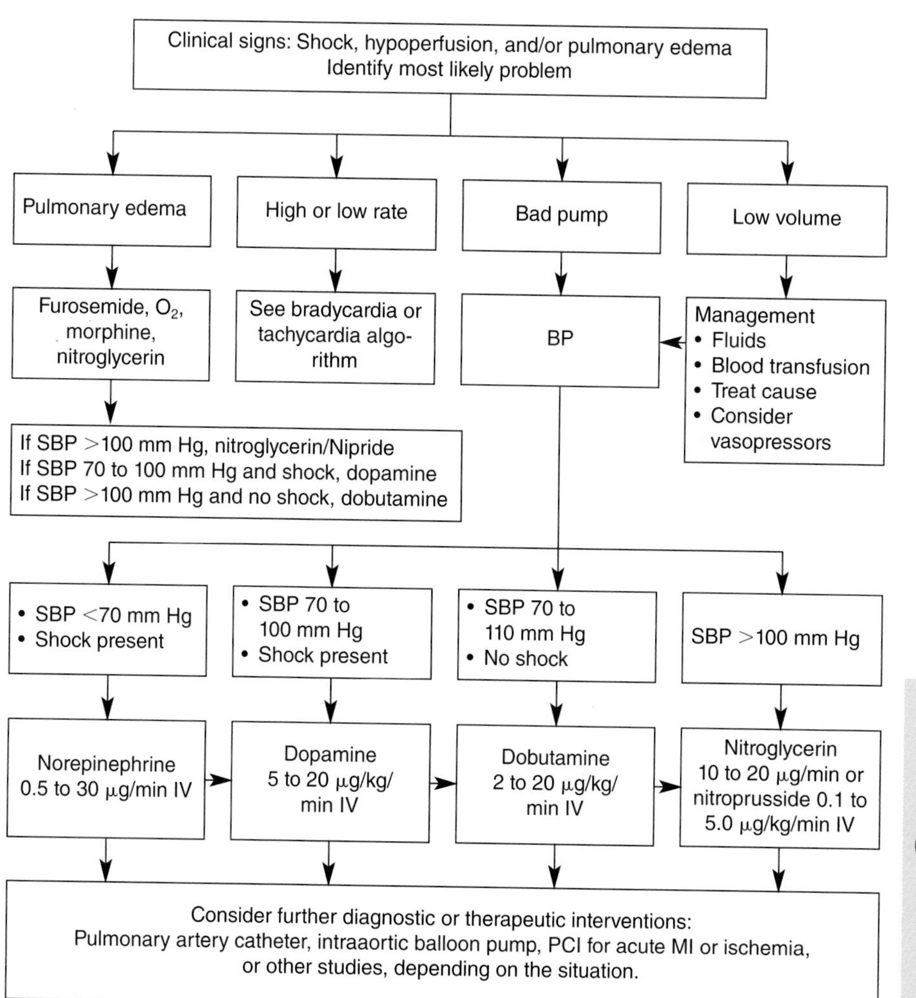

Fig. C-2 Management of pulmonary edema, hypotension, and cardiogenic shock.

C

Interpretation of PCWP

- PCWP correlates with LV filling pressures (LVEDP); see exceptions in following list
- Physiologic LVEDP is rate dependent
  - Bradycardia increases LVEDP; tachycardia decreases LVEDP
- High LVEDP does not always correlate with pulmonary edema
  - No edema with chronically elevated LVEDP (↑ lymph drainage, ↓ vascular permeability)
  - Noncardiogenic pulmonary edema (normal LVEDP) occurs with endothelial injury (such as ARDS) or low-albumin states
- PCWP underestimates LVEDP (preload) in the presence of the following:
  - Decreased LV compliance (with MI, LVH, diastolic dysfunction, and pericardial disease)
  - Severe aortic insufficiency
  - High intrapericardial or intrathoracic pressure (such as with obstructive lung disease, high levels of applied PEEP, or pericardial disease).
  - NOTE: LVEDP is proportional to the gradient between intracardiac and *intrapericardial* pressure; PCWP is proportional to the gradient between intracardiac and *atmospheric* pressure
- PCWP overestimates LVEDP (preload) in presence of the following:
  - Mitral stenosis or regurgitation
  - Catheter in a non–zone III position—overwedged waveform (unnaturally smooth with marked respiratory variation or anterior balloon migration [PCWP >PAD])
  - PEEP or auto-PEEP
  - Increased PA vascular tone (hypoxia, hypovolemia, or dopamine)
  - Catheter whip—especially in hyperdynamic states
  - Catheter tip obstruction (left atrial myxoma, thoracic tumors, or mediastinal fibrosis)
  - Ruptured balloon

Findings From PA Catheterization

Table C-9

Findings	Causes
Giant V waves with obliteration of A waves (balloon inflated) and bifid PA waveform (balloon deflated)	• Acute mitral regurgitation • LA enlargement or LV failure • Acute ventriculoseptal defect
PA diastolic pressure exceeds PCWP by >5 to 7 mm Hg	• Elevated PVR (pulmonary embolism, veno-occlusive disease, hypoxic vasoconstriction, or 1 degree rather than 2 degrees) • Pulmonary parenchymal disorders • Tachycardia
O_2 saturation step-up (>10%) between RA and RV	• Acute ventriculoseptal defect • Primum ASD • Coronary fistula to RV • PDA with pulmonic insufficiency
Elevated RA pressure with prominent *x* and *y* descents (*y* usually >*x*); RA pressure does not decrease with negative intrathoracic pressure (Kussmaul sign)	• RV infarction • Restrictive physiology
Elevated RA pressure with prominent *x* descent and diminished or absent *y* descent; RAP = RVEDP = PAD = mean PAWP; absent Kussmaul sign; pulsus paradoxus	• Pericardial tamponade

Common PA Catheter Problems

Table C-10

Problem	Intervention
Catheter is persistently wedged	• Flush tip • Ensure that balloon is deflated • Pull back to PA tracing then inflate and refloat
Catheter will not wedge	• Ensure that balloon is intact (air returns from balloon) and that tip is not overwedged • Inflate balloon while it is in the PA and advance • Use fluoroscopic guidance • If repeatedly unsuccessful, consider using PAD to estimate PCWP
Ectopy during or after placement	• Pull back catheter to the SVC or advance into the PA • Check electrolytes • Replace or remove the catheter

Choice of Drugs for Patients in Shock

Table C-11

Hemodynamics	Initial Treatment	Comments
PCWP (or CVP) ↓	Aggressive volume expansion	Consider pressors initially, but reevaluate when PCWP ≥18 mm Hg or CVP ≥12 cm H_2O
CO ↓, SVR ↑	Dobutamine	Alternatives include milrinone or dopamine plus nitroprusside
CO ↓, SVR ↔ or ↓	Dopamine	Norepinephrine is a second-line agent
SVR ↓, CO ↑	High dose dopamine or norepinephrine	Add epinephrine or phenylephrine for refractory hypotension

Relative Action of Catecholamine Vasopressors

Table C-12

Drug	Receptor	HR	Inotropy	SVR	Comments
Dopamine (low dose)	DA	0	0	↔ or ↓	Renal and splanchnic vasodilation
Dopamine (high dose)	Beta-1 → alpha-1	↑	↑↑	↑↑	First-line pressor for SBP 70 to 90 mm Hg
Dobutamine	Beta-1, beta-2 >alpha-1	↔ or ↑	↑↑	↓↓	Inotrope and vasodilator; may lower BP
Norepinephrine	Alpha-1, alpha-2, beta-1	↔ or ↑	↑↑	↑↑↑	For hypotension refractory to dopamine
Epinephrine	Alpha-1, alpha-2 beta-1, beta-2	↑↑	↑↑↑	↑↑↑	For refractory cardiac failure (for example, after CABG) or anaphylaxis
Phenylephrine	Alpha-1	0	0	↑↑↑	For refractory hypotension, especially vasculogenic
Isoproterenol	Beta-1, beta-2	↑↑↑	↑↑	↔ or ↑	Primarily increases HR; may cause reflex hypotension

C

Additional Treatment Considerations for Patients in Severe Septic Shock

- Early goal-directed therapy based on hemodynamic parameters[1]
  - Titration of CVP to 8 to 12 cm H_2O
  - Pressors for MAP <65 mm Hg and vasodilators for MAP >90 mm Hg
  - Transfusion to hematocrit >30% if central venous O_2 saturation <70%
  - Inotropic agents if central venous O_2 saturation remains <70%
- Activated protein C (drotrecogin alfa)
- Corticosteroids for relative adrenal insufficiency[2,3]
  - For critically ill patients with hypotension unresponsive to fluids, consider hydrocortisone 50 mg IV q6 hours ± fludrocortisone 50 μg PNGT qd until results of ACTH stimulation test are available

References

1. Rivers E, Nguyen B, Havstad S, et al. Early goal-directed therapy in the treatment of severe sepsis and septic shock. N Engl J Med 345:1368-1377, 2001.
2. Annane D, Sébille V, Charpentier C, et al. Effect of treatment with low doses of hydrocortisone and fludrocortisone on mortality in patients with septic shock. JAMA 288:862-871, 2002.
3. Cooper MS, Stewart PM. Corticosteroid insufficiency in acutely ill patients. N Engl J Med 348:727-734, 2003.

APPENDIX

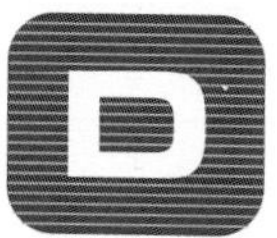

NEUROLOGY AND NEUROSURGERY

D

NEUROOPHTHALMOLOGY

Anisocoria

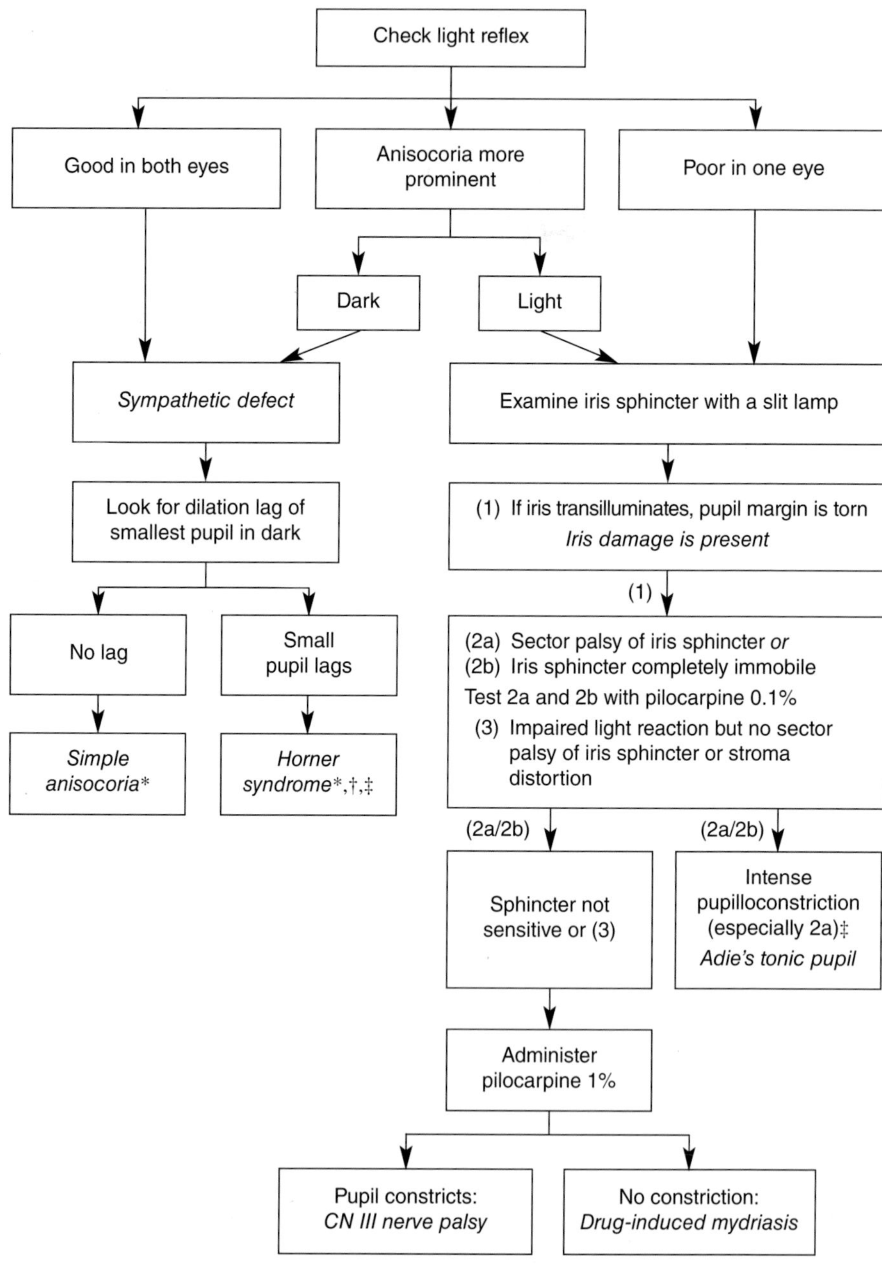

Fig. D-1 Evaluation of anisocoria (asymmetric pupils), assuming no CNS trauma.
*Administration of 2% cocaine causes both pupils to dilate if simple anisocoria is present and causes failure of small pupil to dilate with Horner syndrome.
†Administering 1% hydroxyamphetamine (24 hours later) dilates the pupil if the lesion is preganglionic (consider CT scan of the chest and MRI scan of the brain/neck if there are other signs); the pupil does not dilate if the lesion is postganglionic (benign) Horner syndrome.
‡Horner syndrome is characterized by ptosis, miosis, facial anhydrosis (sympathetic interruption), and Adie's tonic pupil in accommodation (especially in young women with reduced DTRs).

Acute Narrow-Angle Glaucoma

Clinical Features

- Headache, vomiting, and eye pain
- Red eye or perilimbal infection
- Conjunctival edema with cell and flare in anterior chamber
- Middilated, poorly reactive pupil
- Intraocular pressure often >50 mm Hg

Treatment

- Pilocarpine 2% to 4% 2 drops q15 minutes for 2 hours or until pupillary constriction
- Pilocarpine 1 drop to unaffected eye
- Timolol (Timoptic) 0.1% 1 drop
- Acetazolamide 500 mg IV, IM, or po
- Mannitol 0.5% 1g/kg IV
- Laser or surgical iridectomy

Central Retinal Artery Occlusion

Causes

- Cardiac, carotid, or vascular disease
- Hyperviscosity, diabetes, or sickle cell disease

Clinical Features

- Sudden, painless, unilaterally decreased vision
- Afferent pupil defect (no direct reaction to light *and* reaction when light is shone in contralateral eye)
- Narrow retinal arterioles or "boxcars" from segmentation of arteriolar blood
- Infarcted retina turns gray
- Cherry-red macula resulting from thin retina with clear view of underlying vessels

Treatment

- Best to start within 2 hours (attempt up to 48 hours)
- Globe pressure/massage (5 seconds on and 5 seconds off) for 5 to 30 minutes
- ↑ P_{CO_2} by breathing into a bag or 95% O_2/5% CO_2 mixture
- Paracentesis by an ophthalmologist

Iritis

Definition: Acute inflammation of anterior uvea

Clinical Features

- Worsening vision, perilimbal redness, photophobia (consensual photophobia) with or without ↑ IOP
- Slit lamp reveals cell and flare in anterior chamber

Treatment

1. IV antibiotics if infection
2. Homatropine 2% or 5% 1 drop q6 hours
3. Prednisolone 1% 1 drop q6 hours
4. Systemic nonsteroidal agents
5. Consult an ophthalmologist

Temporal Arteritis

Box D-1

History	Examination
Mean age: 70 years	Decreased temporal artery pulse: 46%
Polymyalgia rheumatica: 39%	Tender temporal artery: 27%
Headache: 68%	Indurated, red temporal artery: 23%
Jaw claudication: 45%	Large artery bruit: 21%
Unilateral vision loss: 14%	Afferent pupil, cranial nerve palsies, pale, and swollen disc
Claudication, eye pain, and fever: <5%	
Diagnosis	**Management**
ESR >50 mm in most cases	Prednisone 60 to 80 mg po once a day
Artery biopsy (not emergent)	Ophthalmology consultation

Mydriatics/Cycloplegics

Table D-1

Drug Trade Name	Duration	Effects*	Indication	Comments
Atropine 0.5% to 3%	2 weeks	M, C	Dilation	Caution if narrow angle glaucoma
Cyclopentolate HCl (Cyclogyl) 0.5% to 2%	24 hours	M, C	Dilation (for example, for examination)	Same as atropine
Homatropine 2% to 5%	10 to 48 hours	M, C	Dilation	Same as atropine
Phenylephrine HCl (Neo-Synephrine) 0.12% to 10%	2 to 3 hours	M	Dilation, no cycloplegia	CAUTION: cardiac disease, glaucoma, or hypertension
Scopolamine HBr (Hyoscine) 0.25%	2 to 7 days	M, C	Strong cycloplegia	Same caution as phenyl-ephrine HCl with dizziness and disorientation
Tropicamide (Mydriacyl) 0.5% to 1%	6 hours	M, C	Dilation, cycloplegia	Same as atropine, only weak cycloplegia

The usual dose of medications listed is 1 drop qd to q8h. Higher doses may be used for specific diseases (for example, acute-angle glaucoma).

**M*, Mydriasis (pupillodilation); *C*, cycloplegia.

WEAKNESS

Acute Weakness (Upper Motor Neuron or Lower Motor Neuron)

- UMN lesions cause damage to the cortex (for example, stroke), brainstem, or spinal cord
- LMN lesions damage the anterior horn cells, neuromuscular junction, or muscle (for example, muscular dystrophies)

Table D-2 Differentiation of UMN From LMN Disease

Category	UMN Disease	LMN Disease
Muscular deficit	Muscle groups	Individual muscles
Reflexes	↑ (± acutely ↓)	Decreased/absent
Tone	↑ (± acutely ↓)	Decreased
Fasciculations	Absent	Present
Atrophy	Absent/minimal	Present

Assessment of Acute Muscle Weakness

- Assess ventilation: FVC should be ≥15 ml/kg and maximum inspiratory force >15 cm H_2O

Table D-3 Assessment of Acute Muscle Weakness

	Spinal Cord	Peripheral Neuropathy	Myoneural Junction	Muscle Disease
Clinical	Lower limbs weak Absent lower DTR Sharp sensory level Bladder/bowel incontinence	Generally weak General areflexia Stocking/glove sensory loss Bladder/bowel OK	Cranial nerves generally weak Fasciculations No sensory loss Bladder/bowel OK	Generally weak Weak proximally Muscles tender No sensory loss Bladder/bowel OK
Examples*	Transverse myelitis Cord tumor/bleed, abscess or disc herniation	Guillain-Barré syndrome Porphyria, arsenic toxic neuropathy Tick paralysis	Myasthenia gravis Organophosphate toxicity Botulism	Polymyositis Alcohol/endocrine myopathy Electrolyte abnormalities (K^+, Na^+, Ca^{++})

*This list of examples is not complete.

D

Guillain-Barré Syndrome

Definition: Autoimmune destruction of peripheral nerves after infection

- 85% to 95% of patients have full recovery weeks to months after weakness progression stops

Clinical Features

- Recent viral illness in 50% to 67%
- Weakness begins symmetrically in the legs and ascends to the arms and trunk
- Weak onset and rapid decline in, or absent, DTRs
- Face involvement in 25% to 50% of patients
- Hypesthesias or paresthesias in 33% of patients
- Mill-Fischer variant: Weakness begins in face and descends with ophthalmoplegia and ataxia

Diagnosis

- Primarily based on clinical features
- CSF: Protein normal or >400 mg/L
- CSF: WBC normal or monocytosis
- Slowing nerve conduction on studies

Management

- 28% require ventilatory support
- Plasmapheresis and/or steroids
- Watch for infection and embolism (consider SC heparin)

Myasthenia Gravis

Definition: Autoimmune disease in which antibodies destroy acetylcholine receptors at the myoneural junction

- Thymus abnormalities (thymoma in 10% to 25%) are often present

Clinical Features

- Ptosis, diplopia, and blurring (common)
- Dysarthria, dysphagia, jaw muscle weakness, and head drooping
- Asymmetric weakness
- Either truncal or extremity weakness
- Weakness worsens with repetition
- Heat worsens and cold improves weakness (cold pack improves ptosis)

Myasthenic Crisis

- Difficulty swallowing and respiratory insufficiency, because of worsening disease with weakness
- Precipitants: Infection, antibiotics (aminoglycosides, tetracycline, clindamycin), CNS depressants, beta-blockers, quinidine, procainamide, lidocaine, and metabolic changes (↑ K^+, ↑ Mg^{++}, ↓ K^+, ↓ Ca^{++})

Cholinergic Crisis

- Overdose of anticholinesterase medications
- Weakness occurs along with SLUDGE (salivation, lacrimation, urination, defecation, GI upset, and emesis)

Crisis Management

- Tensilon test: Edrophonium (Tensilon) 1 to 2 mg IV while on cardiac monitor; if no adverse response, give 8 mg IV; improvement indicates myasthenic crisis; worsening indicates cholinergic crisis
- Assess ventilation: FVC should be ≥15 ml/kg, and maximum inspiratory force should be >15 cm H_2O
- Look for and treat precipitants
- Admit all patients with either a myasthenic crisis or a cholinergic crisis

D

ALCOHOL WITHDRAWAL SYNDROMES[1]

- Normal ethanol clearance is 20 mg/dl/hour; more rapid in chronic alcoholics
- Symptoms may occur before the ethanol level reaches zero

Table D-4 Alcohol Withdrawal Syndromes

Syndrome	Timing*	Percentage of Patients†	Symptoms
Minor or early withdrawal	• Onset 8 hours • Peak 24 to 36 hours	≥80%	• Irritability/agitation but no delirium • Sleep disturbance, hypervigilance • ↑ HR, ↑ BP, ↑ temperature, or tremor
Hallucinosis	• Onset 8 hours • Peak 24 to 72 hours	25%	• Visual more than auditory hallucinations • Sensorium typically intact • Does not predict delirium tremens
Withdrawal seizures	• Onset 8 to 24 hours • Peak 24 hours	25%	• Generalized tonic-clonic seizures (partial seizures suggest alternative diagnosis) • May occur singly or in clusters, but status epilepticus uncommon • More common in patients with history of seizures
Delirium tremens	• Onset 48 hours • May occur for up to 2 weeks	5%	• Occurs in chronic alcoholics only, rare if age <30 years • Often precipitated and/or masked by medical illness • Delirium and clouded consciousness • Hyperadrenergic state (↑ HR, ↑ BP, ↑ temperature, tremor, and sweating) • Mortality 1% to 5% (historically 20%) • Complications: arrhythmia, sepsis, aspiration, volume depletion, and electrolyte disturbances

*Since last drink of alcohol.
†Percentage of patients with chronic alcoholism admitted to hospital, not given prophylactic treatment.

PSYCHIATRY

Folstein Mini–Mental Status Examination

*MMSE Sample Items**

- Orientation to time: "What is the date?"
- Registration: "Listen carefully. I am going to say three words. You say them back after I stop. Ready? Here they are . . . APPLE (pause), PENNY (pause), TABLE (pause). Now repeat those words back to me." (Repeat up to 5 times, but score only the first trial.)
- Naming: "What is this?" (Point to a pencil or pen.)
- Reading: "Please read this and do what it says." CLOSE YOUR EYES

Differentiating Delirium, Dementia, and Psychosis

Table D-5

Feature	Delirium	Dementia	Psychosis
Age of onset	Any	Usually older	13 to 40 years
Psychiatric history	Usually absent	Usually absent	Present
Emotion	Labile	Normal or labile	Flat affect
Vital signs	Abnormal	Normal	Normal
Onset	Sudden	Gradual	Sudden
Twenty-four hour course	Fluctuates	Stable	Stable
Consciousness	Altered	Clear	Clear
Attention	Disordered	OK unless severe	Can be disordered
Cognition	Disordered	Impaired	Selective
Hallucinations	Visual or sensory	Rare	Auditory
Delusions	Fleeting	Rare	Sustained, grand
Orientation	Impaired	Often impaired	Rarely impaired
Psychomotor	↑, ↓, or shifting	Normal	Variable
Speech	Incoherent	Perseveration and difficulty finding words	Normal, slow, or rapid
Involuntary movement	Asterixis or tremor	Often absent	Usually absent
Physical illness or drug toxicity	Drug toxicity	Either (especially patients with Alzheimer disease)	Neither

From Murphy BA. Delirium. Emerg Med Clin North Am 18:243-252, 2000.

SPINAL CORD

Spinal Cord Injury Syndromes

Anterior Cord Syndrome

- Flexion or vertical compression injury to anterior cord or spinal artery
- Complete motor paralysis
- Hyperalgesia with preserved touch and proprioception (position sense)
- Loss of pain and temperature sense
- Most likely cord injury to require surgery

Complete Cord Injury

- Flaccid below the injury level
- Warm skin, ↓ BP, and ↓ HR
- Sensation may be preserved
- Decreased sympathetics, with or without priapism
- Absent DTRs
- If duration >24 hours, will be permanent

Central Cord Syndrome

- Hyperextension injury
- Motor weakness in hands more than arms
- Legs are unaffected or less affected
- Variable bladder/sensory dysfunction
- Prognosis is generally good, and most do not require surgery

Brown-Séquard Syndrome

- Hemisection of cord
- Ipsilateral weakness
- Ipsilateral loss of proprioception
- Loss of contralateral pain/temperature

Posterior Cord Syndrome

- Pain and tingling in the neck and hands
- One third have upper extremity weakness
- Mild form of central cord syndrome

Steroid Protocol for Patients With Acute Spinal Cord Injury

Box D-2

Indications	Acute spinal cord injury presenting within 8 hours of injury
Contraindications*	Age <13 years (controversial)
	Isolated nerve root injury
	Cauda equina syndrome
	Penetrating cord trauma
	Life-threatening illness/injury independent of spinal cord injury
Protocol	Methylprednisolone (Solu-Medrol) 30 mg/kg IV over 15 minutes, then wait 45 minutes
	If <3 hours since injury, methylprednisolone 5.4 mg/kg/hour over 23 hours
	If 3 to 8 hours since injury, methylprednisolone 5.4 mg/kg/hour over 47 hours

Compiled from Bracken MB, Shepard MJ, Collins WF. A randomized, controlled trial of methylprednisolone or naloxone in the treatment of acute spinal-cord injury. Results of the Second National Acute Spinal Cord Injury Study. N Engl J Med 322:1405-1411, 1990; Bracken MB, Shepard MJ, Holford TR, et al. Administration of methylprednisolone for 24 or 48 hours or tirilazad mesylate for 48 hours in the treatment of acute spinal cord injury. Results of the Third National Acute Spinal Cord Injury Randomized Controlled Trial. National Acute Spinal Cord Injury Study. JAMA 277:1597-1604, 1997.

*Patients who were pregnant or taking steroids were excluded from the original study (pregnancy and steroid use may be relative contraindications).

Conus Medullaris or Cauda Equina Syndrome

Cause: Loss of spinal space as a result of trauma, central disc herniation at L3-S1, ankylosing spondylitis, rheumatoid arthritis, epidural hematoma, or cancer

- *Conus medullaris syndrome* has a sudden onset with bilateral perineal and thigh pain
  - Motor loss is symmetric
  - Mild fasciculations may be present
  - Sensory loss is in saddle distribution
  - Bladder/rectal/sexual function is severely impaired
- *Cauda equina syndromes* are unilateral and gradual in onset, with severe, asymmetric pain in the thighs, perineum, back, and legs
  - Motor loss is asymmetric and severe; fasciculations are absent
  - Sensory loss in the saddle area—may be unilateral
  - Bladder/rectal/sexual functions have mild impairment
  - Evaluate with CT or MRI and consult a spine surgeon

Subarachnoid Hemorrhage

- Saccular (berry) aneurysms are the most common cause of subarachnoid hemorrhage (more common than AV malformations, mycotic aneurysms, anticoagulation, or vasculitis)
- Risk factors: personal or family history, preeclampsia, polycystic kidney disease, atherosclerosis, hypertension, alcohol, cigarettes, aspirin, and cocaine
- Mean age at rupture is 40 to 60 years
- 56% occur while resting, 25% while working, and 10% while sleeping

Clinical Features

Table D-6

Feature	Incidence
Any headache	70%
Warning (sentinel) headache	55%
Neck pain or stiffness	78%
Altered mental status	53%
Third cranial nerve deficit	9%
Seizure	3% to 25%
Focal deficit	19%
No headache, deficit, or nuchal rigidity	11%

From Adams HP Jr, Kassell NF, Tarner JC, et al. CT and clinical correlations in recent aneurysmal subarachnoid hemorrhage: a preliminary report of the Cooperative Aneurysm Study. Neurology 33:981-988, 1983.

Hunt and Hess Classification

Table D-7

Grade	Characteristics	Normal CT Scan
I	Asymptomatic, minimal headache Mild nuchal rigidity	15%
II	Moderate to severe headache Nuchal rigidity Cranial nerve deficits only	7%
III	Drowsy, confused, or mild focal deficit	4%
IV	Stupor, mild/moderate hemiparesis, early decerebrate or vegetative changes	1%
V	Deep coma Decerebrate rigidity Moribund appearance	0%

Diagnosis	Treatment
CT scans are abnormal in more than 95% of patients if onset is within the previous 12 hours	↓ Systolic BP to ≤160 mm Hg or MAP to ≤110 mm Hg
CT scans are abnormal in 77% of patients if onset is more than 12 hours previously	Nimodipine (Nimotop) 60 mg po q6h to decrease vasospasm
CSF >100,000 RBCs/μl (mean), although any number of RBCs can be found	Fosphenytoin/phenytoin prophylaxis
Xanthochromia (traumatic spinal taps do not cause acute xanthochromia)	Neurosurgical consultation
ECG: peaked, deep, or inverted T waves, ↑ QT, or large U waves	Early angiography and surgical intervention per neurosurgeon

D

STROKE

- Ischemic strokes (85%) are caused by thrombus, embolus, or hypoperfusion
- Hemorrhagic strokes (15%) are intracerebral or subarachnoid (Table D-8)

Common Stroke Syndromes[2]

Table D-8

Syndrome	Arteries	Common Findings
Anterior circulation	Internal carotid Middle cerebral Anterior cerebral	Left: aphasia, right limb/face weakness Right: left visual neglect, denial of deficit, left limb/face weakness, poor visuospatial function
Posterior circulation	Posterior cerebral	Left: right hemianopsia, large lesions may include inability to read but able to write and spell Right: left hemianopsia
Brainstem-cerebellum	Vertebral Basilar	Vertigo Cranial nerve findings (especially extraocular movement) Palsies Quadriparesis Ataxia Nystagmus Crossed signs (ipsilateral cranial nerve palsies and contralateral limb weakness or sensory loss) Coma
Lacunar motor stroke	Penetrating artery in pons or internal capsule	Pure hemiparesis
Lacunar sensory stroke	Penetrating artery in thalamus or posterior limb of internal capsule	Pure hemisensory symptoms

Common Aneurysm Sites

Table D-9

Location (Junction or Bifurcation)	Signs of Leak or Rupture
Internal carotid–posterior communicating artery	Ipsilateral CN III nerve palsy
Anterior communicating artery	Bilateral leg weakness, numbness, and Babinski reflex
Middle cerebral bifurcation	Contralateral face or hand weakness, aphasia (left) or visual neglect (right)
Basilar bifurcation	Bilateral vertical gaze palsies, Babinski sign, and coma
Vertebral–posterior inferior communicating artery junction	Vertigo, lateral medullary syndrome

Unusual Causes of Stroke

Table D-10

Condition	History	Evaluation
Carotid or vertebral artery dissection	Neck injury or pain Horner syndrome ipsilateral to dissection and contralateral to stroke	MRI (including T1 axial images of the neck) MR angiography Contrast angiography
Aortic dissection	Chest or back pain	TEE MRI Chest CT
Paradoxical emboli	Coexisting DVT or PE ASD or VSD findings	Echocardiogram with bubble contrast
Cardiac source emboli	Atrial fibrillation LV dysfunction Recent MI Rheumatic heart disease	Echocardiogram (preferably TEE
Endocarditis (bacterial or marantic)	Fever IVDU End-stage cancer Heart murmur	Blood cultures Echocardiogram
Cholesterol emboli	Recent angiography Livedo Ischemic digital lesions	Retinal examination Eosinophilia ↓ Complement
Venous sinus thrombosis	Postpartum OCP use Hypercoagulability	MR venogram Angiography
CNS vasculitis	SLE Behçet disease Recent ophthalmic zoster	Angiography Brain or meningeal biopsy
Antiphospholipid antibody syndrome	Raynaud disease Recurrent spontaneous abortion Previous thromboembolism	Anticardiolipin antibody Lupus anticoagulant
Thrombotic thrombocytopenic purpura	Thrombocytopenia Azotemia Purpura Fever	Blood smear Renal or skin biopsy
Drug-induced vasospasm	Drug abuse (cocaine or amphetamines)	Toxicology screening Angiography

From Sigurdsson AP, Feldman E. Stroke. In Samuels MA, ed. Hospitalist Neurology. Boston: Butterwor Heinemann, 1999.

National Institutes of Health Stroke Scale (Version 10-03)

Table D-11

1a. LOC		Points
Alert		0
Rouses to obey, respond, answer		1
Responds to pain		2
Autonomic reflexes or no response		3
1b. LOC		
Questions (ask age and current month)	Both correct	0
	One correct	1
	Incorrect	2
1c. LOC		
Commands (make fist and close eyes)	Obeys both	0
	Obeys one	1
	Incorrect	2
2. Best gaze		
Normal		0
Partial palsy		1
Forced deviation or total gaze paresis not overcome by oculocephalic reflex		2
3. Best visual		
No loss		0
Partial hemianopsia		1
Complete hemianopsia		2
Bilateral hemianopsia		3

4. Facial palsy	Points
None	0
Minor asymmetry with smile	1
Partial (near total paralysis low face)	2
Complete	3
5. Best motor arm*	
No drift in 10 seconds	0
Drift without hitting bed/support for 10 seconds	1
Drifts completely down in 10 seconds	2
No effort, limb falls immediately	3
No movement	4
6. Best motor leg†	
No drift in 5 seconds	0
Drifts without hitting bed/support for 5 seconds	1
Drifts completely down in 5 seconds	2
No effort, limb falls immediately	3
No movement	4
(6a. left leg; 6b. right leg)	
7. Limb ataxia‡	
Absent	0
Present in one limb	1
Present in two limbs	2
Absent (0) if cannot understand or paralysis	

From the National Institute of Neurological Disorders and Stroke. Available at *www.ninds.nih.gov.*

*Arm drift: One arm pronates from a 90 degree or 45 degree elevation (10 second test).

†Leg drift: While supine, one leg falls to the bed from a 30 degree elevation (5 second test).

‡Test finger to nose and heel to shin on both sides. The patient has ataxia only if results are out of proportion to weakness.

Continued

D

Table D-11—cont'd

8. Sensory		**10. Dysarthria†**	
Normal	0	Normal	0
Partial loss with sharp pinprick	1	Mild/moderate: Understand slurring	1
Not aware of being touched	2	Severe: Unintelligible	2
9. Best language*		**11. Extinction/inattention (neglect)**	
No aphasia	0	None	0
Mild/moderate aphasia: Loss of fluency or comprehension		Visual, tactile, auditory, spatial, personal inattention or extinction to bilateral stimulation in one of senses tested	1
Can identify material or content of pictures	1	Profound hemi-inattention or extinction to >1 mode (does not recognize hand or orients to only one side of space)	2
Severe aphasia: Fragmented expression			
Cannot identify material from patient response	2		
Mute, aphasia: No comprehension	3		

*Aphasia: Disturbance in processing language. The patient often uses inappropriate words or nonfluent sentences. Test *receptive* aphasia by having the patient follow simple commands, and test *expressive* aphasia by having the patient identify objects.

†Dysarthria: Slurring from paralysis or incoordination of muscles used for speech.

Management of Blood Pressure in Patients With Acute Ischemic Stroke

Table D-12

Blood Pressure*	Management
NOT ELIGIBLE FOR THROMBOLYTICS	
Systolic BP <220 *or* Diastolic BP <120	Only treat if end-organ damage (for example, aortic dissection, MI, pulmonary edema, or hypertensive encephalopathy) Treat symptoms (such as headache, nausea, vomiting, pain, or agitation) as needed Treat acute complications (such as hypoxia, ↑ ICP, seizures, or hypoglycemia) as needed
Systolic BP >220 *or* Diastolic BP <120	Labetalol 10 to 20 mg IV over 1 to 2 minutes; may repeat or double q10 min to maximum total dose of 300 mg *or* Nicardipine 5 mg/hour IV infusion initially, titrate to desired effect by increasing 2.5 mg/hour q5 min to maximum of 15 mg/hour GOAL: 10% to 15% reduction of blood pressure
Diastolic BP >140	Nitroprusside 0.5 μg/kg/minute IV as initial dose with continuous BP monitoring GOAL: 10% to 15% reduction of blood pressure
ELIGIBLE FOR THROMBOLYTIC THERAPY: PRETREATMENT	
Systolic BP >185 *or* Diastolic BP >110	Labetalol 10 to 20 mg IV over 1 to 2 minutes; may repeat once *or* Nitropaste 1 to 2 inches If BP is not reduced and maintained with systolic BP <185 *and* diastolic BP <110, do not give thrombolytics

From Adams HP Jr, Adams RJ, Brott T, et al. Guidelines for the early management of patients with ischemic stroke: a scientific statement from the Stroke Council of the American Stroke Association. Stroke 34:1056-1083, 2003. Available at *www.strokeaha.org.*

*BP values are given in mm Hg.

Continued

Table D-12—cont'd

Blood Pressure*	Management
Thrombolytic Therapy: After Treatment	
Check BP q15 min for 2 hours, then q30 min for 6 hours, then q60 min for 16 hours	
Diastolic BP >140	Nitroprusside 0.5 μg/kg/minute as initial dose and titrate to desired BP
Systolic BP >230 *or* Diastolic BP >120	Labetalol 10 mg IV over 1 to 2 minutes; may repeat *or* double q10 min to maximum total dose of 300 mg *or* give initial bolus and then start drip at 2 to 8 mg/min *or* Nicardipine 5 mg/hour IV infusion initially, titrate to desired effect by increasing 2.5 mg/hour q5 min to maximum of 15 mg/hour If BP not controlled by these, consider nitroprusside
Systolic BP 180 to 230 *or* Diastolic BP 105 to 120	Labetalol 10 mg IV over 1 to 2 minutes; may repeat or double q10 min to maximum total dose of 300 mg *or* give initial bolus and then start drip at 2 to 8 mg/min

*BP values are given in mm Hg.

Use of Thrombolytic Agents (rTPAs) in Patients With Acute Ischemic Stroke

- rTPA: Tissue plasminogen activator (streptokinase is NOT used for acute stroke)
- Facilities administering rTPA should be able to manage intracranial bleeding
- Some published studies on fibrinolytic therapy for stroke patients treated at community hospitals show worse outcomes than traditional therapy[3-5]; fibrinolytic therapy for stroke patients should be performed in the context of a well-established hospital protocol

Indications

- Age 18 to 80 years
- Onset of symptoms ≤3 hours before treatment initiated
- No evidence of bleeding or major early infarct in CT scans
- Acute focal neurologic deficits, excluding contraindications

Contraindications

Box D-3

Any current, or previously known or suspected CNS bleed	CT scan showing major early infarct signs*
CNS surgery, trauma, or stroke in last 3 months	Use caution if NIH stroke scale is >20 (see Table D-11)
Subarachnoid bleed suspected	Use caution if mild or rapidly improving deficit (for example, NIH stroke scale ≤5)
Noncompressible arterial puncture in past 7 days	Pregnant or lactating females
Myocardial infarction in past 3 months	**KNOWN BLEEDING DIATHESIS INCLUDING:**
Recent spinal tap	Warfarin use or PT >15 seconds (INR >1.5)
Blood glucose <50 or >400 mg/dl	Platelets <100,000/ml
Uncontrolled HTN after treatment (BP ≥185/110 mm Hg)	Heparin use ≤48 hours or high PTT
Seizure at onset of stroke	**ISOLATED MILD NEUROLOGIC DEFICIT:**
GI or GU bleeding in past 21 days	Ataxia
Non–CNS major surgery in past 14 days	Sensory loss
CNS neoplasm or aneurysm	Dysarthria
Active bleed or acute trauma (for example, fracture)	Mild weakness

Compiled from Practice advisory: thrombolytic therapy for acute ischemic stroke: summary statement. Report of the Quality Standards Subcommittee of the American Academy of Neurology. Neurology 47:835-839, 1996; Adams HP Jr, Adams RJ, Brott T, et al. Guidelines for the early management of patients with ischemic stroke: a scientific statement from the Stroke Council of the American Stroke Association. Stroke 34:1056-1083, 2003.

*Edema, sulcal effacement, mass effect, or possible hemorrhage.

Protocol for rTPA Administration

- Administer rTPA 0.9 mg/kg (maximum dose 90 mg) with 10% given as IV bolus followed by infusion of remaining drug over 60 minutes
- Monitor arterial BP during ensuing 24 hours as follows:
  1. Monitor q15 minutes for the first 2 hours
  2. Then monitor q30 minutes for the next 6 hours
  3. Then monitor q60 minutes for the next 16 hours
  4. Treat BP as needed

Cranial Nerves

Table D-13

Nerve	Function
I Olfactory	Smell
II Optic	Vision
III Oculomotor	Sphincter muscle of iris, ciliary muscle Superior, inferior, and medial rectus muscles; inferior oblique muscle; levator palpebrae muscle
IV Trochlear	Superior oblique muscle
V Trigeminal	Muscles of mastication and tensor tympani muscle Tactile, pain, and thermal sensation from the face, oral and nasal cavities, and part of the dura
VI Abducent	Lateral rectus muscle
VII Facial	Lacrimal gland Muscles of facial expression and stapedius muscle Tactile sensation to skin of ear Taste from anterior one third of tongue
VIII Vestibulocochlear	Equilibrium Hearing

- Do not administer aspirin, heparin, warfarin, ticlopidine, or other antiplatelet or antithrombotic agents within 24 hours of rTPA treatment
- Do not place a central venous line or perform arterial punctures during the first 24 hours
- Do not place a bladder catheter for 30 minutes or an NG tube for 24 hours after infusion

Table D-13—cont'd

Nerve	Function
IX Glossopharyngeal	Innervation to parotid gland
	Stylopharyngeus muscle
	Tactile sensation to outer ear
	Tactile sensation to posterior two thirds of tongue, pharynx, middle ear, and auditory tube
	Input from carotid sinus and body
	Taste from posterior one third of tongue
X Vagal	Viscera of the thoracic and abdominal cavities to the left colic flexure
	Muscles of the larynx and pharynx
	Tactile sensation to the external ear
	Mucous membranes of the pharynx, larynx, esophagus, trachea, and thoracic and abdominal viscera to the left colic flexure
	Taste from the epiglottis
XI Accessory	Intrinsic muscles of the larynx (except cricothyroid muscle)
	Sternocleidomastoid and trapezius muscles
XII Hypoglossal	Intrinsic and extrinsic muscles of the tongue (except palato-glossus muscle)

Brain Death[6-8]

Definition: Irreversible loss of brain function, including brainstem reflexes

Usual Causes

- Head injury
- Subarachnoid or intracerebral hemorrhage
- Encephalitis

Causes in ICU

- Hypoxic-ischemic coma (after resuscitation)
- Ischemic strokes with edema and herniation
- Massive edema caused by fulminant hepatic failure

Diagnostic Criteria (All Must Be Present)

Prerequisites

1. Clinical or CT/MRI scan evidence of an acute, irreversible CNS catastrophe of known cause, compatible with a clinical diagnosis of brain death
2. No severe, confounding medical conditions (electrolyte, acid-base, or endocrine imbalances)
3. No drug intoxication or poisoning
4. Core temperature ≥32° C

Coma or Unresponsiveness

- No motor responses of limbs to painful stimuli (such as nail bed or supraorbital pressure)
- Excludes spinal reflexes, such as the Babinski reflex

Brainstem Reflexes Absent

1. Pupils: no response to bright light; may be between midposition and dilated (4 to 9 mm)
2. Ocular movement: no eye movements with head turning (test only if cervical spine is stable), and no eye movement with 50 ml of ice water in each ear (head of bed elevated to 30 degrees, observe for 1 minute with 5 minutes between sides)
3. Facial sensation and motor response: no corneal reflex, no jaw reflex, and no grimacing to deep pressure on nail bed, supraorbital ridge, and TMJ
4. Pharyngeal and tracheal reflexes: no gag reflex with tongue blade and no cough with vigorous bronchial suctioning

Apnea—Testing Procedure

1. Prerequisites
   - Core temperature ≥36.5° C
   - SBP ≥90 mm Hg
   - Euvolemic or positive fluid balance for 6 hours
   - Pco_2 normal (or ≥40 mm Hg)
   - Po_2 ≥normal
2. Connect a pulse oximeter and disconnect the ventilator
3. Deliver 100% O_2 at 6 L/minute into the trachea (optimally at the level of the carina)
4. Observe for respiratory movements (chest excursions producing tidal volumes)
5. Measure arterial Po_2, Pco_2, and pH after 8 minutes and reconnect the ventilator
6. Test is positive (confirmatory) if respiratory movements are absent and Pco_2 is ≥60 mm Hg (or increased by 20 mm Hg over the baseline)
7. If respiratory movements are observed, the test is negative and should be repeated
8. If, during the test, the patient develops SBP <90 mm Hg, significant O_2 desaturation, or cardiac arrhythmias, reconnect the ventilator and draw immediate ABG
9. Test is positive if Pco_2 is ≥60 mm Hg (or increased by 20 mm Hg); otherwise, the test is indeterminate and confirmatory testing should be considered

Pitfalls in Diagnosing Brain Death (Consider Confirmatory Testing)

- Severe facial trauma
- Preexisting pupillary abnormalities
- Toxic levels of drugs affecting neuromuscular or ocular function (such as anticholinergic, anticonvulsant, or chemotherapeutic agents; sedatives; aminoglycosides; tricyclic antidepressants; or neuromuscular blockers)
- Chronic CO_2 retention (such as COPD, sleep apnea, or morbid obesity)

Observations Compatible With Brain Death (Diagnosis Still Valid)

- Respiratory-like movements (shoulder elevation and back arching) *without* tidal volumes
- Sweating, blushing, and tachycardia
- Normal BP without pressors
- Spinal reflexes (such as the Babinski reflex) or spontaneous limb movements

Confirmatory Laboratory Testing

- Consider repeating the clinical evaluation in all patients after 6 hours if clinical testing cannot be reliably performed or evaluated
- Confirmatory testing is desirable but not mandatory; options include:
  - Angiography (absence of cerebral blood flow)
  - EEG
  - Transcranial Doppler ultrasound screening
  - Technetium brain scan or SSEPs

References

1. Turner RC, Lichstein PR, Peden JG Jr, et al. Alcohol withdrawal syndromes: a review of pathophysiology, clinical presentation and treatment. J Gen Intern Med 4:432-433, 1998.
2. Chung C-S, Caplan LR. Neurovascular disorders. In Goetz CG, Pappert EJ, eds. Textbook of Clinical Neurology. Philadelphia: WB Saunders, 1999.
3. Katzan IL, Furlan AJ, Lloyd LE, et al. Use of tissue-type plasminogen activator for acute ischemic stroke: the Cleveland area experience. JAMA 283:1151-1158, 2000.
4. Practice advisory: thrombolytic therapy for acute ischemic stroke—summary statement. Report of the Quality Standards Subcommittee of the American Academy of Neurology. Neurology 47:835-839, 1996.
5. Adams HP Jr, Adams RJ, Brott T. Guidelines for the early management of patients with ischemic stroke: a scientific statement from the Stroke Council of the American Stroke Association. Stroke 34:1056-1083, 2003. Available at *www.strokeaha.org*.
6. Heuschmann PU, Berger K, Misselwitz B, et al. Frequency of thrombolytic therapy in patients with acute ischemic stroke and the risk of in-hospital mortality: the German Stroke Registers Study Group. Stroke 34:1106-1113, 2003. Available at *www.strokeaha.org*.
7. Practice parameters for determining brain death in adults (summary statement). The Quality Standards Subcommittee of the American Academy of Neurology. Neurology 45:1012-1014, 1995.
8. Wijdicks EF. The diagnosis of brain death. N Engl J Med 344:1215-1221, 2001.

APPENDIX

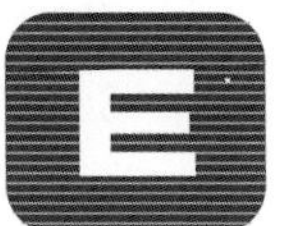

MUSCULOSKELETAL

E

MUSCLE INNERVATION

Table E-1

Muscle	Nerve	Root*
Trapezius	Spinal accessory	C**3-4**
Deltoid	Axillary	C**5**-6
Brachioradialis	Radial	C**5-6**
Extensor carpi radialis longus	Radial	C**6-7**
Triceps	Radial	C6, **7,** 8
Extensor digitorum	Posterior interosseous	C**7**-8
Biceps brachii	Musculocutaneous	C**5**-6
Flexor carpi radialis	Median	C6-**7**
Abductor pollicis brevis	Median	C**8**, T**1**
Opponens pollicis	Median	C8, T**1**
Flexor digitorum profundus 1 and 2	Anterior interosseous	C7-**8,** T1
Flexor digitorum profundus 3 and 4	Ulnar	C7-**8,** T1
Flexor carpi ulnaris	Ulnar	C7-**8,** T1
Interossei (hand)	Ulnar	C**8,** T**1**
Abductor digiti minimi	Ulnar	C**8,** T1
Iliopsoas	Femoral	L2, 3, **4**
Quadriceps femoris	Femoral	L2, **3,** 4
Abductors (leg)	Obturator	L**2, 3,** 4
Gluteus medius/gluteus minimus	Superior gluteal	L4, **5,** S1
Gluteus maximus	Inferior gluteal	L5, S**1,** 2
Hamstrings	Sciatic	L5, S**1,** 2
Gastrocnemius/soleus	Tibial	S**1,** 2
Flexor digitorum	Tibial	L**5,** S1
Interossei (foot)	Medial/lateral plantar	L5, S**1,** 2
Tibialis anterior	Deep peroneal	L**4, 5**
Extensor digitorum	Deep peroneal	L4, **5**

Compiled from Aids to the Examination of the Peripheral Nervous System, 4th ed. Edinburgh: WB Saunders, 2000; and Brazis PW, Biller J, eds. Localization in Clinical Neurology, 4th ed. Philadelphia: Lippincott Williams & Wilkins, 2001.

*Bold denotes the predominant root(s).

SPINAL ROOT AND SELECTED PERIPHERAL NERVE LESIONS

Table E-2

Root	Disc	Muscles	Weakness	Reflex Loss
C4	C3-4	Trapezius, scalene	Shoulder shrugging	None
C5	C4-5	Deltoid, biceps, brachioradialis	Shoulder abduction, external arm rotation, elbow flexion	Biceps, brachioradialis
C6	C5-6	Brachioradialis, biceps, pronator teres, extensor carpi radialis	Elbow flexion, arm pronation, finger and wrist extension	Biceps, brachioradialis
		Radial nerve injuries produce similar findings, except brachioradialis function is normal.		
C7	C6-7	Triceps, pronator teres, extensor digitorum	Elbow extension, finger and wrist extension	Triceps
C8	C7-T1	Flexor digitorum, flexor/abductor pollicis, interossei	Intrinsics of hand (finger abduction, palmar abduction of thumb)	Finger flexor
		Ulnar nerve injuries are similar but also weaken the thumb adductor.		
T10	T9-10		Beevor's sign (umbilicus pulled upward when patient sits up)	
L2	L1-2	Iliopsoas	Hip flexion	Cremaster
L3	L2-3	Iliopsoas, adductors (leg)	Hip flexion, thigh adduction	Knee jerk
L4	L3-4	Quadriceps, sartorius, tibialis anterior	Knee extension, ankle dorsiflexion and inversion	Knee jerk
		• Femoral nerve injury is limited to knee extension. • Associated hip flexion and adduction weakness localizes to plexus.		
L5	L4-5	Glutei, hamstrings, tibialis, extensor hallucis, extensor digiti, peronei	Thigh adduction and internal rotation, knee flexion, plantar flexion and dorsiflexion of ankle and toes	None
		• Deep peroneal nerve weakness is limited to ankle/toe extensor. • Posterior tibial nerve lesions weaken foot inversion.		

Modified from Aids to the Examination of the Peripheral Nervous System, 4th ed. Edinburgh: WB Saunders, 2000; and Brazis PW, Biller J, eds. Localization in Clinical Neurology, 4th ed. Philadelphia: Lippincott Williams & Wilkins, 2001.

Continued

Table E-2—cont'd

Root	Disc	Muscles	Weakness	Reflex Loss
S1	L5-S1	Gluteus maximus, hamstrings, soleus, gastrocnemius, extensor digitorum, flexor digitorum	Hip extension, knee flexion, plantar flexion of ankle and toes	Ankle jerk
S2	S1-2	Interossei	Cupping and fanning of toes	

Modified from Aids to the Examination of the Peripheral Nervous System, 4th ed. Edinburgh: WB Saunders, 2000; and Brazis PW, Biller J, eds. Localization in Clinical Neurology, 4th ed. Philadelphia: Lippincott Williams & Wilkins, 2001.

MOTOR TESTS FOR NERVE INJURY

Table E-3

Nerve	Motor Tests
Median	Lie the dorsum of the hand on a flat surface and palmar abduct the thumb with resistance while palpating the radial border of the thenar eminence (abductor pollicis brevis).
Ulnar	• Abduct fingers, or pinch paper between thumbs and distal index fingers and pull in opposite directions. • If thumb DIP bends (Froment's sign) then there is nerve injury.
Radial	Extend fingers and wrist against resistance.

TENDONS OF THE HAND

Table E-4

Tendon	Test of Function
Interossei	Dorsal (spread hand), palmar (hold paper between fingers) (U)
Lumbricals	Extend wrist and DIP/PIP while pressing down on fingertips (M,U)
Flexor digitorum profundus	Flex DIP while MCP and PIP are extended (M,U)
Flexor digitorum superficialis	Flex PIP while all other digits are extended (M)
Flexor digitorum superficialis (of the index finger)	• Have thumb and index finger pinch or pick up • If FDS is intact, DIP will hyperextend; if not intact, DIP will flex (M)
Flexor carpi radialis/ulnaris	Flex and radially (M) or ulnarly (U) deviate the wrist
Abductor pollicis longus	Extension and abduction of thumb (R)
Extensor pollicis brevis	Extension and abduction of thumb (R)
Extensor carpi radialis longus	Make fist while extending wrist (R)
Extensor carpi radialis brevis	Make fist while extending wrist (R)
Extensor pollicis longus	Lift thumb off of a flat surface while palm is flat and down (R)
Extensor digitorum communis	Extension of fingers at the MCP joint (R)
Extensor indicis proprius	Extension of index finger at the MCP joint with other fingers in a fist (R)
Extensor digiti minimi	Extension of the small finger while making a fist (R)
Extensor carpi ulnaris	Extension and ulnar deviation of the wrist (R)

M, median nerve; *R,* radial nerve; *U,* ulnar nerve.

COMPARTMENT SYNDROMES

Compartment syndromes are caused by a decrease in compartment size (such as from a crush injury) or an increase in contents (such as from swelling or bleeding).

Table E-5

Symptoms	Compartment Pressures (CP)
Pain (especially with passive movement)	Normal: <10 mm Hg
Paresthesia (lose vibratory sense first)	Abnormal: 10 to 30 mm Hg
Pallor or Pulselessness	Compartment syndrome: >30 mm Hg or MAP minus CP <40 mm Hg
Paralysis	

ARTHRITIS

Joint Fluid Analysis

Table E-6

	Normal	Noninflammatory	Inflammatory	Septic
Clarity	Clear	Clear	Cloudy	Purulent/turbid
Color	Clear	Yellow or blood	Yellow	Yellow
WBC/ml	<200	<200	200-50,000	>5000
PMN	<25%	>75%	>75%	>75%
Crystals	Absent	Absent	May be present	Absent
Glucose*	95%-100%	95%-100%	80%-100%	<50%
Culture	Negative	Negative	Negative	Positive >50%
Disease		Osteoarthritis, trauma, rheumatic fever	Gout, pseudogout, spondyloarthropathy RA, Lyme disease, lupus	Nongonococcal and gonococcal septic arthritis

*Ratio of joint fluid to serum glucose × 100%.

Cause of Arthritis Based on Number of Involved Joints

Table E-7

Number of Joints	Causes	
Monoarthritis (1 joint)	Trauma, tumor	Lyme disease
	Infection (septic arthritis)	Avascular necrosis
	Gout or pseudogout	Osteoarthritis (acute)
Oligoarthritis (2-3 joints)	Lyme disease	Gonococcal arthritis
	Rheumatic fever	Ankylosing spondylitis
	Reiter syndrome	Polyarticular gout
Polyarthritis (>3 joints)	Rheumatoid arthritis	Viral (rubella, hepatitis)
	Lupus	Osteoarthritis (acute)

Cause of Migratory Arthritis

- Gonococcal arthritis, viral arthritis
- Rheumatic fever, Lyme disease
- Subacute bacterial endocarditis
- Pulmonary infection
  - Mycoplasma
  - Histoplasmosis
  - Coccidioidomycosis
- Systemic lupus erythematosus
- Drug hypersensitivity (staphylococcus, streptococcus, meningococcus, and Neisseria gonorrhea)
- Henoch-Schönlein purpura

BRACHIAL PLEXUS INJURIES

Brachial plexus injuries are caused by trauma, infection, hematoma, vascular occlusion, or cancer. Sensory loss is generally incomplete/inconsistent.

Table E-8

Injury	Muscles (Sites of Weakness)	Reflex Lost
Upper trunk (Erb-Duchenne syndrome)	Supraspinatus/infraspinatus (shoulder rotation), biceps, deltoid, pronator teres, brachioradialis	Biceps
Middle trunk	Latissimus, triceps, extensor digitorum communis (finger extension), extensor carpi radialis (wrist extension)	Triceps
Low trunk (Klumpke syndrome)	Ulnar nerve muscles (finger flexion/abduction), FDP (second and third fingers), extensor pollicis longus/extensor pollicis brevis (thumb extension/abduction)	Finger flexion
Lateral	Biceps, pronator teres, flexor carpi radialis	Biceps
Posterior	Latissimus dorsi, hand radial nerve (finger extension), deltoid (shoulder abduction)	Triceps
Medial	All ulnar innervated muscles (wrist finger flexion) and median innervated intrinsic hand muscles	Finger flexion

Appendix

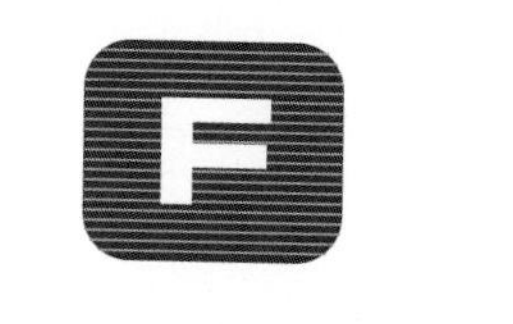

NOTES AND ORDERS

F

ADMIT ORDERS

ADCVAANDIML

A Admit to ward (include pager numbers for house officers)
D Diagnosis
C Condition
V Vital signs (how often they are taken, and include parameters to call house officer)
A Allergies and reactions
A Activity level (e.g., strict bed rest with assist)
N Nursing (e.g., neurologic checks; strict versus routine I/O; O_2 saturation levels; daily weights; blood sugar checks and frequency; any drains, including Foley catheter, nasogastric tube, chest tubes, wound drains, and so forth, and specify whether gravity, low wall intermittent, continuous suction, or bulb suction)
D Diet (e.g., diabetic, renal, npo)
I Intravenous fluids, type and rate
M Medications (e.g., scheduled and prn medications)
L Laboratory results (e.g., specify time to be drawn, stat or routine); also include imaging studies if needed (e.g., CXR after line placement or after intubation)

Also include code status, if known (e.g., full code, DNR).

DAILY SOAP NOTES

S Subjective: what is described by the patient and/or what is reported by nurses over the previous 24 hours.
O Objective: data and factual information—vital signs (range helpful) with 24 hour I/O, lines and tubes with outputs, physical examination, laboratory results (trends are helpful), and imaging results.
A/P Assessment and Plan: Restate the patient's sex, age, and active diagnoses. Provide a plan for each pertinent organ system or problem. Include a plan for transfer or discharge if appropriate.

DEATH NOTES

- Indicate what prompted arrival to patient's bedside (e.g., called by nurse or during the operation)
- Describe pertinent physical examination (e.g., respiratory rate, pulse, blood pressure, neurologic examination)
- Indicate time and date of death or pronouncement of death
- Notify the patient's primary care physician

- Request an autopsy
- Document correspondence with organ donation organizations, if appropriate
- Dictate short death summary

DELIVERY NOTES

On (date and time) this (age and race) female under (no, local, pudendal, or epidural) anesthesia delivered a (male or female) infant weighing (weight) with Apgar scores of (0-10) and (0-10) at 1 and 5 minutes, respectively. Delivery was via (spontaneous or induced vaginal, low transverse C-section, or C-section) into a sterile field. Infant was (bulb) suctioned at (perineum or delivery) and nuchal cord (did or did not) need to be reduced. Cord clamped and cut and infant handed to waiting (pediatrician or nurse). (Cord blood sent for analysis). (Weight) (intact, fragmented, or meconium-stained) placenta with (two- or three-) vessel cord delivered (spontaneously or with manual extraction) at (time). (Amount) of (methylergonovine or oxytocin) given. (Uterus, cervix, vagina, and/or rectum) explored and (midline episiotomy, degree of laceration, uterus, and/or abdominal incision) repaired in a normal fashion with (type) suture. Estimated blood loss (amount in ml). Patient taken to recovery room in stable condition. Infant taken to newborn nursery in stable condition. (Attending physician's name).

DISCHARGE ORDERS

- Dictated by whom and on what date
- Patient name and medical number
- Admission date and discharge date
- Discharge diagnoses
- Procedures/studies performed during admission (including dates)
- Consultations obtained during admission
- Brief summary of patient's history and physical on admission
- Hospital course (helpful if done in list format when multiple issues)
- Disposition and care instructions
- Diet
- Activity
- Wound care
- Restrictions
- Discharge medications
- Follow-up appointments
- Name of person to whom copies of dictation were sent
- Dictated by whom and on what date
- Patient name and medical number

HISTORY AND PHYSICAL

- Chief complaint
  - Reason for visit
  - Duration of problem
  - Other pertinent complaints
- History of present illness
  - Character
  - Onset
  - Location
  - Radiation
  - Duration
  - Intensity
  - Provocative
  - Palliation
- Past medical history
  - General health conditions or illnesses
  - Blood transfusions
  - As appropriate:
    - Childhood illnesses
    - Immunizations
    - Obstetric or gynecologic history
    - Psychiatric history
- Past surgical history (include dates)
- Medications and doses, current and past
- Allergies
- Family history
  - Major illnesses in parents and siblings
  - History of hereditary diseases
- Social history
  - Marital status
  - Children
  - Present occupation and any occupational exposures
  - Education
  - Sexual history
  - Drug history (IVDA, alcohol, and tobacco)
  - Military record
  - Religious practices
- Review of systems
  - General: fever, chills, malaise, fatigue, weight changes
  - Skin: rashes, pruritus, jaundice, bruising, skin cancer, mole changes
  - Head: trauma, masses, dizziness, headache, syncope, seizures
  - Neck: lumps, swelling, suppleness

- Eyes: acuity, blurring, diplopia, photophobia, pain, glaucoma, trauma, discharge
- Ears: hearing loss, tinnitus, pain, vertigo, discharge
- Nose: epistaxis, frequent colds, sinus pain
- Throat and mouth: hoarseness, gum bleeding, ulcers, disturbance of taste, tooth extraction
- Breasts: lumps, pain, discharge, galactorrhea, mammograms, frequency of breast examinations
- Respiratory: wheezing, dyspnea, hemoptysis, cyanosis, cough, night sweats, TB exposure, last CXR, shortness of breath
- Cardiac: orthopnea (number of pillows), edema, palpitations, weakness on exertion, murmurs, HTN, previous myocardial infarction, last ECG
- Circulatory: claudication, cold extremities, edema, numbness, tingling
- Lymph nodes: adenopathy, tenderness, suppuration
- Gastrointestinal: pain, change in bowel habits, jaundice, gallstones, dysphagia, odynophagia, hematemesis, dark urine, history of ulcer, diarrhea, constipation, tarry stools
- Genital: discharge, sores, pain, masses, history of sexually transmitted diseases, abnormal or heavy vaginal bleeding
- Urinary: burning, dysuria, flank pain, urgency, frequency, nocturia, hematuria, stress incontinence
- Neurologic: neurologic deficits; seizures; tremors; memory loss; loss of consciousness, speech, or coordination
- Endocrine: polydipsia; polyuria; polyphagia; heat or cold intolerance; changes in hair, energy levels, or skin
- Hematologic: anemia, bleeding disorders, easy bruising
- Psychiatric: depression, suicidal thoughts or ideation, sleep disturbances, anxiety, phobias

- Physical examination
  - General survey: vital signs; nourishment; grooming; affect; whether alert and oriented to person, place, and time; level of distress or anxiety
  - Skin: color, integrity, temperature, tattoos, edema, presence and description of lesions (size, shape, location, inflammation, tenderness, induration, discharge), hair texture and distribution, clubbing, capillary refill
  - Head: shape, trauma, facial symmetry, characteristics of temporal arteries
  - Eyes: conjunctiva, lid lag, strabismus, exophthalmos, visual acuity and fields, pupils round and reactive to light and accommodation, extraocular movements, funduscopy (red reflex, retina, AV nicking, papilledema, optic disc, macula)
  - Ears: tragal palpation, discharge, otoscopic examination (cerumen, lesions, discharge, foreign body), tympanic membrane (integrity, color, landmarks, mobility, perforation), hearing (air and bone conduction)

- Nose: deformity, patency, smell, pain, septum position, appearance of turbinates, frontal or maxillary sinus pain
- Mouth and throat: inspection (lips, teeth, gums, lesions, ulcers); buccal mucosa; symmetry and movement of tongue, soft palate, and uvula; gag reflex, taste, parotid and submandibular glands
- Neck: mobility; suppleness; position of trachea; thyroid shape, tenderness, or nodules; neck nodes, swallowing, carotid bruits, jugular venous distension
- Chest: size/shape of chest, anteroposterior versus transverse diameter, symmetry of movement with respiration
- Lungs: respiratory rate (depth and regularity), palpation of fremitus, percussion (quality and symmetry, diaphragmatic excursion), auscultation findings (breath sounds, pitch, duration, intensity, vesicular, bronchial, bronchovesicular), friction rub, egophony, whispered pectoriloquy, bronchophony
- Breasts: size, contour, symmetry, texture, masses, scars, tenderness, thickening, nodules, discharge, retraction, or dimpling
- Heart: apical impulse, auscultation (characteristics of S1 and S2, murmurs, clicks, snaps, S3 or S4), palpation (pulsations, thrills, heaves, lifts)
- Vascular: comparison of blood pressure, jugular venous distension, bruits (carotid, temporal, renal, femoral, abdominal aorta), pulses in extremities, lower extremities (temperature, color, hair, skin texture, tenderness)
- Abdomen: shape, contour, visible aorta pulsations, hernia, auscultation (presence and character of bowel sounds in all quadrants), palpation (aorta, organs, masses, muscle resistance), percussion (areas of decreased or increased percussion, costovertebral angle tenderness), liver span
- Male genitalia: circumcision, location of urethral opening, discharge, palpation (testes, epididymides, vas deferens, contour, consistency, tenderness), presence of hernia or scrotal swelling
- Female genitalia: inflammation, scarring, discharge, internal examination (vaginal mucosa, cervix, discharge, odor, lesions), bimanual examination (size; position; tenderness of cervix, vaginal walls, uterus, or adnexa), rectovaginal examination, stress incontinence
- Anus and rectum: sphincter control and tone, hemorrhoids, fissures, skin tags, polyps, prostate (size, contour, consistency, mobility)
- Musculoskeletal: posture, symmetry of muscle mass, range of motion of joints, motor strength
- Neurologic: cranial nerves, cerebellar and motor (gait, balance, coordination, rapid alternating motions), sensory (touch, pain, vibration, temperature, monofilament), superficial and deep tendon reflexes (symmetry, grade)

ICU NOTES

- Lines (central lines, arterial lines, chest tubes and drains–include how many days since placed or changed)
- Drips
- Antibiotics (include which day and anticipated total course date)
- Vital signs
- I/O (fluids and transfusions, UOP and any drain output)
- Ventilator settings
- Laboratory results
- ABG
- Cultures
- Imaging results
- Examination, by system
  - Neurologic
  - Cardiac
  - Pulmonary
  - GI
  - Extremities
- Assessment and plan, by system
  - Neurologic
  - Cardiac
  - Pulmonary
  - GI
  - Renal
  - Hematologic
  - Extremities
  - DVT precautions

OFF-SERVICE NOTES

- Date of admission
- Diagnoses
- Brief pertinent past medical history
- Hospital course (major interventions, events, procedures, studies, and findings)
- Medications (include date and indications for antibiotics)
- Consultants assisting with the patient's care
- Pertinent physical examination
- Assessment and plan

OPERATIVE NOTES

- Time and date of procedure
- Preoperative diagnosis
- Postoperative diagnosis
- Procedure
- Surgeons
- Assistants
- Anesthesia (e.g., local, general with LMA, general endotracheal, regional)
- Name of anesthesiologist or CRNA
- Findings
- Specimens
- Pump or clamp times if appropriate
- Tubes and drains (include how they are secured)
- Estimated blood loss
- Fluids in
- Fluids out
- Complications
- Condition
- Person dictating operative notes

POSTOPERATIVE NOTES

- Subjective: patient statements, nursing comments, pain control
- Objective: vital signs and I/O
- Physical examination: pertinent to the operation, include evaluation of dressing
- Review orders: make necessary changes after postoperative assessment
- Laboratory results: review any laboratory results that were sent during and/or immediately after the operation

POSTPARTUM NOTES

- Subjective: patient statements and nursing comments; pain control, breast tenderness, urination, flatus, bowel movement, vaginal bleeding, leg edema, whether breast or bottle feeding
- Objective: vital signs and I/O
- Physical examination: fundal height and consistency and episiotomy condition—include evaluation of dressing

- Review orders: make necessary changes after postoperative assessment; consider need for RhoGAM and laxatives; contact consultants as necessary
- Laboratory results: review any laboratory results that were sent during and/or immediately after the operation

PROCEDURE NOTES

- Procedure
- Indication
- Type of sterile preparation
- Anesthesia
- Brief description of procedure
- Specimens
- Estimated blood loss (if appropriate)
- Complications
- Postprocedure studies pending (such as CXR after central access)

APPENDIX

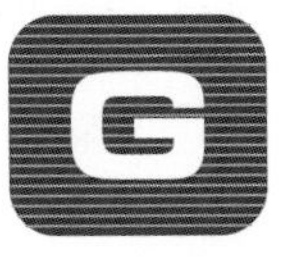

LABS

G

SI LAB VALUE CONVERTER

Table G-1

Lab Value	US Unit	SI Unit	Factor*
CHEMISTRY			
ALT, AST	U/L	μkat/L	0.0167
Alkaline phosphates	U/L	μkat/L	0.0167
Amylase	U/L	μkat/L	0.0167
Bilirubin	mg/dl	μmol/L	17.1
BUN	mg/dl	mmol/L	0.357
Calcium	mg/dl	mmol/L	0.25
Cholesterol	mg/dl	mmol/L	0.0259
Cortisol	mcg/dl	nmol/L	27.6
Creatine kinase	U/L	μkat/L	0.0167
Creatinine	mg/dl	μmol/L	88.4
Glucose	mg/dl	mmol/L	0.0555
LDH	U/L	μkat/L	0.0167
Lipase	U/dl	μkat/L	0.167
Mg^{++}	mEq/L	mmol/L	0.5
5′-NT	U/L	μkat/L	0.0167
Phosphate	mg/dl	mmol/L	0.322
CHEMISTRY—CONT'D			
T_4	mcg/dl	nmol/L	12.9
T_3	mcg/dl	nmol/L	0.0154
Uric acid	mg/dl	mmol/L	59.5
TOXICOLOGY AND DRUG MONITORING			
Acetaminophen	μg/ml	μmol/L	6.62
Amikacin	μg/ml	μmol/L	1.71
Carbamazepine	μg/ml	μmol/L	4.23
Digoxin	ng/ml	nmol/L	1.28
Gentamicin	μg/ml	μmol/L	2.09
Phenytoin	μg/ml	μmol/L	3.96
Salicylate	mg/L	mmol/L	.00724
Theophylline	μg/ml	μmol/L	5.55
Tobramycin	μg/ml	μmol/L	2.14
Valproate	μg/ml	μmol/L	6.93
Vancomycin	μg/ml	μmol/L	0.690

Compiled from Kratz A, Lewandrowski KB. Case records of the Massachusetts General Hospital. Weekly clinicopathological exercises. Normal reference laboratory values. N Engl J Med 339:1063, 1998.

*Factor is used to convert from standard to SI units.

Table G-1—cont'd

Lab Value	US Unit	SI Unit	Factor*	Lab Value	US Unit	SI Unit	Factor*
BLOOD GAS				**HEMATOLOGY**			
$Paco_2$	mm Hg	kPa	0.133	Folate	ng/ml	nmol/L	2.27
Pao_2	mm Hg	kPa	0.133	Hemoglobin	g/dl	mmol/L	0.621
				Iron, TIBC	μg/dl	μmol/L	0.179
				Vitamin B12	pg/ml	pmol/L	0.738

MENINGITIS: TYPICAL CEREBROSPINAL FLUID PARAMETERS

Table G-2

	Normal	Bacteria	Viral	Fungal	TB	Abscess
WBC/ml	0-5	>1000	<1000	100-500	100-500	10-1000
% PMN	0-15	>80	<50	<50	<50	<50
% Lymph	>50	<50	>50	>80	↑ Monocytes	Variable
Glucose	45-65	<40	45-65	30-45	30-45	45-60
Ratio	0.6	<0.4	0.6	<0.4	<0.4	0.6
Protein	20-45	>150	50-100	100-500	100-500	>50
Pressure	6-20	>25-30	Variable	>20	>20	Variable

VIRAL HEPATITIS SEROLOGIES

Table G-3

Scenario	ALT	HAV IgM	HAV IgG	HBs Antigen	GhClgM	GBC IgG
Acute HAV infection	↑↑	+	–			
Previous HAV infection or vaccination	Normal	–	+			
Acute HBV	↑↑			+	+	–
Acute HBV in window period	↑↑			–	+	–
Chronic HBV, active replication	↑			+	–	+
Chronic HBV, precore Mutant	↑			+	–	+
Chronic HBV, minimally replicative (carrier)	Normal			+	–	+
Previous HBV infection	Normal			–	–	+
Previous HBV vaccination	Normal			–	–	–
Acute HCV	↑↑					
Chronic HCV	Normal/↑					
False positive HCV or previous infection eradication	Normal					

*DNA, viral DNA.

HBe Antigen	HBe Antibody	HBs Antibody	HBV DNA*	HCV Antibody	HCV RNA
−	−	−	+		
−	−	−	+/−		
+	−	−	+		
−	−	−	+		
−	+	−	−		
−	−	+/−	−		
−	−	+	−		
				−	+
				+	+
				+	−

PLEURAL FLUID ANALYSIS

Table G-4

Fluid	Specific Gravity	Protein	LDH	Protein Fluid/Serum	LDH Fluid/Serum
Transudate	<1.016	<3.0 g/dl	<200 U/L	<0.5	<0.6
Exudate	>1.016	>3.0 g/dl	>200 U/L	>0.5	>0.6

REPLACEMENT FLUID CONTENTS

Table G-5

Fluid	Na (mEq/L)	K (mEq/L)	Cl (mEq/L)	HCO_3 (mEq/L)	Ca (mEq/L)	Kcal/L (mEq/L)	Glucose (g/L)
½ NS	77	—	77	—	—	—	—
NS	154	—	154	—	—	—	—
D5W1	—	—	—	—	—	170	50
D10W	—	—	—	—	—	340	100
LR	130	4	109	28	3	9	—

NORMAL LABORATORY VALUES

Table G-6 Hematology

WBC	4.5-11.0 x 10^3 per μl
Hemoglobin	M: 13.5-17.5 g/dl F: 12.0-16.0 g/dl
Hematocrit	M: 39%-49% F: 35%-45%
Platelets	150-450 $\times$ 10^3 per ml
Neutrophils	57%-67%
Segmented neutrophils	54%-62%
Bands	3%-5%
Lymphocytes	23%-33%
Monocytes	3%-7%
Eosinophils	1%-3%
Basophils	0%-1%
RBC	M: 4.3-5.7 $\times$ 10^6 per μl F: 3.8-5.1 $\times$ 10^6 per μl
MCV	80-100 fl
MCH	26-34 pg/cell
MCHC	31%-37% hemoglobin/cell
Reticulocyte count	0.5%-1.5%
Hemoglobin A1c	5.0%-7.5%
Haptoglobin	26-185 mg/dl
PT	11-15 seconds
PTT	20-35 seconds
Bleeding time	2-7 minutes
Thrombin time	6.3-11.1 seconds
Fibrinogen	200-400 mg/dl
FDP	<10 μg/ml
ESR	M: <15 F: <20

Table G-7 Chemistries

Sodium	135-145 mEq/L
Potassium	2.5-5.1 mEq/L
Chloride	98-106 mEq/L
Bicarbonate	22-29 mEq/L
Glucose	70-115 mg/dl
BUN	7-18 mg/dl
Creatinine	0.6-1.2 mg/dl
Anion gap	7-16 mEq/L
Osmolality	275-295 mOsm/kg
Calcium, total	8.4-10.2 mg/dl
Calcium, ionized	4.65-5.28 mg/dl
Phosphate	2.7-4.5 mg/dl
Magnesium	1.3-2.1 mEq/L
Protein, total	6.0-8.0 g/dl
Albumin	3.5-5.5 g/dl
Alpha-fetoprotein	<10 ng/ml
Bilirubin, total	0.2-1.0 mg/dl
Bilirubin, conjugated	0-0.2 mg/dl
Lipase	10-140
Amylase	25-125 U/L
C-peptide	0.70-1.89 ng/ml
Cholesterol, total	<200 mg/dl
Cholesterol, LDL	<130 mg/dl
Cholesterol, HDL	M: >29 mg/dl F: >35 mg/dl
Triglycerides	M: 40-160 mg/dl F: 35-135 mg/dl
Lactate, venous	5.0-20.0 mg/dl
Uric acid	M: 3.5-7.2 mg/dl F: 2.6-6.0 mg/dl
Ammonia	10-50 μmol/L
Alkaline phosphate	M: 38-126 U/L F: 70-230 U/L
LDH	90-190 U/L
SGOT/AST	7-40 U/L
SGPT/ALT	7-40 U/L
GGT	M: 9-50 U/L F: 8-40 U/L
CPK	M: 38-174 U/L F: 26-140 U/L
CPK MB	<5%
Iron	M: 65-175 μg/dl F: 50-170 μg/dl
TIBC	25-450 μg/dl
Iron saturation	M: 20%-50% F: 15%-50%
Ferritin	M: 20-250 ng/ml F: 10-120 ng/ml
Vitamin B_{12}	100-700 pg/ml
Folate	3-16 ng/ml
Copper	M: 10-140 μg/dl F: 80-155 μg/dl
Zinc	70-150 μg/dl
PSA	<4.0 ng/ml
Acid phosphatase	<0.8 U/L
CEA	<2.5 ng/ml Smoker: <5.0 ng/ml
CA-125	<35 U/ml

Table G-7 Chemistries—cont'd

ABG pH	7.35-7.45
ABG $Paco_2$	35-45 mm Hg
ABG Pao_2	80-100 mm Hg
ABG HCO_3	21-27 mEq/L
Oxygen saturation	>95%
Base excess	± 2 mEq/L
Aldosterone	Supine: 3-10 ng/dl Upright: 5-30 ng/dl
Cortisol	0800 hours: 6-23 μg/dl 1600 hours: 3-15 μg/dl 2200 hours: <50% of 0800 hours
Estrogen	Follicular: 60-200 pg/ml Luteal: 160-400 pg/ml Menopausal: <130 pg/ml
FSH	Follicular: 1-9 mU/ml Ovulation: 6-26 mU/ml Luteal: 1-9 mU/ml Menopausal: 30-118 mU/ml
Gastrin	<100 pg/ml
Growth hormone	M: <2 ng/ml F: <10 ng/ml M >60 years: <10 ng/ml F >60 years: <14 ng/ml
LH	Follicular: 1-12 mU/ml Midcycle: 16-104 mU/ml Luteal: 1-12 mU/ml Menopausal: 16-66 mU/ml
Progesterone	Follicular: 0.15-0.7 ng/ml Luteal: 2.0-25.0 ng/ml
PTH	10-65 pg/ml
Testosterone	Free: 52-280 pg/ml Total: 300-1000 ng/dl
T_4, total	5.0-12.0 μg/dl
T_4, free	0.8-2.3 ng/dl
T_3, total	100-200 ng/dl
TBG	15-34 μg/ml
TSH	<10 μU/ml >60 yr: M 2.7-3 μU/ml >60 yr: F 2.0-26.8 μU/ml
CSF	
Pressure	70-180 mm (supine)
WBC	0-5 mononuclear cells/μl
Protein	15-45 mg/dl
Glucose	40-70 mg/dl
Synovial Fluid	
WBC	<200 cells per μl
Protein	<3.0 g/day
Glucose	>40 mg/dl
Uric acid	<8.0 mg/dl
LDH	<serum LDH
Toxicology	**(Toxic Values)**
Acetaminophen	>200 μg/ml
CO hemoglobin	>20% saturation
Ethanol	>100 mg/dl (intoxicated) >300 mg/dl (coma) >500 mg/dl (respiratory depression and death)
Ethylene glycol	>20 mg/dl
Lead	100 μg/dl

G

Continued

Table G-7 Chemistries—cont'd

Methanol	>200 mg/L
Salicylate	>300 mg/ml (trough)
URINE	
Specific gravity	1.002-1.030
Osmolality	50-1400 mOsm/kg
Creatinine	M: 14-26 mg/kg/day F: 11-20 mg/kg/day
Creatinine clearance	M: 90-136 ml/min/ 1.73 m^2 F : 80-125 ml/min/ 1.73 m^2
Urea nitrogen	12-20 g/day
Sodium	40-220 mEq/day
Potassium	25-125 mEq/day
Calcium	100-300 mg/day
Phosphate	0.4-1.3 g/day
Uric acid	250-750 mg/day
Amylase	1-17 U/hr
Glucose	<0.5 g/day
Albumin	10-100 mg/day
Protein	10-150 mg/day
5-HIAA	2-6 mg/day
17-Ketosteroids	M: 8-22 mg/day F: 6-15 mg/day
17-Ketogenic steroids	M: 5-23 mg/day F: 3-15 mg/day
17-Hydroxy-corticosteroids	M: 3-10 mg/day F: 2-8 mg/day
Homovanillic acid	1.4-8.8 mg/day
Metanephrine, total	0.05-1.2 μg/mg

SERUM DRUG LEVELS

Table G-8

Drug	Therapeutic	Toxic
Carbamazepine	4-12 μg/ml	>12 μg/ml
Digoxin	0.8-2.0 ng/ml	>2.0 ng/ml
Ethosuximide	40-100 μg/ml	>150 μg/ml
Lidocaine	1.5-6.0 μg/ml	>6 μg/ml
Lithium	0.6-1.2 mEq/L	>1.5 mEq/L
N-acetyl procainamide	5-30 μg/ml	>40 μg/ml
Phenobarbital	15-40 μg/ml	>35 μg/ml
Phenytoin	10-20 μg/ml	>20 μg/ml
Procainamide	3-10 μg/ml	>10 μg/ml
Quinidine	1.5-5 μg/ml	>5 μg/ml
Theophylline	10-20 μg/ml	>20 μg/ml
Valproic acid	50-100 μg/ml	>100 μg/ml

SERUM ANTIBIOTIC LEVELS

Table G-9

Drug	Peak	Trough
Amikacin	25-35 μg/ml	<10 μg/ml
Gentamicin	4-6 μg/ml	<2 μg/ml
Tobramycin	4-6 μg/ml	<2 μg/ml
Vancomycin	20-40 μg/ml	<10 μg/ml

Appendix

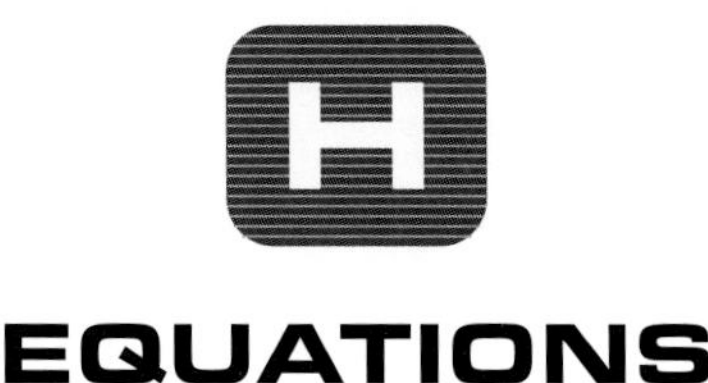

EQUATIONS

MEDICAL STATISTICS

Table H-1

	Disease Present	Disease Absent
Test positive	True positive (TP)	False positive (FP)
Test negative	False negative (FN)	True negative (TN)

Table H-2

Statistic	Calculation	Meaning
Prevalence (prior probability)	(TP + FN)/(ALL)	All patients with disease/all patients
Sensitivity	TP/(TP + FN)	True positive/all diseased
Specificity	TN/(FP + TN)	True negative/all healthy
False positive rate	1 − Specificity	
False negative rate	1 − Sensitivity	
Positive predictive value	TP/(TP + FP)	True positive/all positive
Negative predictive value	TN/(FN + TN)	True negative/all negative
Accuracy	(TP + TN)/(ALL)	True results/all patients
Likelihood ratio (positive results)	$\frac{\text{Sensitivity}}{1 - \text{Specificity}}$	
Likelihood ratio (net results)	$\frac{1 - \text{Sensitivity}}{\text{Specificity}}$	
Pretest odds ratio	$\frac{\text{Pretest probability}}{1 - \text{Pretest probability}}$	
Posttest odds ratio	Pretest odds ratio × Likelihood ratio	
Posttest probability	$\frac{\text{Posttest odds ratio}}{\text{Posttest odds ratio} + 1}$	

Table H-3

Likelihood Ratio	Change From Pretest to Posttest Probability
<0.1 or >10	Large, often conclusive
0.1-0.2 or 5-10	Moderate
0.2-0.5 or 2-5	Small, sometimes important
0.5-2	Rarely important

Compiled from Jaeschke R, Guyatt GH, Sackett DL. Users' guides to the medical literature. III. How to use an article about a diagnostic test. B. What are the results and will they help me in caring for my patients? The Evidence-Based Medicine Working Group. JAMA 271:703, 1994.

HEMODYNAMIC EQUATIONS

Blood pressure: $MAP = \frac{SBP + (2 \times DBP)}{3} = DBP + \frac{SBP - DBP}{3}$

Fick cardiac output:

$$CO = \frac{O_2 \text{ consumption}}{\text{Arterial } O_2 \text{ content} - \text{Venous } O_2 \text{ content}} =$$

$$\frac{10 \times VO_2 \text{ (ml/min/m}^2\text{)}}{\text{Hb (g/dl)} \times 1.39 \times (\text{Arterial } O_2 \text{ saturation [\%]} - \text{Venous } O_2 \text{ saturation [\%]})}$$

Cardiac index: $CI = \frac{CO}{BSA}$ (Normal is 2.5 to 4.2 L/min/m^2)

Stroke volume: $SV = \frac{CO}{HR}$

$$\text{Pulmonary vascular resistance (PVR)} = \frac{80 \times (\text{Mean PA pressure} - \text{Mean PCWP})}{\text{Cardiac output (L/min)}}$$

$$\text{Systemic vascular resistance (SVR)} = \frac{80 \times (\text{MAP [mm Hg]} - \text{RA pressure [mm Hg]})}{\text{Cardiac output (L/min)}}$$

Body surface area (BSA)[1] in m^2 = Height (cm)$^{0.718}$ × Weight (kg)$^{0.43}$ × 74.5 =

$$\sqrt{(\text{Height [cm]} \times \text{Weight [kg]}) \div 3600}$$

H

Reference

1. Winshall JS, Lederman RJ. Tarascon Internal Medicine and Critical Care Pocketbook, 4th ed. Lompoc, CA: Tarascon, 2007, p 9.

Appendix

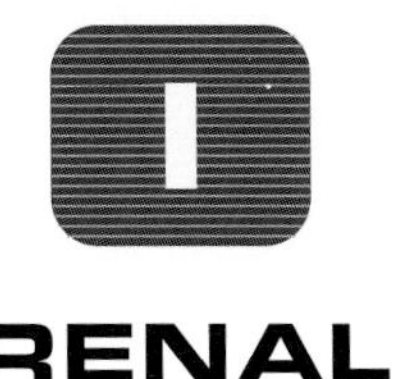

RENAL

I

OTHER RENAL EQUATIONS

$$\text{mmol/L} = \frac{\text{mg/dl} \times 10}{\text{Molecular weight}}$$

$$\text{mEq/L} = \text{mmol/L} \times \text{Valence}$$

mOsm/kg = mmol/L × n (where *n* is the number of dissociable particles per molecule)

$$\text{Calculated osmolarity} = 2 \times \text{Na (mEq/L)} + \frac{\text{BUN (mg/dl)}}{2.8} + \frac{\text{Glucose (mg/dl)}}{18} + \frac{\text{EtOH (mg/dl)}}{4.6} + \frac{\text{Isopropanol (mg/dl)}}{6} + \frac{\text{Methanol}}{3.2} + \frac{\text{Ethylene glycol}}{6.2} \text{ (Normal 275 to 290 mOsm/kg)}$$

Anion gap = Na − Cl − HCO_3

Urinary anion gap = Na + K − Cl − HCO_3 (May ignore HCO_3 if pH <6.5)

Free water deficit = 0.4 × Lean body weight × ([Plasma (Na^+) ÷ 140] − 1)

$$\text{Creatinine clearance} = \frac{U_{Cr} \times V}{P_{Cr}} = \frac{\text{Urine creatinine (mg/dl)} \times \text{Urine volume (ml/day)}}{\text{Plasma creatinine (mg/dl)} \times \text{1440 min/day}}$$

$$\text{Creatinine clearance} \approx \frac{140 - \text{Age (years)}}{\text{Serum creatinine (mg/dl)} \times 72} \times \text{Weight (kg) } (\times 0.85 \text{ if female})$$

Creatinine clearance (MDRD estimation) =

$$170 \times Cr \times Age\ (years)^{-0.18}\ (\times 0.762 \text{ if female})\ (\times 1.18 \text{ if black}) \times BUN^{-0.17} \times Albumin^{0.32}$$

$$\text{Fractional excretion of sodium (FENa)} = \frac{\text{Urine Na} \times \text{Plasma Cr}}{\text{Urine Cr} \times \text{Plasma Na}}$$

$$\text{Transtubular } K^{+} \text{ gradient (TTKG)} = \frac{U_K \times Posm}{P_K \times Uosm}$$

RULES OF THUMB

- Estimated 24-hour urinary protein excretion (g/day) ≈ spot urine protein/creatinine ratio
- Potassium and pH: K^+ increases 0.6 mEq/L for each pH drop of 0.1
- Sodium and glucose: Na^+ decreases 1.6 mEq/L per 100 mg/dl increase in glucose
- Calcium and albumin: Ca^{2+} decreases 0.8 mg/dl for each 1 g/dl ↓ in albumin

FENa[1]

$$\text{FENa (\%)} = \frac{U_{Na} \times P_{Cr}}{P_{Na} \times U_{Cr}} \times 100$$

- FENa is a measure of sodium avidity of the renal tubule (represents % of filtered sodium that is excreted in the urine).
- Normal value varies with Na^+ intake, GFR, and volume status, but is typically ≤1%.
- Useful clinically in acute renal failure to differentiate between prerenal azotemia (FENa <1%) and acute tubular necrosis (FENa >2%). A FENa of 1% to 2% is indeterminate.

Effective Intravascular Volume Status

Table I-1

FENa	Hypovolemic	Normal or Volume Overloaded
$<1\%$	• Prerenal azotemia • Cirrhosis or hepatorenal syndrome • Congestive heart failure	• Nonoliguric ATN (10% of cases) • ATN with underlying CHF or cirrhosis • Drugs: ACE-I, NSAIDs • Acute glomerulonephritis or vasculitis • Acute interstitial nephritis* • Acute renal allograft rejection • Intratubular obstruction: myoglobin (rhabdomyolysis), contrast media • Acute extrarenal obstruction* (FENa depends on duration/severity)
$>2\%$	• Diuretics • Chronic renal failure	• Oliguric ATN • Nonoliguric ATN (90% of cases) • Obstruction

*Seen in only some cases.

Pearls

- FENa is more useful in oliguric renal failure than in nonoliguric renal failure.
- Variability of FENa in nonoliguric patients without renal failure makes it a poor measure of volume status (unless it is *very* low, such as $<0.1\%$ to 0.2%).

ACID-BASE DISORDERS

Anion gap = Na − Cl − HCO_3 (Normal = 8 to 16 mEq/L)

Osmolality gap = Measured osmolality − Calculated osmolality (Normal = 0 to 10 mOsm/L)

Calculated Osmolality = 2 × Na^+ + (glucose/18) + (BUN/2.8) + (ethanol/4.6) + (methanol/2.6) + (ethylene glycol/5) + (acetone/5.5) + (isopropanol/5.9)

Causes of Increased Anion Gap

- **M**ethanol
- **U**remia
- **D**iabetes
- **P**araldehyde
- **I**ron, INH
- **L**actate
- **E**thanol, ethylene glycol
- **S**alicylates, starvation

Causes of Decreased Anion Gap

- Lithium bromide
- Multiple myeloma
- Albumin loss in nephritic syndrome

Causes of Increased Osmolality Gap

- Alcohols (methanol, ethylene glycol, isopropanol)
- Sugar (glycerol, mannitol)
- Ketones (acetone)

ACID-BASE RULES OF THUMB

Table I-2

		Acidosis	Alkalosis
Respiratory	Acute	$\Delta pH = -0.008 \times \Delta Paco_2$ $\Delta HCO_3^- = 0.1 \times Paco_2$ ($\pm$ 3)	$\Delta pH = 0.008 \times \Delta Paco_2$ $\Delta HCO_3^- = -0.2 \times \Delta Paco_2$ (usually not to less than 18 mEq/L)
	Chronic	$Paco_2 = 2.4 \times (HCO_3^-) - 22$ $\Delta HCO_3^- = 0.35 \times \Delta Paco_2$ ($\pm$ 4)	$\Delta HCO_3^- = -0.4 \times \Delta Paco_2$ (usually not to less than 18 mEq/L)
Metabolic		$Paco_2 = 1.5 \times (HCO_3^-) + 8 \pm 2$ $Paco_2 \equiv$ Last two digits of pH $\Delta Paco_2 = 1.2 \times \Delta HCO_3^-$	$Paco_2 = 0.9 \times (HCO_3^-) + 9 \pm 2$ $\Delta Paco_2 = 0.6 \times \Delta HCO_3^-$

Compiled from Schrier RW. Renal and Electrolyte Disorders, 5th ed. Philadelphia: Lippincott-Raven, 1997; and Rose BD, Post TW, Rose B. Clinical Physiology of Acid-Base and Electrolyte Disorders, 5th ed. New York: McGraw-Hill, 2001.

KIDNEY/RENAL DISORDERS

Table I-3 Studies Useful in Determining Causes of Acute Renal Failure

Test	Prerenal	Renal	Postrenal
Urine sodium (mEq/L)	<20	>40	>40
FENa*	$<1\%$	$>2\%$	$>2\%$
Renal failure index (RFI)†	<1	>2	>2
Urine osmolality (mOsm/L)	>500	<300	<400
Urine/serum creatinine ratio	>40	<20	<20
Serum BUN/creatinine ratio	>20	<10-20	<10-20
Renal size by ultrasound	Normal	Normal	Normal or ↑
Radionuclide renal scan	↓ uptake ↓ excretion	Uptake OK ↓ excretion	Uptake OK ↓ excretion

$$*\text{FENa} = 100 \times \frac{\text{Urine Na}^+/\text{Plasma Na}^+}{\text{Urine creatinine/Plasma creatinine}}$$ (Normal FENa is 1%-2%)

$$\dagger\text{RFI} = \frac{\text{Urine Na}^+}{\text{Urine creatinine/Serum creatinine}}$$

CALCULATION OF CREATININE CLEARANCE (CLcr)

- Male CLcr $= \dfrac{(140 - \text{Age [years]}) \times \text{Weight (kg)}}{\text{Serum creatinine (mg/dl)} \times 72}$
- For women, use the equation for men and multiply the result by 0.85
- Normal creatinine clearance is ~100 ml/min

I

EVALUATION OF HEMATURIA

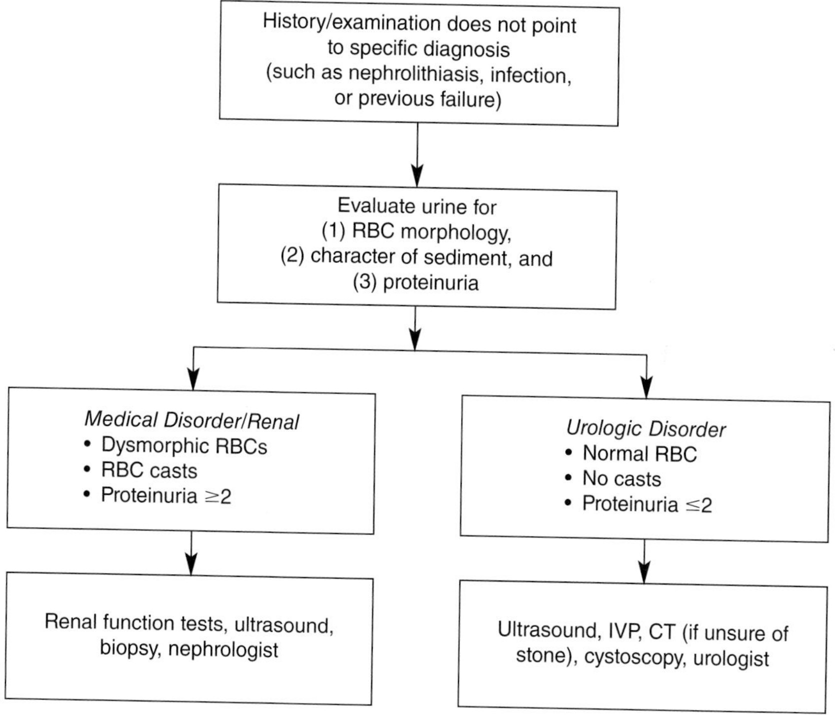

Fig. I-1

Reference

1. Zarich S, Fang LS, Diamond JR. Fractional excretion of sodium. Exceptions to its diagnostic value. Arch Intern Med 145:108, 1985.

APPENDIX

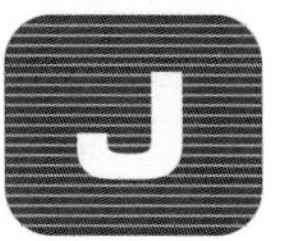

HEMATOLOGY

J

DIFFERENTIAL DIAGNOSIS FOR ANEMIA

Table J-1

Microcytic (MCV <81 μm³)	Normocytic (MCV 81 to 100 μm³): High reticulocyte count*	Normocytic (MCV 81 to 100 μm³): Normal or ↓ reticulocytes	Macrocytic (MCV >100 μm³)
• Low iron RDW >14% • Thalassemia RDW <14% • Chronic inflammation • Sideroblastic anemia • Lead poisoning • Vitamin B6 deficiency	• Subacute or chronic blood loss • Autoimmune hemolysis • Cardiac valves • DIC or HUS • Enzyme deficient G6PD • Spherocytosis • Hemoglobinopathy (such as sickle cell disease)	• Acute blood loss • Chronic disease • Renal insufficiency • Bone marrow suppression (from medications, viral infections, or cancer)	• Folate/B12 deficiency • Liver disease • Hypothyroidism

*Reticulocyte count $\times \frac{\text{Measured hematocrit}}{\text{Normal hematocrit}}$

SICKLE CELL DISEASE

Diagnostic Studies

- A routine Hb test is recommended in most cases to assess the severity o change of anemia.
- White blood cell count often will have elevated results because of sickle crisi alone.
- Obtain a CXR and pulse oximetry if the patient has a cough, shortness of breath or fever.
- Evaluate for crisis precipitant (such as infection or dehydration).
- Consider a reticulocyte count if aplastic crisis is suspected. Mean reticulocyte count for sickle cell patients is 12%; in aplastic crisis it may be <3% to 5%.
- Urine specific gravity is not a useful test for dehydration, because it may be low from isosthenuria (inability to concentrate urine).

Admission Criteria

- Acute chest syndrome—pain/pulmonary infiltrate from infection or pulmonary infarction
- Stroke, priapism, serious bacterial infection, aplastic crisis, hypoxia, acidosis
- Unable to take fluids orally or inadequate pain control in the ED
- Pregnancy, patients with uncertain diagnoses, persistently abnormal vital signs

Managing Complications

Table J-2

Symptom	Treatment
Abdominal pain	• Patients with sickle cell disease have an increased risk of developing cholecystitis, mesenteric ischemia, or perforated viscus. Splenic sequestration is rare in adults. Consider CT scan, ultrasound, and surgical consultation (especially if pain is not typical of normal crisis).
Aplastic crisis	• Exclude reversible causes (medications) and transfuse for severe anemia (Hb <6 to 7 g/dl) or cardiopulmonary distress.
Pain crisis	• Administer O_2 at 2 to 4 L. • Give IV one-half NS at 150 to 200 ml/hr (if mild pain, ± hydration po). • Administer IV narcotics titrated to pain relief (po if mild pain).
Priapism	• Treat as pain crisis. • Exchange transfusion to keep HbS <30% before surgery. • Obtain a urology consultation for aspiration or alternate procedure.
Acute chest syndrome	• Admit all patients with a pulmonary infiltrate to the hospital. • Pulmonary infarct caused by vasoocclusion may become infected. • Treat as pain crisis with IV antibiotics. Do not anticoagulate. • Avoid angiography, because it worsens sickling.
Sepsis	• Admit all patients with invasive bacterial infections.
Sickle cell stroke	• Obtain CT ± spinal tap, and administer IV NS. • Exchange transfusion—keep HbS <30% of total blood volume.

J

HYPERVISCOSITY SYNDROME

Causes

- Increased serum proteins with sludging and decreased circulation
- Common causes include macroglobulinemia, myeloma, and CML

Clinical Features

- Fatigue, headache, and somnolence
- Decreased vision, seizure, deafness, MI, and CHF
- Retinal bleed and exudates

Diagnosis

- WBC (especially blasts) >100,000 cells/mm^3
- Increased serum viscosity—Ostwald viscometer
- Serum protein electrophoresis

Management

- IV NS, plasmapheresis
- Two-unit phlebotomy with NS, packed red blood cell replacement

BLOOD PRODUCTS

Table J-3

Product	Volume (ml)	Indications	Comments
Whole blood (WB)	400-500	• Massive transfusion in acute blood loss	• RBCs plus plasma • Rarely used
Packed red blood cells	250-350	• Increase O_2 carrying capacity if there is evidence or risk of end-organ ischemia • Maintain volume and O_2 capacity if acute blood loss • *Not* indicated solely to maintain target Hb/hematocrit or for volume repletion (isovolemic anemia is well tolerated if no cardiac, pulmonary, or cerebrovascular disease)	• Massive transfusion may cause hypothermia, low Ca^{2+}, high K^+, and dilutional thrombocytopenia • For critically ill patients, restrictive transfusion practice (such as a Hb of 7-9 mg/dl versus 10-12 mg/dl) may reduce mortality • In acute MI, transfusion to hematocrit 30%-33% may reduce mortality

Table J-3—cont'd

Product	Volume (ml)	Indications	Comments
Platelet concentrates	200-250 (per 5-unit to 6-unit pool)	• Bleeding and platelets <100,000/ml • Procedure and platelets <50,000/ml • Prophylactic if platelets <10,000/ml • Bleeding and qualitatively abnormal platelets (for example, uremia, ASA) • Serious bleeding after GP IIb/IIIa inhibitor therapy	• Six-unit pool should raise count by 50,000-60,000/ml, less if alloimmunized • May support platelets in patients refractory to SDPs • Contraindicated in consumptive coagulopathy (HIT, HUS/TTP, HELLP)
Single-donor platelets	200-250	• Same as platelet concentrates but fewer donor exposures (alloimmunization, infection)	• No data to support routine use for alloimmunization prevention
Fresh frozen plasma	200-250	• Bleeding if multiple factor deficiency (massive transfusion, liver disease) • DIC or TTP • Reversal of warfarin • Factor XI deficiency	• Contains factors II, VII, IX, X, XI, XII, and XIII • Dose: 15 ml/kg for massive transfusion, 3-5 ml/kg to reverse warfarin (titrate to PT)
Cryoprecipitate	100-200 (per 10-unit pool)	• Replacement of fibrinogen when acutely low (<100 mg/dl) or qualitatively abnormal • Serious bleeding after thrombolytic therapy • Factor VIII or VWF replacement if concentrate is not available	• Contains factor VIII, VWF, fibronectin, and fibrinogen • Fibrinogen in 10-unit pool equates to 4 units FFP (but is roughly 2% of the volume)

Compiled from Churchill WH. Transfusion therapy. In Federman D, ed. Scientific American Medicine. New York: Scientific American, 2001; Hebert PC, Wells G, Blajchman MA, et al. A multicenter, randomized, controlled clinical trial of transfusion requirements in critical care. Transfusion requirements in critical care investigators, Canadian Critical Care Trials Group. N Engl J Med 340:409, 1999; Wu WC, Rathore SS, Wang Y, et al. Blood transfusion in elderly patients with acute myocardial infarction. N Engl J Med 345:1230, 2001; and TRAPS Group. Leukocyte reduction and UV irradiation to platelets to prevent alloimmunization and refractoriness to platelet transfusions. N Engl J Med 337:1861, 1997.

TYPES OF RED BLOOD CELLS

- Packed red blood cells (PRBCs)
  - Most plasma has been removed
  - For general use
- Leukopoor[1]
  - Most WBCs have been removed
  - Used if there have been previous febrile transfusion reactions or multiple transfusions
  - May prevent CMV infection
- Washed
  - Plasma has been virtually removed
  - Used if there have been previous allergic reactions
- Irradiated
  - Hematopoietic progenitor cells are killed to prevent graft-versus-host disease
  - For related donors or patients with suppressed marrow
- Emergency release (no crossmatch)
  - O-negative in women of childbearing age, and O-positive in all others (if O-negative is not available)
  - Immune reaction in 5% if ABO compatible but antibody screen incomplete

TRANSFUSION RISKS

Table J-4

Adverse Outcome*	Risk Per Unit Transfused
Hepatitis B	1:220,000
Hepatitis C	1:600,000
HTLV 1 or 2	1:600,000
HIV 1 or 2	1:1,800,000
Bacterial contamination—platelets Bacterial contamination—red blood cells	1:25,000 1:250,000
Fatal hemolytic transfusion reaction	1:500,000
Fatal acute lung injury (ARDS)	1:3,000,000

Compiled from Goodnough LT, Brecher ME, Kanter MH, et al. Transfusion medicine. First of two parts—blood transfusion. N Engl J Med 340:438, 1999; and Busch MP, Kleinman SH, Nemo GJ. Current and emerging infectious risks of blood transfusions. JAMA 289:959, 2003.

*Emerging risks include variant Creutzfeldt-Jakob disease, West Nile virus, and *Trypanosoma cruzi.*

TRANSFUSION REACTIONS

Acute Hemolytic Reaction

- One to four events per million units transfused
- Preformed antibodies against major RBC antigens cause acute intravascular hemolysis
- Symptoms: fever, chills, back pain, N/V, hypotension, renal failure, DIC
- Treatment
  - Stop transfusion immediately
  - Give diphenhydramine and acetaminophen ± hydrocortisone 50 to 100 mg IV
  - Maintain urine output with alkalinized IVF
  - Alert blood bank and send product plus samples for Coombs, bilirubin, LDH, free Hb, and DIC screens

Delayed Hemolytic Reaction

- One event per 1000 units transfused
- One to 25 days after transfusion
- Symptoms similar to acute reaction but often less severe
- Treatment: same as acute reaction if warranted by symptoms

Nonhemolytic Febrile Reaction

- Common (one to two events per 100 units transfused)
- Platelets >PRBCs
- Onset ≤5 hours of transfusion
- Fever may be only 1° to 2° F above normal
- Other symptoms: chills, respiratory distress (usually self-limited)
- Differential diagnosis: hemolytic reaction, sepsis, contaminated blood product
- Treatment
  - Stop transfusion and send back to blood bank
  - Blood cultures
  - Antipyretics ± meperidine 50 to 75 mg IV
  - Consider leukocyte-reduced products if patient has had two or more febrile reactions

Allergic Reaction

- Most common reaction (three to four events per 100 units transfused)
- Immune response to plasma proteins
- Symptoms: pruritus, urticaria, bronchospasm, anaphylaxis (more likely if recipient is IgA deficient)
- Treatment
  - Diphenhydramine
  - Unnecessary to stop transfusion if mild, but consider slowing infusion
  - If severe or recurrent reactions, use washed RBCs

Transfusion-Related Acute Lung Injury (TRALI)

- ARDS-like condition
- One to 10 events per 100,000 units transfused, with 3% to 5% mortality
- Bilateral pulmonary infiltrates within 4 hours of transfusion
- Diagnosis of exclusion (assess for CHF and sepsis)
- Treatment is same as for ARDS; usually responds within 24 hours

Posttransfusion Purpura (PTP)

- Rare
- Severe thrombocytopenia 5 to 10 days after transfusion (usually RBC transfusion)
- Caused by antiplatelet alloantibodies

HEPARIN-INDUCED THROMBOCYTOPENIA[2,3]

Type I: Nonimmune Mechanism

- Platelets rarely <100,000/ml
- Occurs in ~30% of patients given heparin
- Onset 1 to 2 days after heparin exposure
- Resolves spontaneously without complications

Type II: Immune-Mediated Platelet Activation

- Less common than type I
- Platelets usually <100,000/ml
- Onset is typically 4 to 8 days after heparin exposure, but may be delayed up to 3 weeks after heparin is discovered, more rapidly if previous exposure
- Persists until all heparin is stopped, including LMWH and heparin-coated catheters

HIT With Thrombosis Syndrome (HITTS)

- HIT type II with thrombotic or thromboembolic complications (30% to 50% of cases)

Clinical Manifestations (Type II)[4]

- Early
  - Increasing heparin resistance
  - Erythematous plaques or skin necrosis at heparin injection site
  - Pseudoembolism: fever, dyspnea, ↑ HR or BP, cardiopulmonary arrest, or transient global amnesia 5 to 30 minutes after heparin bolus
- Thrombocytopenia: typically 30,000/ml to 70,000/ml or a 50% decrease from baseline (consider alternative diagnosis if platelets <20,000/ml)

- Thromboembolism (white clot syndrome)
  - Venous >arterial by 4:1
  - Events commonly occur at site of preexisting pathology (such as from surgery or a vascular device)
    - Venous: DVT, PE, limb gangrene, cerebral sinus thrombosis
    - Arterial: limb ischemia, stroke, MI, graft closure, mesenteric or renal infarction
    - Other: intracardiac thrombus, prosthetic valve thrombosis, A-V fistula occlusion
    - Hemorrhage: uncommon unless infarcted tissue (such as adrenal)

Diagnosis

1. Timing: onset 4 to 8 days after heparin exposure or within 8 to 10 hours if previous heparin exposure.[5]
2. Resolves after heparin is discontinued.
3. Exclusion of other causes.
4. Confirm with serotonin release assay, ELISA (highly sensitive, less specific), or heparin-induced platelet aggregation (highly specific, less sensitive). A negative result on two tests usually excludes diagnosis.

J

Differential Diagnosis

- Sepsis, DIC/TTP, HELLP
- Immune: ITP, SLE, after transfusion
- Ethanol, splenomegaly
- Infections: HIV, EBV, hepatitis
- Drugs: Chemotherapy, quinidine, NSAIDs, sulfa, GP IIb/IIIa inhibitors
- Marrow suppression
- Pseudothrombocytopenia (platelet clumping): Examine smear and redraw in citrate or heparin-containing tube

Treatment (HIT Type II or HITTS)

1. Discontinue *all* heparin (including LMW heparin and line flushes). Platelet count should rise in 24 to 48 hours, with return to normal by 4 to 5 days.
2. Avoid platelet transfusion; it may induce thromboembolic complications.
3. Given the high risk of late thromboembolic complications, consider prophylactic anticoagulation with lepirudin or argatroban unless the patient has a high risk of bleeding.
4. If HITTS is established, use lepirudin or argatroban as an anticoagulant. Treatment should continue until thrombosis resolves and platelet count normalizes or a therapeutic level of warfarin is attained.
5. With acute HITTS, do not give warfarin without concomitant therapy with lepirudin or argatroban, because it may predispose the patient to venous limb gangrene. Delay starting warfarin until the platelet count reaches >100,000/ml.

COAGULATION DISORDERS

Table J-5 Causes of a Prolonged PT or aPTT

	aPTT Normal	aPTT Prolonged
PT Normal	If bleeding: • Platelet disorder (quantitative or qualitative) • Von Willebrand disease • Factor XIII deficiency • Nonspecific vascular	Inherited: • Deficiency of VWF or factors VIII, IX, XI, or XII* Acquired: • Heparin or direct thrombin inhibitor (lepirudin, argatroban) • Lupus anticoagulant (LAC)* • Inhibitor of VWF or factors VIII, IX, XI, or XII* See Fig. J-1
PT Prolonged	Inherited: • Factor VII deficiency Acquired: • Vitamin K deficiency • Warfarin (iatrogenic or self-inflicted) • Liver disease • Inhibitor of factor VII (very rare)	Inherited: • Deficiency of prothrombin, fibrinogen, or factors V or X • Combined factor deficiency Acquired: • Liver disease • DIC • Excessive heparin/warfarin • Inhibitor of prothrombin (LAC), fibrinogen, or factors V or X (X is associated with amyloidosis)

Reproduced with permission from Coutre S. Acquired inhibitors of coagulation. In Basow DS, ed. UpToDate. UpToDate: Waltham, MA, 2008. Copyright 2008, UpToDate, Inc. For more information visit *www.uptodate.com*.
*Most lupus anticoagulant and factor XII deficiency are not associated with clinical bleeding.

Evaluation of an Isolated, Prolonged aPTT

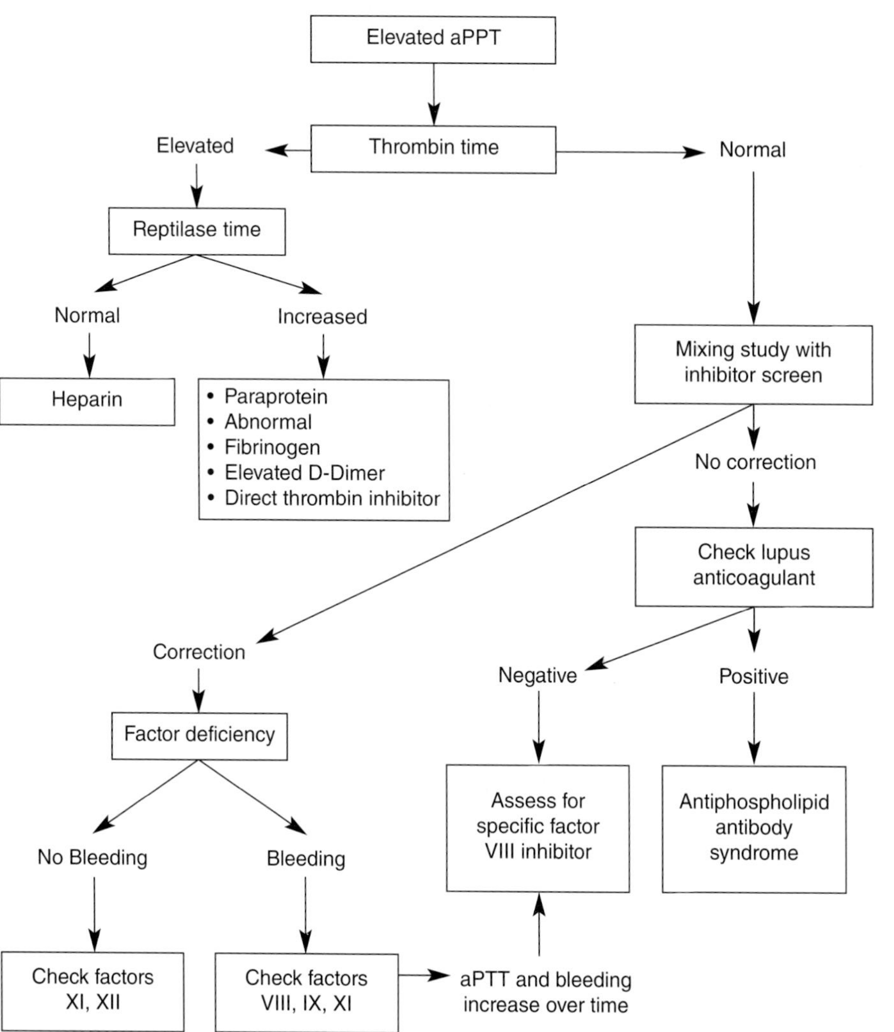

Fig. J-1

J

ACQUIRED INHIBITORS

Factor VIII Inhibitors[6]

- Causes
- Pregnancy or postpartum
- Drug reactions
- Connective tissue disease or antiphospholipid antibody syndrome
- Malignancy (solid tumors)
- Clinical
- Prolonged aPTT, normal PT
- May cause severe bleeding from GU and GI tracts into soft tissues (hematomas)
- Alternatively, may have hypercoagulable state (for example, antiphospholipid antibody syndrome)
- Workup
  1. Exclude heparin (prolonged thrombin time, normal reptilase time; aPTT should correct with protamine)
  2. Mixing studies (aPTT should not correct)
  3. Rule out lupus anticoagulant
  4. Quantify inhibitor with Bethesda assay
- Treatment for bleeding
- Control bleeding with DDAVP or recombinant factor VIII for low-titer inhibitor, otherwise use porcine factor VIII (if no porcine inhibitor), activated prothrombin complex concentrate (Autoplex, FEIBA), or recombinant factor VIIa concentrate
- Prednisone ± cyclophosphamide or intravenous immunoglobulin (IVIG) to eliminate inhibitor

Factor II (Prothrombin) Inhibitors

- Cause: most commonly seen in patients with antiphospholipid antibody syndrome who present with bleeding
- Clinical
  - PT and aPTT prolonged
  - ± LAC
  - Bleeding may be severe
- Treatment
  - FFP
  - Other treatments listed for acquired factor VIII inhibitors

Factor V Inhibitors

- Cause: most arise after exposure to fibrin glue or bovine thrombin
- Clinical
  - Prolonged aPTT and PT, but normal thrombin time
  - Bleeding variable

- Diagnosis: mixing/inhibitors studies
- Treatment for bleeding
  - Platelet transfusions and plasma exchange
  - Immunosuppression not usually needed

MANAGING PATIENTS WITH HIGH INR VALUES

Table J-6

Indications	Treatment*†
INR above the therapeutic range but <5, no significant bleeding	Lower the dose or omit the next dose. Resume therapy at a lower dose when INR is therapeutic. If INR is only slightly above therapeutic values, dose reduction may not be needed.
INR >5 but <9, no significant bleeding	1. Omit the next dose or two, monitor INR more frequently, and resume therapy at a lower dose when INR is therapeutic. 2. Alternatively, omit a dose and give vitamin K1 (1-2.5 mg orally) especially if the patient is at increased risk for bleeding. 3. If a patient requires rapid reversal before urgent surgery, give vitamin K1 (2-4 mg po). If INR remains high at 24 hours, give an additional dose of vitamin K1 (1-2 mg po)
INR >9, no significant bleeding	Omit warfarin; give vitamin K1 (3-5 mg po); closely monitor INR; if INR is not substantially reduced in 24-48 hours, monitor INR more often, giving additional vitamin K1 if necessary. Resume therapy at a lower dose when INR is therapeutic.
INR >20, serious bleeding	Omit warfarin; give vitamin K1 (10 mg by slow IV infusion), supplemented with fresh plasma or prothrombin complex concentrate, depending on urgency; vitamin K1 injections can be repeated every 12 hours.
Life-threatening bleeding	Omit warfarin; give prothrombin complex concentrate with vitamin K1 (10 mg by slow IV infusion). Repeat if necessary, depending on the INR.

From Baumann MH, Strange C, Heffner JE, et al. Management of spontaneous pneumothorax: an American College of Chest Physicians Delphi consensus statement. Chest 119:590-602, 2001.

*If continued warfarin therapy is indicated after high doses of vitamin K1, heparin may be administered until the effects of vitamin K1 are reversed and the patient becomes responsive to warfarin.

†All recommendations are grade 2c, which means (1) the risk-to-benefit ratio is unclear, (2) supporting evidence is derived from observational studies, and (3) the strength of the recommendation is very weak, and other alternatives may be equally reasonable.

MANAGEMENT OF BLEEDING IN PATIENTS ON DIALYSIS

- Direct pressure in bleeding from shunt (dialysis unit will have shunt clamps)
- DDAVP 0.3 μg/kg in 50 ml NS IV over 30 minutes
- Consider protamine IV if recent dialysis

CAUSES OF ABNORMAL RESULTS FROM BLEEDING TESTS

Table J-7

Lab Value	Causes
Thrombocytopenia ↓ platelet count (<150,000/ml)	Heparin, ↓ platelet production, splenic sequestration, platelet destruction (such as from drugs, collagen vascular disease, ITP, DIC, TTP, or HUS)
Platelet dysfunction (with normal count)	Adhesion defects (such as from von Willebrand disease) or aggregation defects (such as thrombasthenia), renal failure
↑ BT (>9 minutes)	All platelet disorders, DIC, ITP, uremia, liver failure, aspirin
↑ PTT (>35 seconds)	Coagulation pathway defects (common factors II, V, X, intrinsic VIII, IX, XI, XII), DIC, liver failure, heparin
↑ PT (>12-13 seconds)	Coagulation pathway defects (common factors II, V, X, extrinsic VII) DIC, liver failure, warfarin
↑ TT (>8-10 seconds)	DIC, liver failure or uremia, heparin
↓ fibrinogen, ↑ FSP	ITP, liver failure, DIC

References

1. Heddle NM, Blajchman MA. The leukodepletion of cellular blood products in the prevention of HLA-alloimmunization and refractoriness to allogeneic platelet transfusions. Blood 85:603, 1995.
2. Brieger DB, Mak KH, Kottke-Marchant K, et al. Heparin-induced thrombocytopenia. J Am Coll Cardiol 31:1449, 1998.
3. Warkentin TE. Heparin-induced thrombocytopenia: pathogenesis and management. Br J Haematol 121:535, 2003.
4. Warkentin TE. Clinical presentation of HIT. Semin Hematol 35:9, 1998.
5. Warkentin TE, Kelton JG. Temporal aspects of heparin-induced thrombocytopenia. N Engl J Med 344:1286, 2001.
6. Bossi P, Cabane J, Ninet J, et al. Acquired hemophilia due to factor VIII inhibitors in 34 patients. Am J Med 105:400, 1998.

APPENDIX

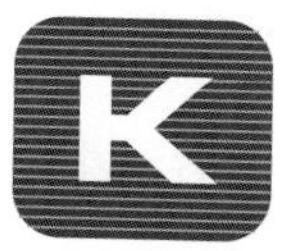

INFECTIOUS DISEASES

K

COMPARISON OF ANTIMICROBIAL SPECTRA

The information provided here is generalized. There are major differences among countries, areas, and hospitals, depending on antibiotic usage patterns. Verify usage patterns for the location. The most common microbes are listed in bold.

Table K-1 Penicillins, Carbapenems, Aztreonam, and Fluoroquinolones

	Penicillins		Antistaphylococcal Penicillins			Amino Penicillins			Antipseudomonal Penicillins				Carbapenems					Fluoroquinolones						
Organisms	**Penicillin G**	**Penicillin V**	**Methicillin**	**Nafcillin/Oxacillin**	**Cloxacillin[NUS]/Dicloxacillin**	**Ampicillin/Amoxicillin**	**Amoxicillin/Clavulanate**	**Ampicillin/Sulbactam**	**Ticarcillin**	**Ticarcillin/Clavulanate**	**Piperacillin/Tazobactam**	**Piperacillin**	**Doripenem**	**Ertapenem**	**Imipenem**	**Meropenem**	**Aztreonam**	**Ciprofloxacin**	**Ofloxacin**	**Pefloxacin[NUS]**	**Levofloxacin**	**Moxifloxacin**	**Gemifloxacin**	**Gatifloxacin**
Gram-positive																								
Streptococcus groups A, B, C, and G	+	+	+	+	+	+	+	+	+	+	+	+	+	+	+	+	0	±	±	0	+	+	+	+
Streptococcus pneumoniae	+	+	+	+	+	+	+	+	+	+	+	+	+	+	+	+	0	±	±	0	+	+	+	+
Viridans streptococcus	±	±	±	±	±	±	±	±	±	±	±	±	+	+	+	+	0	0	0		+	+	+	+
Streptococcus milleri	+	+	+	+	+	+	+	+	+	+	+	+	+	+	+	+	0	0	0		+	+	+	+
Enterococcus faecalis	+	+	0	0	0	+	+	+	±	±	+	+	±	0	+	±	0	*	*	0	+	+	+	+
Enterococcus faecium	±	±	0	0	0	+	+	+	±	±	±	±	0	0	±	0	0	0	0	0	0	±	±	±
***Staphylococcus aureus* (MSSA)**	**0**	**0**	**+**	**+**	**+**	**0**	**+**	**+**	**0**	**+**	**+**	**0**	**+**	**+**	**+**	**+**	**0**	**+**	**+**	**+**	**+**	**+**	**+**	**+**
***Staphylococcus aureus* (MRSA)**	**0**	**0**	**0**	**0**	**0**	**0**	**0**	**0**	**0**	**0**	**0**	**0**	**0**	**0**	**0**	**0**	**0**	**0**	**0**	**0**	**0**	**±**	**±**	**±**
***Staphylococcus aureus* (CA-MRSA)**	**0**	**0**	**0**	**0**	**0**	**0**	**0**	**0**	**0**	**0**	**0**	**0**	**0**	**0**	**0**	**0**	**0**	**±**			**±**	**±**	**±**	**±**
Staphylococcus epidermidis	0	0	+	+	+	0	0	0	±	±	+	0	+	+	+	+	0	+	+	+	+	+	+	+

From Gilbert DN, Moellering RC Jr, Eliopoulos GM, et al, eds. The Sanford Guide to Antimicrobial Therapy 2010. Sperryville, VA: Antimicrobial Therapy, 2010.

*Most strains are lacking clinical trials or are 30% to 60% susceptible, can be used in UTI, not in systemic infection.

+, Usually effective clinically or >60% susceptible; ±, clinical trials lacking or 30% to 60% susceptible; *0,* not effective clinically or <30% susceptible; *blank,* data not available; *CA-MRSA,* community-associated methicillin-resistant *S. aureus; MRSA,* methicillin-resistant *S. aureus; MSSA,* methicillin-sensitive *S. aureus; NUS,* not available in the United States.

Table K-1 Penicillins, Carbapenems, Aztreonam, and Fluoroquinolones

	Penicillins		Antistaphylococcal Penicillins			Amino Penicillins			Antipseudomonal Penicillins				Carbapenems					Fluoroquinolones						
Organisms	**Penicillin G**	**Penicillin V**	**Methicillin**	**Nafcillin/Oxacillin**	**Cloxacillin[NUS]/Dicloxacillin**	**Ampicillin/Amoxicillin**	**Amoxicillin/Clavulanate**	**Ampicillin/Sulbactam**	**Ticarcillin**	**Ticarcillin/Clavulanate**	**Piperacillin/Tazobactam**	**Piperacillin**	**Doripenem**	**Ertapenem**	**Imipenem**	**Meropenem**	**Aztreonam**	**Ciprofloxacin**	**Ofloxacin**	**Pefloxacin[NUS]**	**Levofloxacin**	**Moxifloxacin**	**Gemifloxacin**	**Gatifloxacin**
Corynebacterium jeikeium	0	0	0	0	0	0	0	0	0	0		0		0	0		0	0	0					
Listeria monocytogenes	+	0	0	0	0	+		+	+			+	+	±	+	+	0	+	0	0	+	+	+	+
Gram-negative																								
Neisseria gonorrhoeae	0	0	0	0	0	0	+	+	+	+	+	+	+	+	+	+	+	+†	+†	+†	+†	+†		+†
Neisseria meningitidis	+	0	0	0	0	+	+	+	+	+	+	+	+	+	+	+	+	+	+	+	+	+		+
Moraxella catarrhalis	0	0	0	0	0	0	+	+	0	+	+	±	+	+	+	+	+	+	+	+	+	+	+	+
Haemophilus influenzae	0	0	0	0	0	±	+	+	±	+	+	±	+	+	+	+	+	+	+	+	+	+	+	+
Escherichia coli	0	0	0	0	0	±	+	+	±	+	+	+	+	+	+	+	+	+	+	+	+	+	+	+
Klebsiella sp.	0	0	0	0	0	0	+	+	0	+	+	+	+	+	+	+	+	+	+	+	+	+	+	+
Escherichia coli/Klebsiella sp. ESBL+	0	0	0	0	0	0	0	0	0	±	±	0	+	+	+	+	0	+	+	+	+	+	+	+
Escherichia coli/Klebsiella sp. KPC+	0	0	0	0	0	0	0	0	0	0	0	0	0	0	±	±	0							
Enterobacter sp.	0	0	0	0	0	0	0	0	+	+	+	+	+	+	+	+	+	+	+	+	+	+		+

†Prevalence of quinolone-resistant gonococcus varies worldwide from <1% to 30.9% in Europe and >90% in Taiwan. In the United States in 2006, it was 6.7% overall, and, as a result, the CDC no longer recommends fluoroquinolones for first-line therapy of gonococcus. (Centers for Disease Control and Prevention. Update to CDC's sexually transmitted diseases treatment guidelines, 2006: fluoroquinolones no longer recommended for treatment of gonococcal infections. MMWR Morb Mortal Wkly Rep 56:332-336, 2007; Martin IM, Hoffmann S, Ison CA, et al. European Surveillance of Sexually Transmitted Infections (ESSTI): the first combined antimicrobial susceptibility data for *Neisseria gonorrhoeae* in Western Europe. J Antimicrob Chemother 58:587-593, 2006; Hsueh PR, Tseng SP, Teng LJ, et al. High prevalence of ciprofloxacin-resistant *Neisseria gonorrhoeae* in Northern Taiwan. Clin Infect Dis 40:188-192, 2005; Wang SA, Harvey AB, Conner SM, et al. Antimicrobial resistance for *Neisseria gonorrhoeae* in the United States, 1988-2003: the spread of fluoroquinolone resistance. Ann Intern Med 147:81-88, 2007).

+, Usually effective clinically or >60% susceptible; ±, clinical trials lacking or 30% to 60% susceptible; *0,* not effective clinically or <30% susceptible; *blank,* data not available; *ESBL,* extended-spectrum beta-lactamase; *KPC, K. pneumonia* carbapenemase; NUS, not available in the United States.

Continued

Table K-1 Penicillins, Carbapenems, Aztreonam, and Fluoroquinolones—cont'd

	Penicillins		Antistaphylococcal Penicillins			Amino Penicillins			Antipseudomonal Penicillins				Carbapenems					Fluoroquinolones						
Organisms	Penicillin G	Penicillin V	Methicillin	Nafcillin/Oxacillin	Cloxacillin[NUS]/Dicloxacillin	Ampicillin/Amoxicillin	Amoxicillin/Clavulanate	Ampicillin/Sulbactam	Ticarcillin	Ticarcillin/Clavulanate	Piperacillin/Tazobactam	Piperacillin	Doripenem	Ertapenem	Imipenem	Meropenem	Aztreonam	Ciprofloxacin	Ofloxacin	Pefloxacin[NUS]	Levofloxacin	Moxifloxacin	Gemifloxacin	Gatifloxacin
Gram-negative—cont'd																								
Serratia sp.	0	0	0	0	0	0	0	0	+	+	+	0	+	+	+	+	+	+	+	+	+	+		+
Salmonella sp.	0	0	0	0	0	±	+	+	+	+	+	+	+	+	+	+		+	+	+	+	+		+
Shigella sp.	0	0	0	0	0	±	+	+	+	+	+	+	+	+	+	+	+	+	+	+	+	+		+
Proteus mirabilis	0	0	0	0	0	+	+	+	+	+	+	+	+	+	+	+	+	+	+	+	+	+		+
Proteus vulgaris	0	0	0	0	0	0	+	+	+	+	+	+	+	+	+	+	+	+	+	+	+	+	+	+
Providencia sp.	0	0	0	0	0	0	+	+	+	+	+	+	+	+	+	+	+	+	+	+	+	+		+
Morganella sp.	0	0	0	0	0	0	±	+	+	+	+	+	+	+	+	+	+	+	+	+	+	+		+
Citrobacter sp.	0	0	0	0	0	0	0	0	+	+	+	+	+	+	+	+	+	+	+	+	+	+		+
Aeromonas sp.	0	0	0	0	0	0	+	+	+	+	+	+	+	+	+	+	+	+	+		+	+		+
Acinetobacter sp.	0	0	0	0	0	0	0	+	0	±	±	0	±	0	±	±	0	±	±		±	±	±	±
Pseudomonas aeruginosa	**0**	**0**	**0**	**0**	**0**	**0**	**0**	**0**	**+**	**+**	**+**	**+**	**+**	**0**	**+**	**+**	**+**	**+**	**±**		**±**	**±**		**±**
Burkholderia (Pseudomonas) cepacia	0	0	0	0	0	0	0	0	0				±	0	0	+	0	0	0			0		0
Stenotrophomonas (Xanthomonas) maltophilia	0	0	0	0	0	0	0	0		±	±	±	0	0	0	0	0	0	0	0	±	+		
Yersinia enterocolitica	0	0	0	0	0	0	±	±	±	+		+	+		+		+	+	+	+	+	+		+
***Legionella* sp.**	**0**	**0**	**0**	**0**	**0**	**0**	**0**	**0**	**0**	**0**	**0**	**0**	**0**	**0**	**0**	**0**	**0**	**+**	**+**	**+**	**+**	**+**	**+**	**+**
Pasteurella multocida	+	+	0	0	0	+	+	+	+	+		+	+	+	+		+	+	+	+	+	+		+
Haemophilus ducreyi	+					0	+	+																

+, Usually effective clinically or >60% susceptible; ±, clinical trials lacking or 30% to 60% susceptible; *0,* not effective clinically or <30% susceptible; *blank,* data not available; *NUS,* not available in the United States.

Table K-1 Penicillins, Carbapenems, Aztreonam, and Fluoroquinolones—cont'd

Organisms	Penicillins		Antistaphylococcal Penicillins			Amino Penicillins			Antipseudomonal Penicillins				Carbapenems					Fluoroquinolones						
	Penicillin G	Penicillin V	Methicillin	Nafcillin/Oxacillin	Cloxacillin[NUS]/Dicloxacillin	Ampicillin/Amoxicillin	Amoxicillin/Clavulanate	Ampicillin/Sulbactam	Ticarcillin	Ticarcillin/Clavulanate	Piperacillin/Tazobactam	Piperacillin	Doripenem	Ertapenem	Imipenem	Meropenem	Aztreonam	Ciprofloxacin	Ofloxacin	Pefloxacin[NUS]	Levofloxacin	Moxifloxacin	Gemifloxacin	Gatifloxacin
Miscellaneous																								
Chlamydophila sp.	0	0	0	0	0	0	0	0	0	0	0	0	0	0	0	0	0	+	+	+	+	+	+	+
Mycoplasma pneumoniae	**0**	**0**	**0**	**0**	**0**	**0**	**0**	**0**	**0**	**0**	**0**	**0**	**0**	**0**	**0**	**0**	**0**	**+**	**+**	**+**	**+**	**+**	**+**	**+**
Anaerobes																								
Actinomyces	+	±	0	0	0	+	+	+				+		+	+		0	0	±			+		+
Bacteroides fragilis	**0**	**±**	**0**	**0**	**0**	**0**	**+**	**+**	**0**	**+**	**+**	**0**	**+**	**+**	**+**	**+**	**0**	**0**	**0**	**0**	**0**	**+**		**±**
Prevotella melaninogenica	+	0	0	0	0	+	+	+	+	+	+	+	+	+	+	+	0	0	±		+	+		+
Clostridium difficile	**+‡**							**+‡**				**+‡**	**+**	**+**	**+**	**+**	**0**	**0**			**0**	**0**		**0**
***Clostridium* (not *difficile*)**	**+**	**+**				**+**	**+**	**+**	**+**	**+**	**+**	**+**	**+**	**+**	**+**	**+**	**0**	**±**	**±**		**+**	**+**		**+**
Peptostreptococcus sp.	+	+	+	+	+	+	+	+	+	+	+	+	+	+	+	+	0	±	±		+	+		+

‡There is no clinical evidence that penicillins or fluoroquinolones are effective for *C. difficile* enterocolitis (but they may cover this organism in mixed intraabdominal and pelvic infections).

+, Usually effective clinically or >60% susceptible; ±, clinical trials lacking or 30% to 60% susceptible; *0*, not effective clinically or <30% susceptible; *blank*, data not available; *NUS*, not available in the United States.

K

Table K-2 Cephalosporins

												Oral Agents							
	1st Generation	2nd Generation			3rd and 4th Generations (including anti-MRSA)							1st Generation		2nd Generation			3rd Generation		
Organisms	Cefazolin	Cefotetan	Cefoxitin	Cefuroxime	Cefotaxime	Ceftizoxime	Ceftriaxone	Ceftobiprole	Ceftaroline	Ceftazidime	Cefepime	Cefadroxil	Cephalexin	Cefaclor/Loracarbef*	Cefprozil	Cefuroxime Axetil	Cefixime	Ceftibuten	Cefpodoxime/Cefdinir/Cefditoren
Gram-positive																			
Streptococcus groups A, B, C, and G	+	+	+	+	+	+	+	+	+	+	+	+	+	+	+	+	+	+	+
S. pneumoniae†	+	+	+	+	+	+	+	+	+	+†	+	+	+	+	+	+	+	±	+
Viridans streptococcus	+	+	+	+	+	+	+	+	+	±†	+	+	+	+	0	+	+	0	+
E. faecalis	0	0	0	0	0	0	0	+	+	0	0	0	0	0	0	0	0	0	0
***S. aureus* (MSSA)**	**+**	**+**	**+**	**+**	**+**	**+**	**+**	**+**	**+**	**±**	**+**	**+**	**+**	**+**	**+**	**+**	**0**	**0**	**+**
***S. aureus* (MRSA)**	**0**	**0**	**0**	**0**	**0**	**0**	**0**	**+**	**+**	**0**	**0**	**0**	**0**	**0**	**0**	**0**	**0**	**0**	**0**
***S. aureus* (CA-MRSA)**	**0**	**0**	**0**	**0**	**0**	**0**	**0**	**+**	**+**	**0**	**0**	**0**	**0**	**0**	**0**	**0**	**0**	**0**	**0**
S. epidermidis	±	±	±	±	±	±	±	+	+	±	±	±	±	±	±	±	0	0	±
C. jeikeium	0	0	0	0	0	0	0			0		0	0	0	0	0	0	0	
L. monocytogenes	**0**	**0**	**0**	**0**	**0**	**0**	**0**			**0**	**0**	**0**	**0**	**0**	**0**	**0**	**0**	**0**	**0**

From Gilbert DN, Moellering RC Jr, Eliopoulos GM, et al, eds. The Sanford Guide to Antimicrobial Therapy 2010. Sperryville, VA: Antimicrobial therapy, 2010.

*A 1-carbacephem is best classified as a cephalosporin.

†Ceftazidime is 8 to 16 times less active than cefotaxime/ceftriaxone, effective only against penicillin-sensitive strains (Barry AL, Brown SD, Novick WJ. In vitro activities of cefotaxime, ceftriaxone, ceftazidime, cefpirome, and penicillin against Streptococcus pneumoniae isolates. Antimicrob Agents Chemother 39:2193-2196, 1995). Oral cefuroxime, cefprozil, and cefpodoxime are most active in vitro versus resistant *S. pneumoniae* (Bradley JS, Kaplan SL, Klugman KP, et al. Consensus: management of infections in children caused by *Streptococcus pneumoniae* with decreased susceptibility to penicillin. Pediatr Infect Dis J 14:1037-1041, 1995).

+, Usually effective clinically or >60% susceptible; ±, clinical trials lacking or 30%-60% susceptible; *0,* not effective clinically or <30% susceptible; *blank,* data not available; *CA-MRSA,* community-associated methicillin-resistant *S. aureus; MRSA,* methicillin-resistant *S. aureus, MSSA,* methicillin-sensitive *S. aureus.*

Table K-2 Cephalosporins—cont'd

												Oral Agents							
	1st Generation	2nd Generation			3rd and 4th Generations (including anti-MRSA)							1st Generation		2nd Generation			3rd Generation		
Organisms	Cefazolin	Cefotetan	Cefoxitin	Cefuroxime	Cefotaxime	Ceftizoxime	Ceftriaxone	Ceftobiprole	Ceftaroline	Ceftazidime	Cefepime	Cefadroxil	Cephalexin	Cefaclor/Loracarbef*	Cefprozil	Cefuroxime Axetil	Cefixime	Ceftibuten	Cefpodoxime/Cefdinir/Cefditoren
Gram-negative																			
N. gonorrhoeae	+	±	±	±	±	±	+	+	+	±	+	0	0	±	±	±	+	±	+
N. meningitidis	**0**	**±**	**±**	**+**	**+**	**±**	**+**	**+**	**+**	**±**	**+**	**0**	**0**	**±**	**±**	**±**	**±**	**±**	
M. catarrhalis	±	+	+	+	+	+	+	+	+	+	+	0	0	±	+	+	+	+	+
H. influenzae	+	+	+	+	+	+	+	+	+	+	+		0	+	+	+	+	+	+
E. coli	**+**	**+**	**+**	**+**	**+**	**+**	**+**	**+**	**+**	**+**	**+**	**+**	**+**	**+**	**+**	**+**	**+**	**+**	**+**
Klebsiella sp.	+	+	+	+	+	+	+	+	+	+	+	+	+	+	+	+	+	+	
E. coli/Klebsiella sp. ESBL+	0	0	0	0	0	0	0	0	0	0	0	0	0	0	0	0	0	0	0
E. coli/Klebsiella sp. KPC+	0	0	0	0	0	0	0	0	0	0	0	0	0	0	0	0	0	0	0
Enterobacter sp.	0	±	0	±	+	+	+	+	+	+	+	0	0	0	0	0	0	±	0
Serratia sp.	0	+	0	0	+	+	+	+	+	+	+	0	0	0	0	0	±	±	0
Salmonella sp.					+	+	+	+	+	+	+	0	0				+	+	+
Shigella sp.					+	+	+			+	+	0	0				+	+	+
Proteus mirabilis	+	+	+	+	+	+	+	+	+	+	+	+	+	+	+	+	+	+	+
Proteus vulgaris	0	+	+	+	+	+	+	+	+	+	+	0	0	0	0	0	+	+	±
Providencia sp.	0	+	+	0	+	+	+	+	+	+	+	0	0	0	0	+	+	+	
Morganella sp.	0	+	+	±	+	+	+	+	+	+	+	0	0	0	0	±	0	0	0
Citrobacter freundii	0	0	0	0	+	0	+			0	+	0	0	0	0	0	0	0	0
Citrobacter diversus	0	±	±	±	+	+	+	+	+	+	+	0	0	0	0		+	+	+
Citrobacter sp.	0	±	±	±	+	+	+	+	+	+	+		0	±	0	±	+	+	+

*A 1-carbacephem is best classified as a cephalosporin.

+, Usually effective clinically or >60% susceptible; ±, clinical trials lacking or 30%-60% susceptible; *0,* not effective clinically or <30% susceptible; *blank,* data not available; *ESBL,* extended-spectrum beta-lactamase; *KPC, K. pneumonia* carbapenemase.

Continued

K

Table K-2 Cephalosporins—cont'd

												Oral Agents							
	1st Generation	2nd Generation			3rd and 4th Generations (including anti-MRSA)							1st Generation		2nd Generation			3rd Generation		
Organisms	**Cefazolin**	**Cefotetan**	**Cefoxitin**	**Cefuroxime**	**Cefotaxime**	**Ceftizoxime**	**Ceftriaxone**	**Ceftobiprole**	**Ceftaroline**	**Ceftazidime**	**Cefepime**	**Cefadroxil**	**Cephalexin**	**Cefaclor/Loracarbef***	**Cefprozil**	**Cefuroxime Axetil**	**Cefixime**	**Ceftibuten**	**Cefpodoxime/Cefdinir/Cefditoren**
Gram-negative—cont'd																			
Aeromonas sp.	0	+	±	+	+	+	+	+	+	+	+						+	+	
Acinetobacter sp.	0	0	0	0	0	0	0	±		±	±	0	0	0	0	0	0	0	
Pseudomonas aeruginosa	**0**	**0**	**0**	**0**	**±**	**±**	**±**	**+**	**±**	**+**	**+**	**0**	**0**	**0**	**0**	**0**	**0**	**0**	**0**
Burkholderia (Pseudomonas) cepacia	0	0	0	0	±	±	±	0	0	+	±	0	0	0	0	0	0	+	
Stenotrophomonas (Xanthomonas) maltophilia	0	0	0	0	0	0	0	0	0	±	0	0	0	0	0	0	0	0	
Y. enterocolitica	0	±	±	±	+	+	+			±	+						+	+	
***Legionella* sp.**	**0**	**0**	**0**	**0**	**0**	**0**	**0**	**0**	**0**	**0**	**0**	**0**	**0**	**0**	**0**	**0**	**0**	**0**	**0**
P. multocida		+		+	+	+	+				+		0				+		+
H. ducreyi			+		+	+	+			+							+		
Anaerobes																			
Actinomyces						+	+												
B. fragilis	**0**	**±‡**	**+**	**0**	**0**	**±**	**0**	**0**	**0**	**0**	**0**		**0**	**0**	**0**	**0**	**0**	**0**	
Prevotella melaninogenica		+	+	+	+	+	±	±		+	0			+	+	+	+		
C. difficile			**0**		**0**	**0**		**0**			**0**								
***Clostridium* (not *difficile*)**		**+**	**+**	**+**	**+**	**+**	**+**	**+**		**+**					**+**	**+**	**0**		
Peptostreptococcus sp.		+	+	+	+	+	+	+		+	+		+	+	+	+	+		

*A 1-carbacephem is best classified as a cephalosporin.
‡Cefotetan is less active against *Bacteroides ovatus*, *B. distasonis*, and *B. thetaiotaomicron.*
+, Usually effective clinically or >60% susceptible; ±, clinical trials lacking or 30%-60% susceptible; *0*, not effective clinically or <30% susceptible; *blank*, data not available.

Table K-3 Other Antimicrobial Agents

Organisms	Gentamicin	Tobramycin	Amikacin	Chloramphenicol	Clindamycin	Erythromycin	Azithromycin	Clarithromycin	Telithromycin	Doxycycline	Minocycline	Tigecycline	Vancomycin	Teicoplanin[NUS]	Telavancin	Fusidic acid[NUS]	Trimethoprim	Trimethoprim-sulfamethoxazole	Nitrofurantoin	Fosfomycin	Rifampin	Metronidazole	Quinupristin/dalfopristin	Linezolid	Daptomycin	Colistimehtate (Colistin)
	Aminoglycosides					Macrolides			Ketolide	Tetracyclines		Glycylcycline	Glycopeptides/ Lipoglycopeptides						Uninary Tract Agents		Miscellaneous					
Gram-positive																										
Streptococcus groups A, B, C, and G	0	0	0	+	+	±	±	±	+	±	+	+	+	+	+	±	+	+*	+		+	0	+	+	+	0
S. pneumoniae	0	0	0	+	+	+	+	+	+	+	+	+	+	+	+	±	±	+	+		+	0	+	+	+†	0
E. faecalis	S	S	S	±	0	0	0	0	±	0	0	+	+	+	+	+	+	+*	+	+	±	0	0	+	+	0
E. faecium	S	0	0	±	0	0	0	0	0	0	0	+	±	±	+		0	0	+	±	0	0	+	+	+	0
***S. aureus* (MSSA)**	+	+	+	±	+	±	+	+	+	±	+	+	+	+	+	+	±	+	+		+	**0**	+	+	+	**0**
***S. aureus* (MRSA)**	**0**	**0**	**0**	**0**	**0**	**0**	**0**	**0**	**0**	±	±	+	+	+	+	+	±	+	+		+	**0**	+	+	+	**0**
***S. aureus* (CA-MRSA)**					±	±	±	±	±	+	+	+	+	+	+	+	+	+	+		+	**0**	+	+	+	**0**
S. epidermidis	±	±	±	0	0	±	0	0	0	0	0	+	+	±	+	+	+	±			+	0	+	+	+	0
C. jeikeium	0	0	0	0	0	0	0	0	0	0	0	+	+	+	+	+	0	0	0		+	0	+	+	+	0
L. monocytogenes	**S**	**S**	**S**	+		+	+	+	+	+	+	+	+	+	+		+	+			+	**0**	+	+	±	**0**

From Gilbert DN, Moellering RC Jr, Eliopoulos GM, et al, eds. The Sanford Guide to Antimicrobial Therapy 2010. Sperryville, VA: Antimicrobial Therapy, 2010.

Antimicrobials such as azithromycin have high tissue penetration, and some, such as clarithromycin, are metabolized to more active compounds, hence in vivo activity may exceed in vitro activity.

*Although active in vitro, trimethoprim-sulfamethoxazole is not clinically effective for group A *Streptococcus pharyngitis* or for infections caused by *E. faecalis.*

†Although active in vitro, daptomycin is not clinically effective for pneumonia caused by *S. pneumoniae.*

+, Usually effective clinically or >60% susceptible; ±, clinical trials lacking or 30%-60% susceptible; *0,* not effective clinically or <30% susceptible; *S,* potential synergy in combination with penicillin, ampicillin, vancomycin, or teicoplanin; *blank,* data not available; *CA-MRSA,* community-associated methicillin-resistant *S. aureus; MRSA,* methicillin-resistant *S. aureus; MSSA,* methicillin-sensitive *S. aureus; NUS,* not available in the United States.

Continued

Table K-3 Other Antimicrobial Agents—cont'd

	Aminoglycosides					Macrolides			Ketolide	Tetracyclines		Glycylcycline	Glycopeptides/Lipoglycopeptides						Urinary Tract Agents		Miscellaneous					
Organisms	**Gentamicin**	**Tobramycin**	**Amikacin**	**Chloramphenicol**	**Clindamycin**	**Erythromycin**	**Azithromycin**	**Clarithromycin**	**Telithromycin**	**Doxycycline**	**Minocycline**	**Tigecycline**	**Vancomycin**	**Teicoplanin[NUS]**	**Telavancin**	**Fusidic acid[NUS]**	**Trimethoprim**	**Trimethoprim-sulfamethoxazole**	**Nitrofurantoin**	**Fosfomycin**	**Rifampin**	**Metronidazole**	**Quinupristin/dalfopristin**	**Linezolid**	**Daptomycin**	**Colistimehtate (Colistin)**
Gram-negative																										
N. gonorrhoeae	0	0	0	+	0	±	±	±	+	±	±	+	0	0	0	+	0	±	+	+	+	0	+		0	0
N. meningitidis	**0**	**0**	**0**	**+**	**0**	**+**	**+**		**+**	**+**	**+**		**0**	**0**	**0**	**+**	**±**	**+**			**+**	**0**	**0**	**0**	**0**	**0**
M. catarrhalis	+	+	+	+	0	+	+	+	+	+	+	+						+			+	0	+	±	0	
H. influenzae	+	+	+	+	0	±	+	+	+	+	+	+					±	±			+	0	±	±	0	
Aeromonas	0			+						+	+	+	0	0	0			+			0	0			0	
E. coli	**+**	**+**	**+**	**+**	**0**	**0**	**0**	**0**	**0**	**+**	**+**	**+**	**0**	**0**	**0**	**0**	**+**	**±**	**+**	**+**	**0**	**0**	**0**	**0**	**0**	**+**
Klebsiella sp.	+	+	+	±	0	0	0	0	0	±	±	+	0	0	0	0	±	±	±	±	0	0	0	0	0	+
E. coli/Klebsiella sp. ESBL+	+	+	+	±	0	0	0	0	0	±	±	+	0	0	0	0	±	±			0	0	0	0	0	+
E. coli/Klebsiella sp. KPC+													0	0	0	0							0	0	0	+
Enterobacter sp.	+	+	+	0	0	0	0	0	0	0	0	+	0	0	0	0	±		±	±	0	0	0	0	0	+
Salmonella sp.				+	0	0	±	0	0	±	±	+	0	0	0	0	±	±	+		0	0	0	0	0	
Shigella sp.	+	+	+	+	0	0	±	0	0	±	±	+	0	0	0	0	±	±	+		0	0	0	0	0	
Serratia marcescens	+	+	+	0	0	0	0	0	0	0	0	+	0	0	0	0	0	±	0	±	0	0		0	0	0
Proteus vulgaris	+	+	+	±	0	0	0	0	0	0	0	±	0	0	0	0	0	0	0	±	0	0		0	0	0
Acinetobacter sp.	0	0	±	0	0	0	0	0	0	0	0	±	0	0	0	0	0	±			0	0		0	0	+
Pseudomonas aeruginosa	**+**	**+**	**+**	**0**	**0**	**0**	**0**	**0**	**0**	**0**	**0**	**0**	**0**	**0**	**0**	**0**	**0**	**0**	**0**		**0**	**0**	**0**	**0**	**0**	**+**

+, Usually effective clinically or >60% susceptible; ±, clinical trials lacking or 30%-60% susceptible; *0,* not effective clinically or <30% susceptible; *blank,* data not available; *ESBL,* extended-spectrum beta-lactamase; *KPC, K. pneumonia* carbapenemase; *NUS,* not available in the United States.

Table K-3 Other Antimicrobial Agents—cont'd

	Aminoglycosides				Macrolides			Ketolide	Tetracyclines		Glycylcycline	Glycopeptides/Lipoglycopeptides			Urinary Tract Agents					Miscellaneous					
Organisms	**Gentamicin**	**Tobramycin**	**Amikacin**	**Chloramphenicol**	**Clindamycin**	**Erythromycin**	**Azithromycin**	**Clarithromycin**	**Telithromycin**	**Doxycycline**	**Minocycline**	**Tigecycline**	**Vancomycin**	**Teicoplanin[NUS]**	**Telavancin**	**Fusidic acid[NUS]**	**Trimethoprim**	**Trimethoprim-sulfamethoxazole**	**Nitrofurantoin**	**Fosfomycin**	**Rifampin**	**Metronidazole**	**Quinupristin/dalfopristin**	**Linezolid**	**Daptomycin**	**Colistimethate (Colistin)**
Burkholderia (Pseudomonas) cepacia	0	0	0	+	0	0	0	0	0	0	±	±	0	0	0	0	+	+	0		0	0		0	0	0
Stenotrophomonas (Xanthomonas) maltophilia	0	0	0	+	0	0	0	0	0	0	0	+	0	0	0	0	0	+	0			0		0	0	±
Y. enterocolitica	+	+	+	+	0	0	0	0	0	0	0					0		+				0		0	0	
Francisella tularensis	+			+						+								+			+	0		0	0	
Brucella sp.	+			+	0	0	0	0	0	+	+		0	0	0		+	+			+	0		0	0	
***Legionella* sp.**						**+**	**+**	**+**	**+**	**+**	**+**	**+**				**±**	**+**	**+**				**0**			**0**	
H. ducreyi				+	+	+	+						0					±				0			0	
Vibrio vulnificus	±	±	±	+						+	+					0						0			0	
Miscellaneous																										
Chlamydophila sp.	0	0	0	+	±	+	+	+	+	+	+	+				0	0		0		+	0	+	+		
Mycoplasma pneumoniae	**0**	**0**	**0**	**+**	**0**	**+**	**+**	**+**	**+**	**+**	**+**	**+**				**0**						**0**	**+**	**0**		
Rickettsia sp.	0	0	0	+		±			+	+	+		0	0	0	0						0				
Mycobacterium avium			+				+	+		0	0	0										0	0	0		

+, Usually effective clinically or >60% susceptible; ±, clinical trials lacking or 30%-60% susceptible; *0*, not effective clinically or <30% susceptible; *blank*, data not available; *NUS*, not available in the United States.

Continued

Table K-3 Other Antimicrobial Agents—cont'd

	Aminoglycosides					Macrolides			Ketolide	Tetracyclines		Glycylcycline	Glycopeptides/ Lipoglycopeptides						Urinary Tract Agents		Miscellaneous					
Organisms	**Gentamicin**	**Tobramycin**	**Amikacin**	**Chloramphenicol**	**Clindamycin**	**Erythromycin**	**Azithromycin**	**Clarithromycin**	**Telithromycin**	**Doxycycline**	**Minocycline**	**Tigecycline**	**Vancomycin**	**Teicoplanin[NUS]**	**Telavancin**	**Fusidic acid[NUS]**	**Trimethoprim**	**Trimethoprim-sulfamethoxazole**	**Nitrofurantoin**	**Fosfomycin**	**Rifampin**	**Metronidazole**	**Quinupristin/dalfopristin**	**Linezolid**	**Daptomycin**	**Colistimethate (Colistin)**
Anaerobes																										
Actinomyces	0	0	0	+	+	+	+	+		+	+		+		+	+						0				
B. fragilis	**0**	**0**	**0**	**+**	**±**	**0**	**0**	**0**		**±**	**±**	**+**	**0**		**0**		**+**	**0**				**+**		**±**		
P. melaninogenica (B. melaninogenicus)	0	0	0	+	+		+	+		+	+	+	0		0	+						+	+			
C. difficile	**0**	**0**	**0**	**±**									**+**	**+**	**+**							**+**	**±**	**±**		
***Clostridium* (not *difficile*)‡**				**+**		**±**	**+**	**+**		**+**	**+**	**+**	**+**	**+**	**+**	**+**						**+**	**+**	**+**		
Peptostreptococcus sp.	0	0	0	+	+	±	+	±	+	+	+	+	+	+	+	+						+		+		

‡Vancomycin and metronidazole given po are active versus *C. difficile;* vancomycin given IV is not effective.

+, Usually effective clinically or >60% susceptible; ±, clinical trials lacking or 30%-60% susceptible; *0,* not effective clinically or <30% susceptible; *blank,* data not available; *NUS,* not available in the United States.

ACUTE FEVER AND FEVER OF UNKNOWN ORIGIN (FUO)

Table K-4 Cause of Acute Fever in IV Drug Users in the Emergency Department

Specific Infection/Cause*	Frequency
Pneumonia	38%
Viral, pharyngitis/bronchitis	21%
Endocarditis	13%
Pyrogen reaction or unexplained	10%
Cellulitis	5%
Varicella or Tuberculosis	3% each
Partially treated endocarditis or peritonitis	3%
Urinary infection or septic arthritis	2%
Osteomyelitis or GI bleed	1% each

Modified from Marantz PR, Linzer M, Feiner CJ, et al. Inability to predict diagnosis in febrile intravenous drug abusers. Ann Intern Med 106:823, 1987.
*No clinical data could exclude endocarditis; therefore admit all febrile IV drug users.

Table K-5 Causes of Acute Fever in Patients Aged 65 or Older in the Emergency Department (Serious Illness Prevalence = 76%*)

Specific Infection/Cause	Frequency
Pneumonia	25%
Urinary tract infection	22%
Sepsis/bacteremia	18%
Unknown	11%
Diverticulitis, colitis, or cholecystitis	8%
Bronchitis, pharyngitis, or sinusitis	7%
Cellulitis	7%
PE, meningitis, prostate, cancer, or GI bleed	5%
Dehydration, appendix, or bone	1% or less each

Modified from Marco CA, Schoenfeld CN, Hansen KN, et al. Fever in geriatric emergency patients: clinical features associated with serious illness. Ann Emerg Med 26:18, 1995.
*Although fever ≥103° F, RR ≥30, WBC ≥11,000, HR ≥120, and positive CXR results were associated with serious illness, 50% of patients with none of these features had serious illness defined as positive blood culture results, death, need for surgery, admitted for >3 days, or a return ED visit within 72 hours.

FEVER AND NEUTROPENIA

Fever is defined as a single oral temperature at or above 38.3° C (101° F) or at or above 38.0° C (100.4° F) for 1 hour or longer. Neutropenia is marked by a neutrophil count of less than 500 cells/mm^3, or less than 1000 cells/mm^3 with a predicted decrease to less than 500 cells/mm^3.

Table K-6 Clinical Score for Risk of Infection in Febrile Neutropenic Patients*

Symptom	Score
Absent or mild symptoms	5
Moderate symptoms	3
Normal blood pressure	5
Absent COPD	4
Solid tumor or no fungal infection	4
No dehydration	3
Outpatient onset of fever	3
Age <60 years	2

Modified from Klastersky J, Paesmans M, Rubenstein EB, et al. The Multinational Association for Supportive Care in Cancer risk index: A multinational scoring system for identifying low-risk febrile neutropenic cancer patients. J Clin Oncol 18:3038, 2000.

*A total of 21 or more signifies <10% probability of serious infection and potential to use less aggressive management options.

Table K-7 Empiric Antibiotic Choices for Adults With Febrile Neutropenia

Risk	Method	Antibiotic Choices
Low risk*	Oral	• Ciprofloxacin (Cipro) 750 mg po bid and amoxicillin with clavulanate potassium (Augmentin) 875 mg po bid
	IV options	• Cefepime (Maxipime) 2 g IV q8 hr, ceftazidime (Fortaz) 2 g IV q8 hr, imipenem (Primaxin) 0.5-1.0 g IV q6-8 hr, or meropenem (Merrem) 1 g IV q8 hr
High risk†‡	IV options (monotherapy or combination therapy)	• Monotherapy with cefepime, ceftazidime, imipenem, or meropenem (see IV dosing above) or • Aminoglycosides such as gentamicin or tobramycin 1.7 mg/kg IV q8 hr or either AG at 5-7 mg/kg/day plus one of the following: ticarcillin with clavulanate potassium (Timentin) 3.1 g IV q4-6 hr, piperacillin with tazobactam (Zosyn) 3.375-4.5 g IV q4-6 hr, cefepime, ceftazidime, imipenem, or meropenem (see IV dosing above)
	Vancomycin regimen†	• Vancomycin 1 g IV q12 hr (maximum of 2g/day) plus cefepime, ceftazidime, imipenem, or meropenem (see IV options above) • ± Aminoglycosides (see IV options above)

*Only assign low risk and consider outpatient management if no bacterial infection is found. Closely coordinate follow-up with hematologist/oncologist.

†Add vancomycin if there is suspected catheter-related infection, colonization by penicillin-resistant and cephalosporin-resistant pneumococci or methicillin-resistant *S. aureus,* positive blood culture results for gram-positive bacteria before final identification and susceptibility testing, or hypotension or other evidence of cardiovascular impairment.

‡If a worsening course is expected and there is an expected long delay of bone marrow recovery, colony-stimulating factors such as filgrastim or sargramostim may be helpful.

FEVER AND RASH

Table K-8

Infectious Causes	Noninfectious Causes
Petechial Rash and Fever	
Endocarditis	Allergy, thrombocytopenia
Meningococcemia	Scurvy, lupus
Gonococcemia	Henoch Schonlein purpura
Other pathogenic bacteria such as gram-negative enterics	Hypersensitivity vasculitis
Rickettsia (RMSF)	Rheumatic fever, amyloidosis
Enterovirus	
Dengue fever	
Hepatitis B	
Rubella, Epstein-Barr virus	
Rat bite fever	
Epidemic typhus	
Maculopapular Rash and Fever	
Typhoid fever/typhus	Allergy, serum sickness
Secondary syphilis, Lyme disease	Erythema multiforme
Meningococcemia	Erythema marginatum
Mycoplasma, psittacosis	Lupus, dermatomyositis
Rickettsia, leptospirosis	Sweet's syndrome
Ehrlichiosis, *Enterovirus*	Acrodermatitis enteropathica
Parvovirus B19 (fifth disease)	
Human herpesvirus 6	
Rubeola, rubella, arbovirus	
Epstein-Barr virus	
Adenovirus, primary HIV	
Streptobacillus moniliformis	

Compiled from Schlossberg D. Fever and rash. Infect Dis Clin North Am 10:101, 1996; and Levin S, Goodman LJ. An approach to acute fever and rash (AFR) in the adult. Curr Clin Top Infect Dis 15:19, 1995.

Table K-8—cont'd

Infectious Causes	Noninfectious Causes
Vesicobullous Rash and Fever	
Staphylococcemia	Allergy, plant dermatitis
Gonococcemia, *Rickettsia*	Eczema vaccinatum
Herpes, varicella	Erythema multiforme bullosum
Vibrio vulnificus	
Folliculitis *(Staphylococcus, Candida, Pseudomonas)*	
Enterovirus	
Parvovirus B19, HIV, fifth disease	
Erythematous Rash and Fever	
Staphylococcus or *Streptococcus* infection (toxic shock, scarlet fever)	Allergy
Ehrlichiosis	Vasodilation
Streptococcus viridans	Eczema
Clostridium haemolyticum	Psoriasis
Kawasaki disease	Lymphoma
Enterovirus	Pityriasis rubra
	Sézary syndrome
Urticarial Rash and Fever	
Mycoplasma	Allergy
Lyme disease	Vasculitis
Enterovirus	Malignancy
HIV, hepatitis B	Idiopathic
Adenovirus, Epstein-Barr virus	
Strongyloides, trichinosis	
Schistosomiasis	
Onchocerciasis, loiasis	

K

TOXIC SHOCK SYNDROME

Toxic shock syndrome is caused by a toxin (TSST-1) produced by *Staphylococcus aureus.* TSST-1 sources include tampons (50% of cases), nasal packing, wounds, postpartum vaginal colonization, and many others.

Criteria for Diagnosis

The patient must have each of the following:

- Temperature >38.9° C (102° F)
- Systolic BP <90, orthostatic decrease of systolic BP by 15 mm Hg, or syncope
- Rash: diffuse, macular erythroderma with subsequent desquamation
- Involvement of three of the following organ systems discovered either clinically or by laboratory tests:
  - GI: vomiting or profuse diarrhea
  - Muscular: myalgias or CPK ↑ twofold
  - Renal: ↑ BUN plus creatinine doubled, sterile pyuria
  - Hematology: <100,000 platelets/mm^3
  - Liver: AST, ALT ↑ twofold
  - Mucosa: vaginal, conjunctiva, or pharyngeal hyperemia
  - CNS: disoriented, nonfocal examination
- Negative serology for Rocky Mountain spotted fever, leptospirosis, measles, hepatitis B, antinuclear antibody, venereal disease, and mononucleosis, and negative results from blood, urine, and throat cultures.

Management

- Restore intravascular volume with NS (pressors may be needed) and admit to the ICU.
- Obtain blood for CBC, platelets, coagulation studies, electrolytes, liver function tests, culture urine, and blood ± CSF; obtain CXR, arterial blood gas, and ECG.
- Search for focus of infection and remove source (for example, a tampon).
- If bleeding, treat coagulopathy with platelets, fresh frozen plasma, or transfusion.
- Nafcillin or oxacillin 1-2 g IV q4 hr until clinically improved, then oral antistaphylococcal agents (dicloxacillin or first-generation cephalosporin) for 10-14 days. Consider vancomycin if methicillin-resistant *S. aureus* is suspected. NOTE: Antibiotics only reduce the recurrence of toxic shock syndrome and do not treat the actual disease.

DUKE CRITERIA FOR ENDOCARDITIS

Box K-1

Definite	Pathologic criteria: • Microorganisms (demonstrated by culture or histology in vegetation, embolized vegetation, or intracardiac abscess) or • Pathologic lesions (vegetation or intracardiac abscess confirmed by histology showing active endocarditis) Clinical criteria: two major, or one major plus three minor, or five minor
Possible	Clinical criteria: one major plus one minor, or three minor
Rejected (negative predictive value ≥92%)	Firm alternative diagnosis explaining evidence of IE or Resolution of endocarditis syndrome with antibiotic therapy for ≤4 days or No pathologic findings of IE at surgery or autopsy (after antibiotic therapy for ≤4 days) or Does not meet criteria for possible IE

Compiled from Durack DT, Lukes AS, Bright DK. New criteria for diagnosis of infective endocarditis: utilization of specific echocardiographic findings. Duke Endocarditis Service. Am J Med 96:200, 1994; Li JS, Sexton DJ, Mick N, et al. Proposed modifications to the Duke criteria for the diagnosis of infective endocarditis. Clin Infect Dis 30:633, 2000; and Dodds GA, Sexton DJ, Durack DT, et al. Negative predictive value of the Duke criteria for infective endocarditis. Am J Cardiol 77:403, 1996.

Continued

Box K-1—cont'd

Major Criteria	Minor Criteria
Positive blood cultures for IE • Two separate blood cultures with organisms typical for IE* • Persistently positive blood cultures with organism consistent with IE (2 drawn >12 hours apart, or all of 3 or most of ≥4 separate cultures, with the first and last drawn at least 1 hour apart) • Single positive blood culture for *Coxiella burnetii* or antibody titer >1:800 Evidence of endocardial involvement Echocardiogram positive for IE†: oscillating intracardiac mass,‡ or abscess, or new partial dehiscence of prosthetic valve • New valvular regurgitation¶	Predisposing heart condition or IVDU • Fever ≥38.0° C (100.4° F) • Vascular phenomena: major arterial emboli, septic pulmonary infarcts, mycotic aneurysm, intracranial hemorrhage, Janeway lesions, and conjunctival hemorrhages • Immunologic phenomena: Osler's nodes, glomerulonephritis, Roth's spots, and rheumatoid factor • Microbiologic evidence: positive blood culture for organism that causes IE but failure to meet major criteria or serologic evidence of active infection with organism consistent with IE

*Typical organisms include viridans *Streptococcus, Streptococcus bovis,* HACEK group, *S. aureus*, or community acquired *Enterococcus* in the absence of a primary focus.

†Transesophageal echocardiogram (TEE) is recommended for patients with prosthetic valves, for those rated with at least possible IE by clinical criteria, or for those with complicated IE (paravalvular abscess); transthoracic echocardiogram (TTE) first study in other patients.

‡Mass on valve or supporting structures, or in the path of regurgitant jets, or on implanted material—in the absence of an alternative anatomic explanation.

¶An increase or change in a preexisting murmur is not sufficient.

ACUTE INFECTIOUS DIARRHEA

Table K-9

Pathogen	Comments	Fever	Abdominal Pain	Bloody Stools	Nausea/ Vomiting	Fecal WBC
Toxins *(Staphylococcus, Bacillus cereus, Clostridium perfringens)*	Incubation <6 to 24 hours	−	+	−	++	−
Salmonella	Community acquired, foodborne	++	++	+	+	++
Campylobacter	Community acquired, undercooked poultry	++	++	+	+	++
Shigella	Community acquired, person-to-person	++	++	+	++	++
Shiga-toxin–producing *E. coli* (O157:H7)	Foodborne outbreaks, undercooked beef; bloody stool without fever	−	++	++	+	−
C. difficile	Nosocomial, postantibiotic; marked leukocytosis in 50% of cases	+	+	+	−	++
Vibrio	Seafood	±	±	±	±	±
Yersinia	Community acquired, foodborne	++	++	+	+	+
Entamoeba histolytica	Tropical	+	+	++	±	±
Cryptosporidium	Waterborne outbreaks, travel, immunocompromised; symptoms last >10 days	±	±	−	+	−
Cyclospora	Travel, foodborne; profound fatigue	±	±	−	+	−
Giardia	Waterborne, day care, IgA deficiency; symptoms last >10 days	−	++	−	+	−
Norovirus	Winter outbreaks; nursing homes, schools, cruise ships; shellfish	±	++	−	++	−

From Thielman NM, Guerrant RL. Acute infectious diarrhea. N Engl J Med 350:38, 2004.
++, Common; +, occurs; ±, variable; −, atypical or not characteristic.

Noninfectious Differential Diagnosis

- Medications
- Tube feeding
- Inflammatory bowel disease
- Ischemic colitis
- Factitious
- Secretory: villous adenoma, gastrinoma, VIPoma

Treatment

- Antimotility agents (such as loperamide, bismuth subsalicylate) are fine to use for typical traveler's diarrhea or water diarrhea, but avoid with bloody or inflammatory diarrhea (they may prolong fever or predispose a patient to toxic megacolon or hemolytic-uremic syndrome).
- Consider empiric fluoroquinolone for moderate or severe traveler's diarrhea or for febrile community-acquired diarrhea. Add erythromycin or azithromycin if fluoroquinolone-resistant *Campylobacter* infection is suspected (from travel to southeast Asia), or if the patient is severely ill or immunocompromised. Avoid antibiotics if the patient has bloody stools without fever or if there is a suspicion of Shiga-toxin–producing *E. coli* (because it may predispose patients to hemolytic-uremic syndrome).

TREATING *CLOSTRIDIUM DIFFICILE* COLITIS[1,2]

Initial Therapy

- First line: Stop antibiotics if at all possible and observe without treatment if symptoms are mild. If symptoms are severe, give metronidazole 500 mg po tid.
- Second line: Give vancomycin 125 mg po qid. There is no documented benefit over metronidazole, but consider using it if there is no prompt response to metronidazole in severe infections.
- IV: Give metronidazole 500 mg IV q8 hr if NPO; add to vancomycin po for severe infections (IV vancomycin is ineffective).
- Duration: Ten to14 days (longer if receiving long-term antibiotics for another infection).[3]

Recurrent Infections (10% to 25% of Cases)

- Initial relapse: Stop antibiotics if at all possible. Confirm diagnosis. Treat again with metronidazole or vancomycin for 10 to 14 days.
- Multiple relapses: tapering oral vancomycin
  - Week 1: 125 mg qid
  - Week 2: 125 mg bid
  - Week 3: 125 mg qd
  - Week 4: 125 mg qod
  - Weeks 5-6: 125 mg q3 days
  - Weeks 7-10: cholestyramine 4 g po qid
- Alternative therapies: Colestipol (5 g bid) or cholestyramine (4 g tid/qid with oral vancomycin (2-3 hours apart). Give vancomycin (125 mg po qid) plus rifampin (600 mg po bid). Reconstitute bowel flora with *Saccharomyces boulardii,* lactobacillus, or stool enemas.

Indications for Surgery (Required in 1% to 3% of Patients)

- Perforation
- Severe ileus with toxic megacolon
- Refractory septicemia
- Failure of medical treatment

SEPSIS AND SYSTEMIC INFLAMMATORY RESPONSE SYNDROME (SIRS)

SIRS

Two or more of the following:

- Temperature >38° C (100.4° F) or <36° C (96.8° F)
- Heart rate >90 beats/minute
- Respiration rate >20 or $Paco_2$ <32 mm Hg
- WBC >12,000, <4000, or >10% bands

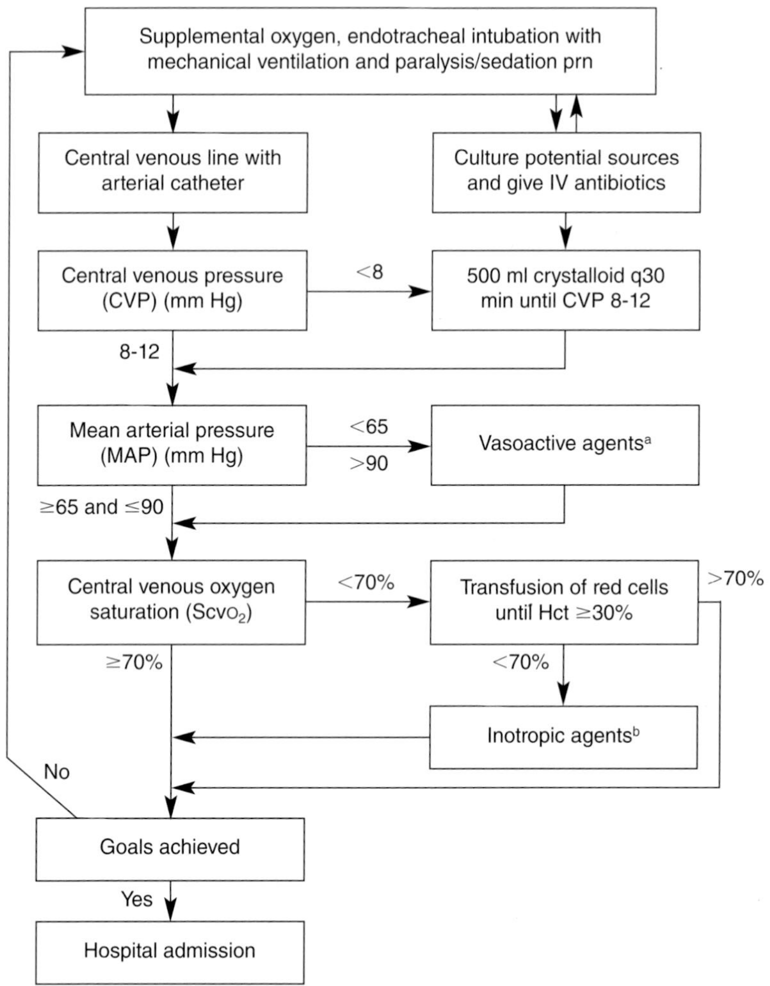

Fig. K-1 Early Goal-Directed Therapy for Severe Sepsis and Septic Shock. Eligibility: two of the four SIRS criteria, and either systolic BP ≥90 mm Hg after one 20-30 ml/kg NS challenge or lactate ≥4 mmol/L. Original exclusion criteria (some are now relative contraindications): age <18 years, acute stroke, pulmonary edema, status asthmaticus, acute coronary syndrome, primary arrhythmia, active GI bleed, seizure, drug overdose, burn or trauma, uncured cancer, immunosuppressed, contraindication to central line, acute surgery needed, or DNR status. a, If MAP >90 mm Hg, vasodilators are given to lower MAP to ≤90 mm Hg. If MAP <65 mm Hg, vasopressors are given to maintain a MAP ≥65 mm Hg. b, Initiate dobutamine at 2.5 μg/kg/min. Increase dose by 2.5 μg/kg/min every 30 minutes until $Scvo_2$ is ≥70% or maximum dose of 20 μg/kg/min is given. Decrease dobutamine dose or discontinue if MAP <65 mm Hg or HR >120 beats/min. (Modified from Rivers E, Nguyen B, Havstad S, et al. Early goal-directed therapy in the treatment of severe sepsis and septic shock. N Engl J Med 345:1368, 2001.)

Table K-10 Antimicrobial Therapy for Sepsis/SIRS

Possible Source	Antimicrobial Agents
Unknown or immunocompromised	Antipseudomonal cephalosporins,* or imipenem 0.5 mg IV q6 hr, or meropenem 1 g IV q8 hr plus either aminoglycoside† or fluoroquinolone,‡ or Zosyn 4.5 g IV q6 hr plus aminoglycoside
Abscess or cellulitis	Imipenem 0.5 g IV q6 hr, or meropenem 1 g IV q8 hr, or Zosyn 4.5 g IV q6 hr; add vancomycin 1 g IV q12 hr if methicillin-resistant *S. aureus* is suspected
Necrotizing fasciitis, gangrene	Penicillin G 4 million units IV q4 hr, or imipenem 0.5-1.0 g IV q6 hr, or meropenem 1 g IV q8 hr, or Zosyn 4.5 g IV q6 hr with aminoglycoside and clindamycin hydrochloride (Cleocin) 600-900 mg IV q8 hr
Pelvic: septic pelvic thrombophlebitis	Metronidazole (Flagyl) 1g IV and antipseudomonal cephalosporin, ampicillin and sulbactam (Unasyn) 3g IV, Zosyn 4.5 g IV, or Timentin 3.1
Pneumonia	See Pneumonia in Table K-11
Urinary	Ceftriaxone 1-2 g IV q24 hr or cefotaxime 1-2 g IV/IM q12 hr or fluoroquinolone If *Pseudomonas,* then cefepime 2 g IV q12 hr, or ceftazidime 1-2 g IV q8 hr, or aminoglycoside, or fluoroquinolone‡
Wound or vascular catheter	Follow the unknown/immunocompromised regimen and add vancomycin 1 g IV q12 hr

*Antipseudomonal cephalosporins include ceftazidime 2 g IV q6 hr, cefoperazone 2-3 g IV q6 hr, and cefepime 2 g IV q12 hr.

†Amikacin has the least *Pseudomonas* resistance, tobramycin has the most intrinsic activity, and gentamicin has the most *Pseudomonas* resistance.

‡Second generation (effective against *Chlamydia, Legionella, Mycoplasma,* and *Pseudomonas,* but not *Streptococcus*): lomefloxacin (Maxaquin), norfloxacin (Noroxin), ofloxacin (Floxin), ciprofloxacin (Cipro) 400 mg IV q8-12 hr. Third generation: levofloxacin (Levaquin) (gram-positive activity). Fourth generation: moxifloxacin (Avelox), gemifloxacin (Factive), gatifloxacin (Tequin) (better anaerobic).

THERAPY: EMPIRIC ANTIMICROBIAL COVERAGE AND SPECIFIC INFECTIONS IN ADULTS

Table K-11

Infection	Treatment*
Abortion, septic	• See Chorioamnionitis
Abscess	• In general, drainage is necessary; see specific site within text for antimicrobials (for example, brain, breast, or parapharyngeal)
Acne vulgaris	• Mild inflammation: Tretinoin (Retin-A) 0.025-0.1% cream gel qhs, or adapalene (Differin) 0.1% cream/gel qhs • Moderate inflammation: Erythromycin 2%-3% or clindamycin (Cleocin) gel bid, and benzoyl peroxide (Benzyl, Desquam) gel/cream qd-bid or Benzamycin Pak (erythromycin 3% plus benzoyl peroxide 5%) gel bid or BenzaClin (benzoyl peroxide 5% plus clindamycin 1%) gel • Severe inflammation: Doxycycline 100 mg po bid, azithromycin pulse therapy (500 mg po qd × 4 days/month × 4 months), or clindamycin 300-450 mg po qid
Balanitis *(Candida)*	• See Vaginitis *(Candida)* ± cover *Streptococcus* or *Trichomonas*
Bite infection—dog, cat, or rat	• Augmentin 875 mg po bid × 10 days (first line listed bites) • Cat: Cefuroxime (Ceftin) 500 mg po bid • Dog: Clindamycin 300 mg po q6 hr plus flouroquinolone† • Rat, cat, or dog: Doxycycline 100 mg po bid × 10 days
Bite infection—human	• Oral: Augmentin 875 mg po bid or penicillin plus cephalosporin × 10-14 days (shorter if prophylaxis) • IV: Unasyn 3 g IV q6 hr, cefoxitin (Mefoxin) 2 g IV q8 hr, Timentin 3.1 g IV q6 hr, Zosyn 3.375-4.5 g IV q8 hr, or clindamycin 600-900 mg IV q8 hr plus ciprofloxacin 400 mg IV q12 hr

Compiled from Ong CS, Keogh AM, Kossard S, et al. Skin cancer in Australian heart transplant recipients. J Am Acad Derm 40:27, 1999; Noble SL, Forbes RC, Stamm PL. Diagnosis and management of common tinea infections. Am Fam Physician 58:163, 1998; Chuang TY, Brashear R, Lewis C. Porphyria cutanea tarda and hepatitis C virus: a case-control study and meta-analysis of the literature. J Am Acad Derm 41:31, 1999; and Lee HS, Chun YS, Hann SK. Nevus depigmentosus: clinical features and histopathologic characteristics in 67 patients. J Am Acad Derm 40:21, 1999.

*The decision to use IV or po regimens is complex. Listed medications are only recommendations. Consult textbooks, recent literature, and experts if uncertain about proper treatment options. Certain diseases (such as fasciitis, gangrene, septic arthritis, and osteomyelitis) may require surgical treatment. Drug doses may need to be changed or selections altered depending on cultures, renal function, and underlying disease.

†Fluoroquinolones such as ciprofloxacin 250-500 mg po bid, gatifloxacin 400 mg qd, levofloxacin 250-500 mg po qd, moxifloxacin, ofloxacin 200-400 po bid, and sparfloxacin 400 mg po day 1, then 200 mg po qd.

Table K-11—cont'd

Infection	Treatment*
Brain abscess	• Primary: Cefotaxime 2 g IV q4 hr or ceftriaxone 2 g IV q12 hr, and metronidazole 7.5 mg/kg IV q6 hr • Add vancomycin if related to trauma, surgery, or recent admission (methicillin resistance suspected)
Breast abscess	• Lactating *(S. aureus):* Nafcillin or oxacillin 2 g IV q4 hr or cefazolin (Ancef) 1 g IV q8 hr • Not lactating (usually anaerobic): Clindamycin 300 mg IV/po q6 hr, or lactating regimen and metronidazole 7.5 mg/kg q6 hr
Breast infection	• See Mastitis
Bronchitis	• Augmentin 500-875 mg po bid × 7-10 days, azithromycin 500 mg po qd × 3 days, clarithromycin (Biaxin) 500 mg po bid × 7-14 days, Biaxin XL 1 g po qd × 7 days, or fluoroquinolone†
Cat scratch disease	• Azithromycin 500 mg po × 1 plus 250 mg po × 4 days
Cellulitis—uncomplicated healthy patient	• Oral: Dicloxacillin or cephalexin (Keflex) 250-500 mg po qid × 10 days, levofloxacin 500 mg qd × 7-10 days, azithromycin 500 mg po × 1 day, then 250 mg po × 4 days, or clarithromycin 500 mg po bid × 10 days • IV: Nafcillin 1-1.5 g IV q4-6 hr or cefazolin 1 g IV q8 hr
Cellulitis—diabetic, alcohol, methicillin-resistant *S. aureus* (MRSA)	• Oral: Augmentin 875 mg po bid or IV/IM 3G cephalosporins‡ • IV, mild to moderate disease: Unasyn 3 g IV q6 hr, ceftazidime 2 g IV q8 hr, cefoperazone 2 g IV q6 hr, or cefepime 2 g IV q12 hr • IV, severe disease: Imipenem 0.5-1 g IV q6-8 hr or meropenem 1 g IV q8 hr • MRSA: Linezolid (Zyvox) 600 mg IV/PO q12 hr × 10-14 days
Cellulitis—lake/sea water (IV regimen differs if salt or fresh water cause)	• Oral: Sulfamethoxazole and trimethoprim (Septra DS) 1 po bid × 10 days or flouroquinolone† × 10 days • If salt water: Aminoglycosides and doxycycline 200 mg IV × 1 plus 50-100 mg IV q12 hr • If fresh water: Ciprofloxacin 400 mg IV q12 hr or ceftazidime 2 g IV q8 hr and gentamicin

*The decision to use IV or po regimens is complex. Listed medications are only recommendations. Consult textbooks, recent literature, and experts if uncertain about proper treatment options. Certain diseases (such as fasciitis, gangrene, septic arthritis, and osteomyelitis) may require surgical treatment. Drug doses may need to be changed or selections altered depending on cultures, renal function, and underlying disease.
†Fluoroquinolones such as ciprofloxacin 250-500 mg po bid, gatifloxacin 400 mg qd, levofloxacin 250-500 mg po qd, moxifloxacin, ofloxacin 200-400 po bid, and sparfloxacin 400 mg po day 1, then 200 mg po qd.
‡Third-generation cephalosporins such as cefotaxime, ceftizoxime, and ceftriaxone.

Continued

Table K-11—cont'd

Infection	Treatment*
Chancroid	• Azithromycin 1 g po or ceftriaxone 250 mg IM
Chlamydia—urethritis or simple cervicitis	• Azithromycin 1 g po, doxycycline 100 mg po bid, or erythromycin 500 mg qid × 7-10 days (treat gonorrhea)
Chorioamnionitis	• Cefoxitin 2g IV q6-8 hr, Unasyn 3.0 g IV q6 hr, or Zosyn 3.375-4.5 g IV q8 hr, plus doxycycline 100 mg IV over 1-4 hr bid, then switch to 100 mg po when stable or • Cleocin 600-900 mg IV q8 hr, and ceftriaxone 1 g IV q12 hr or gentamicin 1.7 mg/kg IV q8 hr or 5 mg/kg/24 hr
Conjunctivitis	• Ciprofloxacin (Ciloxan) 1-2 gtt q2 hr (while awake) × 2 days, then q4 hr × 5 days, or ofloxacin (Ocuflox) 2 gtt q2-4 hr × 2 days, then 2 gtt qid × 5 days, or either gentamicin (Garamycin) or tobramycin (Tobrex), 1-2 gtt q2-4 hr (or ointment applied bid-tid), or erythromycin (Ilotycin) applied q3-4 hr
Corneal ulcer	• Ciloxan 2 gtt q15 min × 6 hr, then q30 min × 1 day, then q1 hr × 1 day, then q4 hr × 3-14 days, or Ocuflox 1-2 gtt q30 min (while awake) × 2 days (awaken and instill q4-6 hr at night), then 1-2 gtt q1 hr × 5 days, then 1-2 gtt qid × 3 days
Dental infection	• Oral therapy: Augmentin 875 mg po bid, clindamycin 300-450 mg po qid, penicillin (↑ resistance) 500 mg po qid, or erythromycin 250-500 mg po qid × 10 days • IV therapy: Clindamycin 600 mg IV q6 hr, Unasyn 1.5-3g IV q6 hr, or cefotetan 2g IV q12 hr
Diarrhea *(Clostridium difficile)*	• Metronidazole 500 mg po tid × 10-14 days or vancomycin 125 mg po qid × 10-14 days • If patient cannot take po: Metronidazole 500 mg IV q6 hr ± vancomycin 1 to 3 ml/min of 500 mg/L saline solution per small bowel catheter or cecal catheter to maximum of 2 g per day

*The decision to use IV or po regimens is complex. Listed medications are only recommendations. Consult textbooks, recent literature, and experts if uncertain about proper treatment options. Certain diseases (such as fasciitis, gangrene, septic arthritis, and osteomyelitis) may require surgical treatment. Drug doses may need to be changed or selections altered depending on cultures, renal function, and underlying disease.

Table K-11—cont'd

Infection	Treatment*
Diarrhea (*Salmonella, Shigella, Campylobacter, E. coli,* or traveler's diarrhea)	• Ciprofloxacin 500 mg po bid × 5 days or Septra DS 1 po bid × 5 days (for severe symptoms, such as fever or bloody diarrhea, only treat *Salmonella* if the patient is old, septic, immunocompromised, or ill enough to be hospitalized)
Diarrhea (*Vibrio cholerae)*	• Ciprofloxacin 1 g po × 1, doxycycline 300 mg po × 1, or tetracycline 500 mg po qid × 3 days
Diverticulitis—outpatient	• Septra DS 1 po bid or ciprofloxacin 500 mg po bid, and metronidazole 500 mg po qid for at least 7-10 days or • Augmentin 500 mg po tid × 7-10 days
Ehrlichiosis	• Doxycycline 100 mg po bid × 7-14 days
Encephalitis	• See Herpes—encephalitis
Endocarditis IV drug use	• Nafcillin 2g IV q4 hr and gentamicin 1 mg/kg IV q8 hr
Endocarditis—native valve, empiric Rx	• Penicillin G 20 million units IV qd (continuous or divided q4 hr) or ampicillin 2g IV q4 hr, and nafcillin 2g IV q4 hr, and gentamicin 1mg/kg IV q8 hr • Penicillin-allergic: Vancomycin 15 mg/kg IV q12 hr and gentamicin 1 mg/kg IV q8 hr
Endocarditis—prosthetic valve, empiric Rx	• Vancomycin 15 mg/kg IV q12 hr (maximum of 2 g/day), gentamicin 1 mg/kg IV q8 hr, and rifampin 600 mg po qd
Enterococcus faecium	• Vancomycin-resistant: Linezolid 600 mg IV/po q12 hr
Epididymitis—all ages	• Ciprofloxacin 500 mg po bid or ofloxacin 300 mg po bid × 14 days
Epididymitis—≤35 years	• See Pelvic inflammatory disease—outpatient treatment
Epiglottitis	• Ceftriaxone (Rocephin) 2 g IV q24 hr or cefuroxime (Zinacef) 0.75-1.5 g IV q8 hr or Unasyn 3 g IV q6 hr

*The decision to use IV or po regimens is complex. Listed medications are only recommendations. Consult textbooks, recent literature, and experts if uncertain about proper treatment options. Certain diseases (such as fasciitis, gangrene, septic arthritis, and osteomyelitis) may require surgical treatment. Drug doses may need to be changed or selections altered depending on cultures, renal function, and underlying disease.

Continued

Table K-11—cont'd

Infection	Treatment*
Gingivitis—acute necrotizing, ulcerative	• Penicillin 250-500 mg po qid, tetracycline 250 mg po qid, or doxycycline 100 mg po bid × 10 days
Gonorrhea—cervicitis, urethritis, pharyngitis, proctitis (not invasive disease, such as PID or arthritis)	• One dose po of any of the following: Azithromycin 2 g, cefixime 400 mg, ciprofloxacin 500 mg, ofloxacin 400 mg, gatifloxacin 400 mg, lomefloxacin 400 mg, or ceftriaxone 125 mg (also treat *Chlamydia* with azithromycin 1 g po)
Granuloma inguinale	• See Lymphogranuloma venereum, or use Septra DS 1 po bid × 21 days
Helicobacter pylori	• Prevpac as directed or • Amoxicillin 1g, clarithromycin 500 mg, and omeprazole 20 mg po bid × 14 days or • Lansoprazole 30 mg po bid and Pepto Bismol 2 po qid plus metronidazole 500 mg po tid and tetracycline 500 mg po qid × 14 days
Herpes—encephalitis	• Acyclovir (Zovirax) 10 mg/kg IV over 1 hr q8 hr × 2-3 weeks
Herpes—simplex (use oral agents and treat for half of primary time period if recurrent simplex)	• Primary: Acyclovir 400 mg po tid × 10 days or valacyclovir (Valtrex) 1 g po bid × 10 days • Labialis, recurrent: Penciclovir (Denavir) apply topically q2 hr while awake × 4 days • Prophylaxis: Acyclovir 400 mg po bid, famciclovir 250 mg po bid, or valacyclovir 500 mg po qd
Herpes—varicella	• Acyclovir 800 mg po qid × 5 days (use IV dosing if immunocompromised, pneumonia, or third trimester of pregnancy)
Herpes—zoster (if immunocompromised or ill, consider IV therapy)	• Acyclovir 800 mg po 5 × per day × 5-7 days, famciclovir 500 mg po tid × 7 days, or valacyclovir 1 g po tid × 7 days
Impetigo	• Mupirocin topical tid ± (See Cellulitis)

*The decision to use IV or po regimens is complex. Listed medications are only recommendations. Consult textbooks, recent literature, and experts if uncertain about proper treatment options. Certain diseases (such as fasciitis, gangrene, septic arthritis, and osteomyelitis) may require surgical treatment. Drug doses may need to be changed or selections altered depending on cultures, renal function, and underlying disease.

Table K-11—cont'd

Infection	Treatment*
Influenza—treatment (start within 48 hours of symptom onset)	• Influenza A or B: Oseltamivir (Tamiflu) 75 mg po bid × 5 days or zanamivir (Relenza) 2 puffs bid × 5 days • Influenza A only: Rimantadine or amantadine 100 mg po bid × 7 days (100 mg qd if >65 years)
Influenza—prophylaxis	• Influenza A or B: Oseltamivir 75 mg po qd × at least 7 days or • Influenza A: Rimantadine or amantadine 100 mg po qd × 7 days
IV catheter line infection	• Vancomycin 1 g IV q12 hr if sepsis, immunocompromised, or ill
Ludwig's angina	• See Submandibular abscess
Lymphogranuloma venereum	• Doxycycline 100 mg po bid × 21 days or erythromycin 500 mg po qid × 21 days
Mastitis	• Oral: Dicloxacillin or cephalexin 250-500 mg po qid • IV: Cefazolin 1 g IV q8 hr • (see also Breast abscess)
Mastoiditis	• Cefotaxime 1g IV q4 hr or ceftriaxone 1-2g IV q24 hr
Meningitis—bacterial (<50 years and healthy)	• Cefotaxime 2g IV q4-6 hr or ceftriaxone 2g IV q12 hr, and vancomycin 15 mg/kg IV q12 hr and dexamethasone 0.15 mg/kg IV concurrent or 15 min preantibiotic and 0.15 mg/kg IV q6 hr × 4 days
Meningitis—bacterial (>50 years or unhealthy)	• Follow regimen for <50-year-old and add ampicillin 2 g IV q4 hr • Severe penicillin allergy: Septra 15-20 mg/kg/day (divided q6-8 hr) and vancomycin 500-750 mg IV q6 hr
Meningitis exposure *(Neisseria meningitidis, Haemophilus influenzae)*	• *N. meningitidis* exposure: Rifampin 20 mg/kg po q24 hr × 4 days (maximum dose 600 mg), ceftriaxone 250 mg IM, or ciprofloxacin 500 mg × 1 in adult; treat household and day care or nursery contacts within 24 hours of case and older children and/or adults if kissed or shared food or drink; also treat medical personnel exposed to secretions • *H. influenzae* exposure: Rifampin 20 mg/kg po q24 hr × 4 days (maximum dose 600 mg) if a household contact when the household has an unimmunized child <4 years or an immunocompromised child, regardless of vaccine status; or nursery or child care contacts when ≥2 cases of Hib-invasive disease have occurred within 60 days

*The decision to use IV or po regimens is complex. Listed medications are only recommendations. Consult textbooks, recent literature, and experts if uncertain about proper treatment options. Certain diseases (such as fasciitis, gangrene, septic arthritis, and osteomyelitis) may require surgical treatment. Drug doses may need to be changed or selections altered depending on cultures, renal function, and underlying disease.

Continued

Table K-11—cont'd

Infection	Treatment*
Meningitis/ ventriculitis—CSF (shunt or trauma)	• Shunt: Vancomycin 1 g IV q6-12 hr and rifampin 600 mg po q24 hr; use ceftazidime (Fortaz) 2 g IV q8 hr if gram stain is positive for gram-negative bacilli • Trauma: Vancomycin 1 g IV q6-12 hr plus ceftazidime 2 g IV q8 hr
Oroesophageal candidiasis—immuno-compromised	• Fluconazole (Diflucan) 200 mg po/IV on day 1, then 100 mg po/IV qd (oropharynx × 14 days; esophageal × 3 weeks and 2 weeks after symptoms) • Itraconazole (Sporanox), oropharynx: 20 mg swish and swallow × 1-2 weeks; esophageal: 100-200 mg swish and swallow × 3 weeks and 2 weeks after symptoms
Osteomyelitis—healthy	• Nafcillin or oxacillin 2 g IV q4 hr, or cefazolin 2 g IV q8 hr • If osteomyelitis from punctured rubber sole, ceftazidime 2 g IV q8 hr, or cefepime 2 g IV q12 hr
Osteomyelitis—IV drug user, on dialysis, or immuno-compromised	• Nafcillin or oxacillin 2 g IV q4 hr or cefazolin 2 g IV q8 hr, and ciprofloxacin 200-400 mg IV q12 hr or • Ciprofloxacin 200-400 mg IV q12 hr plus vancomycin 1g IV q12 hr
Otitis externa	• Bacitracin/neomycin/polymyxin B and hydrocortisone (Cortisporin Ophthalmic) 4 gtt qid or ciprofloxacin/hydrocortisone (Cipro HC Otic) 3 gtt bid × 7 days or ofloxacin otic 10 gtt bid × 10 days • If severe: Dicloxacillin or cephalexin 500 mg po qid, or diabetic regimen • If diabetes *(Pseudomonas):* Imipenem 0.5-1.0 g IV q6 hr, meropenem 1 g IV q8 hr, Cipro 400 mg IV q12 hr, ceftazidime 2 g IV q8 hr, or antipseudomonal penicillin plus aminoglycoside
Otitis media	• Amoxicillin 250 mg po tid, Augmentin 500-875 mg po bid, cefdinir (Omnicef) 600 mg po qd, cefpodoxime (Vantin) 200 mg po bid, or cefuroxime 250 mg po bid × 10 days • See Otitis externa: diabetic if *Pseudomonas* suspected
Parapharyngeal abscess	• See Submandibular abscess

*The decision to use IV or po regimens is complex. Listed medications are only recommendations. Consult textbooks, recent literature, and experts if uncertain about proper treatment options. Certain diseases (such as fasciitis, gangrene, septic arthritis, and osteomyelitis) may require surgical treatment. Drug doses may need to be changed or selections altered depending on cultures, renal function, and underlying disease.

Table K-11—cont'd

Infection	Treatment*
Parotitis—infectious	• Nafcillin or oxacillin 2 g IV q4 hr or cefazolin 1 g IV q8 hr (ineffective if caused by HIV, mumps, CMV, diabetes, mycobacteria, cirrhosis, malnutrition, or medications)
Peritonitis (spontaneous)	• Cefotaxime 2 g IV q8 hr, Unasyn 3 g IV q6 hr, Timentin 3.1 g IV q6 hr, or Zosyn 4.5 g IV q8 hr • Resistant *E. coli/Klebsiella* sp.: ESBL, extended spectrum B lactamase, and ciprofloxacin 400 mg IV q12 hr or imipenem
Pelvic inflammatory disease—inpatient treatment	• Cefoxitin 2 g IV q6 hr or cefotetan 2 g IV q12 hr, and doxycycline 100 mg po of IV q12 hr × 14 days or • Clindamycin 900 mg IV q8 hr and gentamicin 1.5 mg/kg IV q8 hr; after discharge, doxycycline 100 mg po bid ± clindamycin 450 mg po qid × 14 days
Pelvic inflammatory disease—outpatient treatment	• Ceftriaxone 250 mg IM and doxycycline 100 mg po bid × 10-14 days, or ofloxacin 400 mg po bid × 14 days, or levofloxacin (Levaquin) 500 mg po qd × 14 days • Add metronidazole 500 mg po bid × 14 days to any of the outpatient regimens listed
Pharyngitis—if group A *Streptococcus* is likely)	• Benzathine penicillin (Bicillin L-A) 1.2 million units IM, penicillin VK 500 mg po bid, cephalexin 250-500 mg po qid × 10 days, cefadroxil 0.5-1 g po qd × 10 days, or azithromycin 500 mg po day 1, then 250 mg po × 4 days, or clarithromycin 250 mg po bid × 10 days
Pneumonia—aspiration or lung abscess	• Clindamycin 600-900 mg IV q8 hr, cefoxitin 2 g IV q8 hr, Timentin 3.1g IV q6 hr, or Zosyn 4.5g IV q8 hr
Pneumonia—influenza with mild bacterial superinfection (requires admission, in general)	• Augmentin 2 g po tid, amoxicillin 1 g po tid, cefpodoxime 200 mg po bid, cefprozil (Cefzil) 500 mg po bid, or cefuroxime 250-500 mg po bid or • Moxifloxacin (Avelox) 400 mg po qd, levofloxacin 500 mg po/IV qd, gatifloxacin 400 mg po qd, or gemifloxacin (Factive) 320 mg po qd (each agent should be given for 7 days)

*The decision to use IV or po regimens is complex. Listed medications are only recommendations. Consult textbooks, recent literature, and experts if uncertain about proper treatment options. Certain diseases (such as fasciitis, gangrene, septic arthritis, and osteomyelitis) may require surgical treatment. Drug doses may need to be changed or selections altered depending on cultures, renal function, and underlying disease.

Continued

Table K-11—cont'd

Infection	Treatment*
Pneumonia—inpatient, medical ward admission, community acquired	• Moxifloxacin 400 mg po/IV qd, levofloxacin 750 mg po qd, gatifloxacin 400 mg po/IV qd, or gemifloxacin 320 mg po qd (each agent is given for 7 days) or • Cefotaxime (Claforan) 2 g IV q8 hr or ceftriaxone 1 g IV q12-24 hr or Unasyn 3g IV q6 hr or ertapenem (Invanz) 1 g IV q24 hr, and azithromycin 500 mg po × 1—then 250 mg po qd × 4 or clarithromycin (Biaxin XL) 1 g po qd—then Biaxin 500 mg po bid × 7 days
Pneumonia—inpatient, ICU admission, community acquired—if *Pseudomonas* is not a concern (Methicillin-resistant *S. aureus*)	• Cefotaxime (Claforan) 2 g IV q8 hr, ceftriaxone 1 g IV q12-24 hr, Unasyn 3 g IV q6 hr, or ertapenem 1 g IV q24 hr and • Moxifloxacin 400 mg po/IV qd or levofloxacin 750 mg po/IV qd or gatifloxacin 400 mg po/IV qd or gemifloxacin 320 mg po qd (each agent is given for 7 days), or Zithromax 500 mg po × 1—then 250 mg po qd × 4 or Biaxin XL 1 g po qd × 7 days or Biaxin 500 mg po bid × 7 days • If beta-lactam allergy: Fluoroquinolone and consider clindamycin 600-900 mg IV q8 hr • Methicillin-resistant *S. aureus:* Linezolid 600 mg IV/po q12 hr × 10-14 days
Pneumonia—inpatient, ICU admission, community acquired—if *Pseudomonas* is a concern	• Zosyn 4.5 g IV q8 hr, imipenem 500 mg IV q6 hr, meropenem 1 g IV q8 hr, cefepime (Maxipime) 2 g IV q12 hr *and* ciprofloxacin 400 mg IV q12 hr or • Zosyn, imipenem, meropenem, or cefepime as above for ICU patients, and aminoglycoside,§ moxifloxacin, levofloxacin, gatifloxacin, gemifloxacin, azithromycin, or clarithromycin (see dosing above) • If beta-lactam allergy: Aztreonam 1 g IV q12 hr and either levofloxacin 500 mg po/IV q24 hr alone or moxifloxacin 400 mg IV/po q24 hr or gatifloxacin 400 mg po/IV q24 hr plus aminoglycoside§

*The decision to use IV or po regimens is complex. Listed medications are only recommendations. Consult textbooks, recent literature, and experts if uncertain about proper treatment options. Certain diseases (such as fasciitis, gangrene, septic arthritis, and osteomyelitis) may require surgical treatment. Drug doses may need to be changed or selections altered depending on cultures, renal function, and underlying disease.

§Amikacin has the least *Pseudomonas* resistance, tobramycin has the most intrinsic activity, and gentamicin has the most *Pseudomonas* resistance.

Table K-11—cont'd

Infection	Treatment*
Pneumonia—nursing home	• Treated in nursing home: Moxifloxacin 400 mg po qd or levofloxacin 500 mg po/IV qd or gatifloxacin 400 mg po qd or gemifloxacin 320 mg po qd (each is given for 7 days), or Augmentin 2 g po tid and azithromycin 500 mg po × 1, then 250 mg po qd × 4, Biaxin XL 1 g po qd × 7 days, or Biaxin 500 mg po bid × 7 days • Hospitalized: Treat as per ward or ICU
Pneumonia—outpatient (healthy with no antibiotics in past 3 months)	• Azithromycin 500 mg po × 1, then 250 mg po qd × 4 days, or Biaxin XL 1 g po qd × 7 days, or Biaxin 500 mg po bid × 10-14 days, or doxycycline 100 mg × 14 days
Pneumonia—outpatient (healthy with antibiotic use in past 3 months)	• Moxifloxacin 400 mg po qd, levofloxacin 500 mg po qd, gatifloxacin 400 mg po qd, or gemifloxacin 320 mg po qd (each agent is given for 7 days) or • Azithromycin 500 mg po × 1, then 250 mg po qd or Biaxin XL 1 g po qd × 7 days, plus amoxicillin 1 g po tid or Augmentin 2 g po tid
Pneumonia—outpatient (comorbidity, such as COPD, diabetes, renal or congestive heart failure, or cancer) (no antibiotics in past 3 months)	• Azithromycin 500 mg po × 1, then 250 mg po qd × 4 days, or Biaxin XL 1 g po qd × 7 days, or Biaxin 500 mg po bid × 7 days or • Moxifloxacin 400 mg po qd, levofloxacin 500 mg po qd, gatifloxacin 400 mg po qd, or gemifloxacin 320 mg po qd (each agent is given for 7 days)
Pneumonia—outpatient (comorbidity, such as COPD, diabetes, renal or congestive heart failure, or cancer) (antibiotics in past 3 months)	• Moxifloxacin 400 mg po qd, levofloxacin 500 mg po qd, gatifloxacin 400 mg po qd, or gemifloxacin 320 mg po qd (each agent is given for 7 days) or • Azithromycin 500 mg po × 1, then 250 mg po qd × 4 days or Biaxin XL 1 g po qd × 7 days or Biaxin 500 mg po bid × 7 days, and Augmentin 2 g po tid or amoxicillin 1 g po tid or cefpodoxime 200 mg po bid, cefprozil 500 mg po bid, or cefuroxime 250-500 mg po bid

*The decision to use IV or po regimens is complex. Listed medications are only recommendations. Consult textbooks, recent literature, and experts if uncertain about proper treatment options. Certain diseases (such as fasciitis, gangrene, septic arthritis, and osteomyelitis) may require surgical treatment. Drug doses may need to be changed or selections altered depending on cultures, renal function, and underlying disease.

Continued

Table K-11—cont'd

Infection	Treatment*
Pneumonia *(Pneumocystis carinii)*	• Septra DS 2 tablets po q8 hr or IV Septra 15 mg/kg of trimethoprim if ill q8 hr × 21 days or • Clindamycin 600 mg IV q8 hr or 300-450 mg po qid, and primaquine 15-30 mg of base po qd × 21 days or • Pentamidine (Pentam) 4 mg/kg IV q24 hr × 21 days, or dapsone 100 mg po qd and trimethoprim (Primsol) 5 mg/kg po tid × 21 days, or atovaquone 750 mg po bid × 21 days • Add prednisone taper for 2-3 weeks if Po_2 <70 mm Hg
Prostatitis—≤35 years	• See Pelvic inflammatory disease—outpatient treatment
Prostatitis—>35 years	• Ciprofloxacin 500 mg po bid × 14 days, Septra DS 1 po bid × 14 days, or see Epididymitis—all ages • Chronic prostatitis may require 4 weeks of treatment
Pyelonephritis—healthy	• Oral × 7 days: Ciprofloxacin 250 mg bid, levofloxacin 250-500 mg qd, ofloxacin 200-400 mg bid, lomefloxacin 400 mg qd, gatifloxacin 200-400 mg pd, or moxifloxacin 400 mg qd or • Septra DS po bid or oral cephalosporin (see dosing for Urinary tract infection (pregnant and uncomplicated...)—give each for 14 days • IV: Ampicillin 2 g IV q4 hr and gentamicin, or ciprofloxacin/levofloxacin/gatifloxacin IV (highest po dose IV), or cefotaxime 1 g IV q12 hr, or ceftriaxone 1g IV qd, or Timentin 3.1 g IV q6 hr, or Zosyn 3.375-4.5 mg IV q6-8 hr • If pregnant, use IV cefotaxime or ceftriaxone as listed above
Pyelonephritis—nursing home or Foley catheter	• Ampicillin 2 g IV q4 hr and gentamicin, or IV fluoroquinolone (healthy pyelonephritis dose), or Timentin 3.1 g IV q8 hr, or Zosyn 4.5 g IV q8 hr, or imipenem 0.5-1 g IV q6-8 hr, or meropenem 0.5-1 g IV q8 hr
Retropharyngeal abscess	• See Submandibular abscess

*The decision to use IV or po regimens is complex. Listed medications are only recommendations. Consult textbooks, recent literature, and experts if uncertain about proper treatment options. Certain diseases (such as fasciitis, gangrene, septic arthritis, and osteomyelitis) may require surgical treatment. Drug doses may need to be changed or selections altered depending on cultures, renal function, and underlying disease.

Table K-11—cont'd

Infection	Treatment*
Scabies and head lice	• Permethrin 5% (Elimite) or 1% (Nix); scabies: Massage cream into body and remove within 8-14 hours; scalp lice: Apply lotion to dry hair, saturate for 10 minutes, then rinse off • Crotamiton (Eurax); scabies: Apply with chin down, repeat in 24 hours, and wash off in 48 hours • Lindane (Kwell); scabies: Apply lotion with neck down and wash off in 8-12 hours; lice: Apply lotion or cream to affected areas and wash off in 12 hours or shampoo with 30-60 ml lotion and remove in 4 minutes • Ivermectin (Stromectol) 200 μg/kg po (tabs are 3 or 6 mg) • Malathion 0.5% (Ovide); lice: Apply to dry hair, dry naturally, and wash off in 8-12 hours, repeat in 7-9 days
Sepsis	• Drotrecogin alfa/recombinant human activated protein C 24 μg/kg/hr × 96 hr if ≥3 SIRS features and there is evidence of sepsis-induced organ dysfunction >24 hr
Septic arthritis—no trauma or operation	• Nafcillin or oxacillin 2 g IV q4 hr, and antipseudomonal cephalosporin or ciprofloxacin 400 mg IV bid • If gonorrhea is suspected, use a third-generation cephalosporin
Septic arthritis—after trauma/surgery or prosthetic joint	• Vancomycin 1 g IV q12 hr, and ciprofloxacin 400 mg IV q12 hr or gentamicin 1.7 mg/kg IV q8 h or aztreonam 1 g IV q8 hr or antipseudomonal cephalosporin IV
Septic bursitis	• IV therapy: Nafcillin or oxacillin 2 g IV q4 hr, cefazolin 2 g IV q8 hr, or vancomycin 1g IV q12 hr • Oral therapy: Dicloxacillin 500 mg po qid, or ciprofloxacin 750 mg po bid plus rifampin 300 mg po bid
Sinusitis	• Mild disease: See Otitis media • Severe disease (if well enough for outpatient treatment): Moxifloxacin 400 mg po qd × 10 days, levofloxacin 500 mg po qd × 10-14 days, or gatifloxacin 400 mg po qd × 10 days
Submandibular abscess—surgery often required	• Clindamycin 600-900 mg IV q8 hr, cefoxitin 2 g IV q8 hr, Unasyn 1.5-3.0 g IV q8 hr, Timentin 3.1 g IV q4-6 hr, or Zosyn 3.375-4.5 g IV q6 hr
Syphilis—primary or secondary <1 year	• Penicillin G benzathine (Bicillin LA) 2.4 million units IM, or doxycycline 100 mg po bid × 14 days

*The decision to use IV or po regimens is complex. Listed medications are only recommendations. Consult textbooks, recent literature, and experts if uncertain about proper treatment options. Certain diseases (such as fasciitis, gangrene, septic arthritis, and osteomyelitis) may require surgical treatment. Drug doses may need to be changed or selections altered depending on cultures, renal function, and underlying disease.

Continued

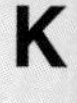

Table K-11—cont'd

Infection	Treatment*
Syphilis—secondary >1 year	• Penicillin G benzathine 2.4 million units IM q week × 3, or doxycycline 100 mg po bid × 28 days
Tinea—capitis and barbae (scalp and beard) (not all agents are FDA approved for these indications)	• Terbinafine (Lamisil) 250 mg po qd × 4-8 weeks, griseofulvin (Grifulvin V) 500 mg po qd × 6 weeks, itraconazole 3-5 mg/kg/day po qd × 6 weeks, or fluconazole 8 mg/kg q week × 8-12 weeks (max 150 mg/week) • Add ketoconazole 2% or selenium sulfide shampoo
Tinea—corporis, cruris pedis (skin, inguinal, feet) (not all oral agents are FDA approved for these indications)	• Topical options: Ciclopirox (Loprox) bid, clotrimazole bid, econazole (Spectazole) qd, miconazole bid, naftifine (Naftin) bid, oxiconazole (Oxistat) qd, or terbinafine bid • If unresponsive to topicals: Fluconazole 150 mg/week × 2-4 weeks, terbinafine 250 mg po qd × 2 weeks (use a longer regimen for tinea pedis), ketoconazole 200 mg po qd × 4 weeks, or griseofulvin 500 mg po qd × 4-6 weeks
Tinea unguium—nails and onychomycosis (not all oral agents are FDA approved for this indication)	• Terbinafine 250 mg po qd × 6 weeks or pulse 500 mg po qd × 1 week on/3 weeks off × 2 months (use longer regimen for toes, shorter for fingers), or fluconazole 150-300 mg/week × ≥3 months, or itraconazole 200 mg po qd × 3 ml or pulse 200 mg po bid × 1 week on/3 weeks off × 2-3 months
Tinea versicolor	• Topical options: Ciclopirox bid, clotrimazole bid, econazole qd, ketoconazole qd, miconazole bid, oxiconazole qd, or terbinafine bid • Oral options: Ketoconazole 400 mg po × 1 or 200 mg/day × 7 days or fluconazole 400 mg po × 1
Trichomonas	• Metronidazole 2 g po × 1 or 500 mg po bid × 7 days
Urinary tract infection (healthy females, nonrecurrent)	• Simple UTI: 3 days po of any of the following (if complicated outpatient, use for 10-14 days): Septra DS 1 bid, ciprofloxacin 250 mg bid, Cipro XR 500 mg po qd, levofloxacin 250 mg qd, lomefloxacin 400 mg qd, norfloxacin 400 mg bid, ofloxacin 200-300 mg bid, or gatifloxacin 200-400 mg qd

*The decision to use IV or po regimens is complex. Listed medications are only recommendations. Consult textbooks, recent literature, and experts if uncertain about proper treatment options. Certain diseases (such as fasciitis, gangrene, septic arthritis, and osteomyelitis) may require surgical treatment. Drug doses may need to be changed or selections altered depending on cultures, renal function, and underlying disease.

Table K-11—cont'd

Infection	Treatment*
Urinary tract infection (pregnant and uncomplicated without pyelonephritis or pregnant asymptomatic bacteriuria)	• Treat 7-10 days for simple infection or 3 days for asymptomatic bacteriuria; choose one of following: Nitrofurantoin (Macrodantin) 50-100 mg po qid, cefadroxil (Duricef) 1 g po bid, cephalexin 500 mg po bid, cefuroxime 125-250 mg po bid, loracarbef (Lorabid) 200 mg po bid, cefixime 400 mg po qd, or cefpodoxime 100 mg po bid
Vaginosis (bacterial)	• Oral: Metronidazole 500 mg or clindamycin 300 mg po bid × 7 days • Intravaginal: Metronidazole gel qd or bid × 5 days or clindamycin vaginal cream qhs × 7 days
Vaginitis *(Candida)*	• Miconazole topical bid × 2 weeks, fluconazole 150 mg po × 1 dose, or itraconazole 200 mg po bid × 1 day
Vascular infection	• Vancomycin 1 g IV q12 hr (such as IV, central line, or dialysis)
Viral encephalitis	• See Herpes
Warts	• Anogenital: Imiquimod (Aldara) 3 × per week qhs until clear (max 16 weeks) (wash off in 6-10 hr), or podofilox (Condylox) bid for 3 consecutive days/week × 4 weeks (only apply 3 days/week), or physician-applied podophyllin 25% applied to wart for 30 minutes first treatment then minimum time for desired result (1-4 hr) q week, or other therapy by physician (cryotherapy, laser, trichloroacetic acid, bleomycin, or surgery) • Cutaneous: Topical salicylic acid (Dr. Scholl's/Duo-Film/Clear Away) bid or q48 hr if plaster or pad application × 4-12 weeks (over the counter), tretinoin topical (Retin-A) 0.025-0.1% qhs for verruca plana (flat warts), or other therapy listed above

*The decision to use IV or po regimens is complex. Listed medications are only recommendations. Consult textbooks, recent literature, and experts if uncertain about proper treatment options. Certain diseases (such as fasciitis, gangrene, septic arthritis, and osteomyelitis) may require surgical treatment. Drug doses may need to be changed or selections altered depending on cultures, renal function, and underlying disease.

References

1. Fekety R. Guidelines for the diagnosis and management of Clostridium difficile–associated diarrhea and colitis. American College of Gastroenterology, Practice Parameters Committee. Am J Gastroenterology 92:739, 1997.
2. Bartlett JG. Clinical practice. Antibiotic-associated diarrhea. N Eng J Med 346:334, 2002.
3. Tedesco FJ, Gordon D, Fortson WC. Approach to patients with multiple relapses of antibiotic-associated pseudomembranous colitis. Am J Gastroenterol 80:867, 1985.

Appendix

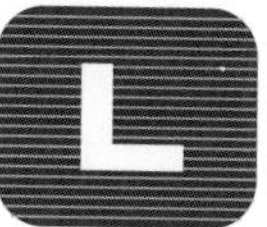

OBSTETRICS AND GYNECOLOGY

L

DIAGNOSIS OF ECTOPIC PREGNANCY IN CLINICALLY STABLE PATIENTS

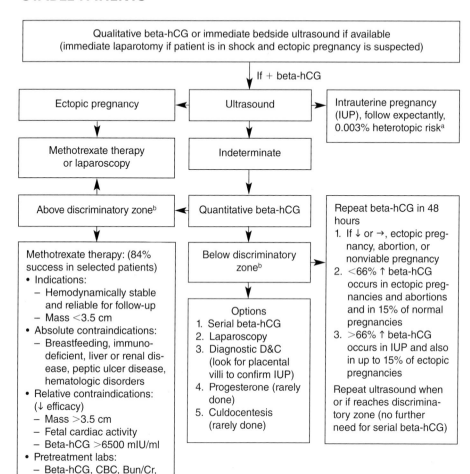

Qualitative beta-hCG or immediate bedside ultrasound if available
(immediate laparotomy if patient is in shock and ectopic pregnancy is suspected)

↓ If + beta-hCG

Ultrasound

- → Ectopic pregnancy → Methotrexate therapy or laparoscopy
- → Intrauterine pregnancy (IUP), follow expectantly, 0.003% heterotopic risk[a]
- → Indeterminate → Quantitative beta-hCG

Quantitative beta-hCG

- → Above discriminatory zone[b] → Methotrexate therapy or laparoscopy
- → Above discriminatory zone[b] → Methotrexate therapy: (84% success in selected patients)
  - Indications:
    - Hemodynamically stable and reliable for follow-up
    - Mass <3.5 cm
  - Absolute contraindications:
    - Breastfeeding, immunodeficient, liver or renal disease, peptic ulcer disease, hematologic disorders
  - Relative contraindications: (↓ efficacy)
    - Mass >3.5 cm
    - Fetal cardiac activity
    - Beta-hCG >6500 mIU/ml
  - Pretreatment labs:
    - Beta-hCG, CBC, Bun/Cr, AST/ALT, type and Rh
  - Dose: (Based on BMI)
    - 50 mg/m² IM
  - Follow-up:
    - Serial beta-hCG on days 0, 4, and 7
    - Expect >15% ↓ on day 4 to 7 (may ↑ day 0 to 4); if not, may repeat
  - Side effects:
    - Nausea, vomiting, diarrhea, stomatitis, and sun sensitivity
- → Below discriminatory zone[b]

Below discriminatory zone[b]

- → Options
  1. Serial beta-hCG
  2. Laparoscopy
  3. Diagnostic D&C (look for placental villi to confirm IUP)
  4. Progesterone (rarely done)
  5. Culdocentesis (rarely done)
- → Repeat beta-hCG in 48 hours
  1. If ↓ or →, ectopic pregnancy, abortion, or nonviable pregnancy
  2. <66% ↑ beta-hCG occurs in ectopic pregnancies and abortions and in 15% of normal pregnancies
  3. >66% ↑ beta-hCG occurs in IUP and also in up to 15% of ectopic pregnancies

  Repeat ultrasound when or if reaches discriminatory zone (no further need for serial beta-hCG)

Fig. L-1 *a,* Concurrent IUP plus ectopic pregnancy. *b,* Discriminatory zone is 1200-1500 mIU/ml for transvaginal ultrasonography and 6500 mIU/ml for transabdominal ultrasonography. (Compiled from Brennan DF. Ectopic pregnancy: Part I: clinical and laboratory diagnosis. Acad Emerg Med 2:1081, 1995.)

ULTRASOUND FINDINGS*

Intrauterine Pregnancy (IUP)

1. Decidual reaction
2. Gestational sac is seen at 4.5 weeks with beta-hCG 1000 to 1400 via transvaginal ultrasonography or 6 weeks with beta-hCG >6500 via transabdominal ultrasonography
3. Yolk sac is seen at 5.5 weeks with beta-hCG >7200; if no fetal pole with sac >18 mm, the pregnancy is likely nonviable
4. Fetal pole/heartbeat is seen at 5.5 to 7 weeks with beta-hCG 10,800 to 17,200; cardiac activity with a 5 mm fetal pole should be visible. It is best not to correlate beta-hCG with viability, because the range is wide

Ectopic Pregnancy (Percent With Finding)

1. Empty uterus, decidual reaction, or pseudosac (10% to 20%)
2. Cul-de-sac fluid (24% to 63%); echogenic indicates blood
3. Adnexal mass (60% to 90%)
4. Echogenic halo around tube (26% to 68%)
5. Fetal heart activity (8% to 23%)

---

*Transvaginal ultrasonography unless otherwise stated.

Table L-1 Quantitative beta-hCG in IUP*

Time	mIU/ml
<1 week	<5-50
1-2 weeks	40-300
2-3 weeks	100-1000
3-4 weeks	500-6000
1-2 months	5000-200,000
2-3 months	10,000-100,000
Second trimester	3000-50,000
Third trimester	1000-50,000

*Time from conception. Median time for beta-hCG to turn negative after spontaneous abortion is 16 days (30 days for elective). Urine HCG + correlates to serum beta-hCG 20 mIU/ml.

Rh ISOIMMUNIZATION

The Kleihauer-Betke test estimates blood transfused into maternal circulation.

$$\text{Fetal whole blood volume (ml)} = \frac{\text{Maternal blood volume (ml)} \times \text{Maternal hematocrit} \times \text{Fetal red cells}}{\text{Newborn hematocrit}}$$

- RhIG/RhoGAM: One vial IM is indicated if fetal RBCs possibly entered the circulation of Rh-negative mother; one RhIG vial contains approximately 300 μg of immune globulin and protects against the transfusion of 30 ml of Rh-positive fetal RBCs
- RhIG (MICRhoGAM, Mini-Gamulin Rh, HypRho-D Mini Dose): A 1/6 dose neutralizes 2.5 ml RBCs; indications: spontaneous or elective first trimester pregnancy termination or ectopic ≤12 weeks*

Indications for RhIG Therapy

Give therapy within 72 hours of event. Indications include an Rh-negative mother and one of the following:

- Delivery of Rh-positive infant
- Abortion or ectopic pregnancy
- Following trauma (even if minor)
- Any transfusion of Rh-positive blood
- Threatened abortion (controversial)*
- Following amniocentesis, chorionic villi, or umbilical blood sampling
- At 28 weeks

PREGNANCY-INDUCED HYPERTENSION, PREECLAMPSIA, AND ECLAMPSIA

Pregnancy-Induced Hypertension

- BP ≥140/90 mm Hg
- Measure BP on two occasions ≥6 hours apart (not practical in the ED)

Preeclampsia

- Hypertension with nondependent edema or proteinuria >20 weeks gestation
- Weight gain >2 lb/week or 6 lb/month is suggestive
- Proteinuria occurs late, >300 mg protein/24 hr (300 mg/day = 1 + dipstick) or >1 g/L in two urines >6 hr apart

---

*The use of RhoGAM is controversial in spontaneous or elective abortion <12 weeks. Some authors recommend its use,[1] whereas others do not.[2]

Severe Preeclampsia

- BP ≥160/110 mm Hg
- Proteinuria ≥2+, Cr >1.2 mg/dl—new
- Oliguria (urine output ≤500 ml/24 hr)
- Elevated AST/ALT
- Platelets <100,000 cells/μl
- Headache, visual change, RUQ or midepigastric abdominal pain, pulmonary edema, or hyperreflexia

HELLP Syndrome

- **H**emolytic anemia, **E**levated **L**iver function tests, **L**ow **P**latelets
- Variant of preeclampsia with upper abdominal pain and/or vomiting
- Minimal hypertension

Eclampsia

- Seizures caused by preeclampsia or ≤7 days of delivery (± later)

TREATMENT OF PREECLAMPSIA/ECLAMPSIA

- The ultimate cure is delivery
- Seizure prophylaxis
  - Load 4 to 6 g $MgSO_4$ IV in 100 ml NS over 30 minutes
  - Maintenance: Add 20 g $MgSO_4$ to 500 ml NS and administer 50 ml/hr (2 g/hr). Continue through labor and 24 hours after delivery
  - Side effects: Flushing, headache, blurring, dizziness, decreased reflexes, and respiratory and cardiac arrest. Monitor patellar reflexes and respirations and keep urine output ≥25 ml/hr. Restrict fluid to a total of 2400 to 3000 ml/24 hr while treating. Follow serum levels every 6 hours or if toxicity is suspected, and keep at 4 to 6 mEq/L
  - Antidote to $MgSO_4$ overdose (causes lethargy, loss of DTRs, respiratory depression, and ultimately CV collapse): Give calcium gluconate (10%) 10 to 20 ml or 1 g slow IV push
  - Contraindications to $MgSO_4$: Myasthenia gravis, maternal cardiovascular disease, renal impairment, or use of nifedipine, beta agonists, and steroids, because use of these drugs with $MgSO_4$ may lead to pulmonary edema/cardiac depression
- Seizure treatment: Check serum magnesium level and bolus 2 to 4 g if needed; barbiturates and benzodiazepines (diazepam 10 mg IV push) are second line, because both may cause fetal depression

- Antihypertensives: Treat to prevent stroke, not cure preeclampsia
  - Indications: Diastolic BP is ≥105 mm Hg
  - Goal: Decreased diastolic BP to 90 to 95 mm Hg (lower if baseline diastolic BP is known to be <75 mm Hg)
  - Hydralazine: Administer 5 mg IV over 1 to 2 minutes; repeat 5 to 10 mg IV q20 to 30 min prn; if a total of 20 mg is given without effect, try a second drug
  - Labetalol: Give 10 mg IV; double q10 min until BP goal or maximum is reached (300 mg total)
  - Diazoxide: Administer 30 mg IV q5 to 15 min prn (maximum dose 150 mg)

DIFFICULT DELIVERIES: BREECH AND SHOULDER DYSTOCIA

The techniques described are for instances when obstetric expertise is unavailable and ED delivery is required. Call for OB backup immediately for these occasions.

Breech Delivery[3]

In cases of frank breech presentation (hips and legs extended) delivery occurs spontaneously and little intervention is warranted. For cases of footling breech presentation, risk is high for umbilical cord prolapse. Delivery maneuvers in these cases are as follows:

- Grasp both feet with index finger between ankles, and pull feet through vulva. Wrap feet in towel, and perform episiotomy
- Apply downward traction until the hips are delivered, with thumbs over sacrum and fingers over hip; continue downward traction
- As scapula emerges, rotate back laterally
- Attempt shoulder delivery only after low scapula and axilla are visible
- First deliver anterior shoulder/arm, then rotate and deliver posterior arm
- If unable, deliver posterior shoulder first by pulling feet up above the mother's groin, guiding two fingers along the humerus and gently sweeping the fetal arm down; the anterior arm may be delivered by depression of the body alone or with finger sweep as with the posterior shoulder
- Rotate occiput anteriorly
- Next, extract the head using the Mauriceau maneuver; apply suprapubic pressure, and gently flex the head by pressing on the maxilla

Maneuvers for Managing Shoulder Dystocia[4]

- Assure generous episiotomy
- First use the McRoberts maneuver (hyperflex the hips—rotate the hips cephalad—and flatten lumbar lordosis) while assistant applies suprapubic pressure; assistant's pressure may be applied anterior to posterior (Mazzanti) or lateral to medial (79% success)

- The Gaskin maneuver (hand/knee position) allows posterior shoulder descent (83% success)
- Wood's screw: Push posterior shoulder anteriorly 180 degrees and deliver the shoulder
- Rubin: Push (adduct) either shoulder to anterior fetal chest 15 to 30 degrees (decrease bisacromial diameter)
- Deliver posterior arm
- Clavicle fracture: Pull upward—anteriorly on the distal clavicle—to decrease bisacromial diameter

THIRD TRIMESTER VAGINAL BLEEDING AND POSTPARTUM HEMORRHAGE

Placental Abruption

Placental abruption is the separation of normal placenta before birth.

Risk Factors

- Hypertension, maternal age >35 years
- Smoking, cocaine use, or trauma
- Causes 30% of third trimester bleeds

Clinical Features

- Vaginal bleeding (dark) (78%)
- Abdominal pain (66%)
- Uterine contractions (17%)
- Fetal death (15%)
- Maternal DIC: Bedside screen: Place 5 ml of maternal venous blood in red top tube, DIC if no clots by 6 minutes

Management

- Avoid digital pelvic examination until placenta previa is excluded
- Ultrasound is only 25% sensitive; diagnosis is primarily clinical
- Concealed hemorrhage (retroplacental) has minimal to no vaginal bleeding and may lead to underestimation of true EBL
- Administer O_2 and IV NS
- Obtain type and crossmatch, PT/PTT, CBC, and fibrinogen
- Administer blood, FFP, and platelets prn
- May require immediate delivery

Placenta Previa

Placenta previa occurs when the placenta is implanted over the cervical os.

Clinical Features and Diagnosis

- Responsible for 20% to 30% of third trimester bleeding
- Sudden, painless vaginal bleeding
- Absence of abdominal pain
- Soft, nontender uterus
- Avoid digital pelvic examination
- Ultrasound is 95% sensitive (transvaginal ultrasound is okay)

Management

- If preterm, consider tocolysis with one of the following:
  - $MgSO_4$ 4 to 6 g IV (slow) plus 2 to 3 g/hr IV
  - Terbutaline 0.25 mg SC q30 min up to 1 mg in 4 hr
  - Terbutaline 2.5 to 5 mg po q4 to 6 hr
  - Ritodrine 0.05 mg/kg/min IV; increase by 0.05 mg/min until effect (typica range is 0.15 to 0.35 mg/min)
- If viable pregnancy (near term), deliver via cesarean section

Postpartum Hemorrhage

Postpartum hemorrhage is the loss of >500 ml of blood in the first 24 hours afte delivery.

Most Common Causes

- Uterine atony
- Retained placental fragments
- Cervical and uterine lacerations

Management

1. IV NS (ensure adequate access, two large-bore IVs), give blood products prn oxygen, and fundal/bimanual massage. Include DIC screen with initial labs.
2. Oxytocin (Pitocin) 10 U IM or 10 to 40 U in 1 L NS at 100 to 200 ml/hr after placental delivery (may decrease BP) or methylergonovine tartrate (Methergine 0.2 mg IM after placenta delivers (may repeat after 15 min). Methergine is contraindicated in patients with hypertension.
3. Give 15-methyl PGF_2-alpha (Carboprost) 0.25 mg IM q15 to 90 min to maximum dose of 2 mg. This may decrease O_2, so apply pulse oximeter. Carbopros is contraindicated in patients with asthma or cardiac disease.
4. Misoprostol (Cytotec/PGE1) 800 μg per rectum, which may take up to 30 minutes for effect.

5. Uterine artery embolization can be considered if the patient is stable. Surgery (uterine curettage or hysterectomy) may be needed for severe bleeding that is unresponsive to medical management.
6. Consider cervical or uterine laceration, uterine rupture, or abnormal placental attachment (placenta accreta, especially if history of previous cesarean) if the patient has continued bleeding.

References

1. Fung Kee Fung K, Eason E, Crane J, et al. Prevention of Rh alloimmunization. J Obstet Gynaecol Can 765, 2003.
2. Weissman AM, Dawson JD, Rijhsinghani A, et al. Non-evidence-based use of Rho(D) immune globulin for threatened abortion by family practice and obstetric faculty physicians. J Reprod Med 47:909, 2002.
3. Cunningham FG, MacDonald PC, Gant NF, et al. Williams Obstetrics. Stamford, CT: Appleton & Lange, 1997, p 501.
4. Romney S. Gynecology and Obstetrics: The Health Care of Women. New York: McGraw-Hill, 1975.

APPENDIX

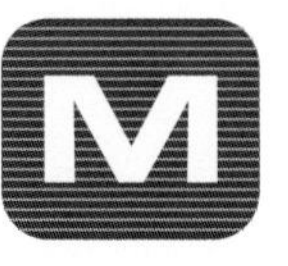

ENDOCRINOLOGY

M

ENDOCRINE DISORDERS

Adrenal Insufficiency

Clinical Features

- Weakness (99%)
- Hyperpigmentation (92%)
- Weight loss (97%)
- Vomiting (70%)
- Anorexia (98%)
- BP <110/70 (85%)
- Abdominal pain (34%)
- Salt craving (22%)
- Diarrhea (20%)
- ↑ K^+
- ↓ Na^+
- Eosinophilia

Adrenal Crisis Therapy

- Give 1 to 2 L NS IV with further IV fluids as needed
- Correct electrolyte abnormalities
- Give hydrocortisone (Solu-Cortef) 200 mg IV plus 100 mg q8 hr or dexamethasone 4 mg IV (will not interfere with ACTH stimulation testing)
- If possible, draw and store blood for steroid level analysis, including baseline serum cortisol and ACTH levels
- Consider broad-spectrum antibiotics (such as ceftriaxone 1 to 2 g IV) if sepsis is suspected
- Perform rapid bedside check of blood sugar
- Treat underlying precipitants such as sepsis, hypothermia, MI, ↓ glucose, bleeding, or trauma; remove medications that ↓ cortisone (such as morphine, chlorpromazine, or barbiturates)

Adrenal Crisis[1,2]

Setting

- Sudden extensive adrenal destruction (such as hemorrhage or infarction), or
- Major physiologic stress (such as surgery, infection, or trauma) in patient with unrecognized primary adrenal insufficiency, or
- Inadequate stress-dose corticosteroids in a patient with known or suspected adrenal insufficiency (such as chronic corticosteroid treatment, even at low doses)
- Uncommon in secondary or tertiary (central) adrenal insufficiency because of preserved mineralocorticoid homeostasis; however, severe or sudden pituitary

dysfunction (such as hemorrhage) may produce hypotension on the basis of glucocorticoid deficiency (mineralocorticoid → intravascular volume; glucocorticoid → vascular tone)
- Septic shock itself may cause relative (reversible) adrenal insufficiency

M

Causes of Adrenal Insufficiency
- Bilateral adrenal destruction:
  - Hemorrhagic (often occult): Anticoagulation, coagulopathy, postoperative
  - Thrombotic: Adrenal vein thrombosis after back injury, thrombotic microangiopathy (DIC, HIT)
  - Metastatic tumor
- Sepsis: Meningococcemia (Waterhouse-Friderichsen syndrome), *Pseudomonas*
- Autoimmune adrenalitis: Idiopathic or polyglandular failure syndrome
- Granulomatous infection: Tuberculosis, histoplasmosis, or other fungi
- HIV: HIV itself, CMV, or MAC
- Drugs:
  - Adrenal suppression (corticosteroids, megestrol, medroxyprogesterone acetate)
  - Inhibition of cortisol synthesis (ketoconazole, etomidate)
  - Accelerated cortisol degradation (phenytoin, rifampin, barbiturates)
- Pituitary apoplexy: Secondary insufficiency (glucocorticoid only)

Manifestations
- Shock: Both hypovolemic and distributive; shock is often out of proportion to severity of acute illness and refractory to fluids and pressors until adrenal hormone replacement is given
- GI symptoms: Nausea and vomiting, anorexia, or abdominal pain (may mimic acute abdomen)
- Fever: Accentuated by low cortisol, but occult infection is common
- CNS: Lethargy, confusion, or coma
- Physical/radiologic findings
  - Hyperpigmentation of mucosa, creases, and sun-spared skin (primary insufficiency only)
  - Small cardiac silhouette on CXR
  - Calcified or enlarged adrenals on CT scan
- Laboratory features: ↓ Na^+, ↑ K^+ (↓ aldosterone), ↑ BUN/Cr, ↓ glucose, ↑ Ca^{2+}, and eosinophilia
- Secondary adrenal insufficiency differs in the following ways
  - ACTH is low to normal
  - There is no hyperpigmentation
  - Mineralocorticoid activity is preserved (no hyperkalemia)
  - The presence of hyponatremia from centrally increased ADH
  - Hypoglycemia is common

Diagnosis

- High-dose ACTH (cosyntropin) stimulation[3]
  - Give 250 μg IV
  - Cortisol ≥18 to 21 μg/dl at baseline or within 60 minutes of injection is highly accurate at ruling out chronic, severe adrenal insufficiency
  - Criteria may miss partial or recent onset insufficiency, especially in critically ill patients
- Random cortisol level[4,5]
  - In patients with critical illness (especially septic shock), relative adrenal insufficiency may occur and contribute to hypotension, etc.
  - A random cortisol level <15 μg/dl is clearly abnormal in critical illness, whereas a random cortisol level >34 μg/dl is clearly sufficient
  - If random cortisol is 15 to 34 μg/dl, check ACTH stimulation and consider abnormal if incremental response is <9 μg/dl
- ACTH level is used to differentiate between primary disease (normal ACTH) and secondary or tertiary disease (low to normal ACTH); check a random sample before empiric corticosteroids

Therapy

1. Rapid volume resuscitation (30% to 50% of normal intravascular volume, typically 2 to 3 L NS) titrated to JVP or pulmonary edema. Replace potassium and glucose prn.
2. Draw baseline cortisol and ACTH level.
3. Give dexamethasone (4 mg IV) to restore vascular tone (will not interfere with ACTH stimulation test).
4. Perform ACTH stimulation test.
5. Start hydrocortisone 100 mg IV q6 to 8 hr. Taper gradually (such as 50% per day) after the patient is stabilized. Separate mineralocorticoid repletion is not required acutely, but fludrocortisone should be added when total daily hydrocortisone <100 mg/day.
6. Identify and treat precipitating illness.
7. If primary adrenal insufficiency, the patient will need chronic repletion with hydrocortisone (typically 20 mg q AM, 10 mg q PM) and fludrocortisone (0.1 mg qd, titrated to K^+).

Laboratory Features of Thyrotoxicosis

Laboratory tests can diagnose hyperthyroidism, but thyrotoxicosis is a clinical diagnosis.

- ↑ free T4, ↑ T3, and ↓ TSH
- ↑ T4 RIA, ↑ FT4 I
- ↑ glucose, ↑ Ca^{2+}, ↓ Hb
- ↑ WBC, ↓ cholesterol

Treatment
- Give supportive care, O_2, and alpha glucose; control fever (avoid aspirin) and treat precipitants
- Inhibit thyroid hormone synthesis
  - Propylthiouracil (PTU) 600 to 900 mg po on day 1, then 300 to 400 mg/day po × 3 to 6 weeks
  - PTU inhibits the conversion of T4 to T3
- Inhibit thyroid hormone release
  - Give K^+ iodide as Lugol solution (8 mg iodide per drop) 1 ml or 20 drops po q8 hr
  - Or give SSKI (40 mg iodide per drop) 2 to 10 drops po daily
  - Or give Na^+ iodide 1 g IV q8 to 12 hr (give over 30 minutes)
  - CAUTION: Administer iodide ≥1 hour after antithyroid medications to prevent use in hormone synthesis
- Blockade of peripheral effects
  - Propranolol 1 mg slowly IV q15 min (maximum of 5 mg) prn to reduce sympathetic hyperactivity and conversion for T4 to T3
  - Begin propranolol 20 to 120 mg po q6 to 8 hr when symptoms improve
- Inhibit conversion of T4 to T3
  - Give hydrocortisone 100 mg IV q8 hr

Hypothyroidism: Myxedema Coma

Precipitants
- Pneumonia, GI bleed
- CHF, cold exposure
- Stroke, trauma, ↓ glucose
- ↓ Po_2, ↑ pCO_2, ↓ Na^+

Drugs
- Phenothiazines
- Lithium
- Narcotics
- Sedatives
- Phenytoin
- Propranolol

Laboratory Tests
- Serum TSH >60 μU/ml
- ↓ total and free T4
- ↓ or ↔ total and free T3

M

Clinical Features

- Vital signs: Temperature is often <90° F, 50% have BP <100/60
- Cardiac: ↓ HR, heart block, low voltage, ST-T changes, ↑ Q-T, effusion
- Pulmonary: Hypoventilation, ↑ PCO_2, ↓ O_2, pleural effusions
- Metabolic: Hyponatremia, hypoglycemia
- Neurologic: Coma, seizures, tremors, ataxia, nystagmus, psychiatric disturbances, depressed or hung-up reflexes
- GI/GU: Ileus, ascites, fecal impaction, megacolon, urinary retention
- Skin: Alopecia; loss of lateral third of eyebrows; nonpitting puffiness around eyes, hands, and pretibial region of legs
- Ear, nose, throat: Tongue enlarges, voice deepens and becomes hoarse

Management

- Administer O_2, rewarm, and treat cause (such as infection or ↓ glucose)
- Give thyroxine 400 to 500 μg slow IV on day one, plus 50 to 100 μg IV qd
  CAUTION: IV thyroxine may cause cardiac arrest; reduce dose if cardiac ischemia or arrhythmias; some experts recommend no IV thyroxine for 3 to 7 days after day one
- Start oral thyroxine 100 to 200 μg po qd when possible
- Hydrocortisone 100 mg IV q8 hr

Hyperthyroidism: Thyroid Storm[6,7]

Underlying Thyroid Disease

- Graves' disease (most common)
- Toxic nodular goiter
- Toxic adenoma
- Factitious thyrotoxicosis
- Excess TSH
- Jod-Basedow phenomenon (iodine-induced)

Precipitants of Thyroid Storm

- Infection (most common)
- Pulmonary embolus
- DKA or HHNC
- Thyroid hormone excess
- Iodine therapy/dye
- Stroke
- Surgery

- Childbirth
- D&C
- Psychiatric stress
- Withdrawal of antithyroid drugs
- Diabetic ketoacidosis
- Sympathomimetic drugs (pseudoephedrine)

Clinical Features of Thyroid Storm (Thyrotoxicosis)

- Hyperkinesis
- Palpable goiter
- Proptosis, lid lag
- Exophthalmos, palsy (palsy of extraocular muscles)
- Temperature >101° F
- Palpitations, dyspnea
- Psychosis, apathy
- Tremor, hyperreflexia
- Weight loss
- Jaundice
- Tachycardia
- Diaphoresis (out of proportion to the apparent infection)
- Cardiopulmonary: ↑ metabolic demand, ↑ O_2 consumption, ↑ cardiac output, ↑ HR, ↑ pulse pressure
  - Hyperdynamic circulation → high-output CHF
  - Myocardial ischemia
  - Arrhythmia (new onset): Atrial fibrillation/flutter, which may be refractory to digoxin
  - Systolic HTN with widened pulse pressure
- Neurologic
  - Delirium, stupor or coma, seizures
  - Myopathy >50%
  - Ophthalmopathy (Graves' disease)
  - Rare complications: Aggravated myasthenia gravis or thyrotoxic hypokalemic periodic paralysis (in Asian men)
- GI: Vomiting, diarrhea, malabsorption
  - Increased gastrin → PUD
  - Abnormal LFTs
- Laboratory features: ↑ glucose, ↑ WBC, ↓ Hct, ↓ platelets, ↓ K^+, ↑ Ca^{2+} (may be severe), ↑ LFTs

Treatment

1. Antithyroid treatment—effective for hyperfunctioning gland (such as with Graves' disease) but not thyroiditis or exogenous thyroid hormone
   - Inhibit new hormone synthesis with PTU (200 to 250 mg po/ng q4 hr) or methimazole (20 mg po/ng q4 hr); PTU is preferred because it blocks peripheral T4 to T3 conversion; the IV form is not available in the United States, but it may be given as a retention enema
   - Inhibit hormone secretion with iodine: SSKI or Lugol solution (8 gtt po q6 hr). CAUTION: Use at least 2 hours after methimazole or PTU (iodine monotherapy can exacerbate thyrotoxicosis). *Iodine allergy:* Give lithium carbonate 300 mg po q6 hr to keep lithium level approximately 1 mEq/L
2. Block peripheral action and conversion of thyroid hormone
   - Give a beta-adrenergic blockade such as propranolol (0.5 to 1 mg IV/min to a total of 2 to 10 mg titrated to HR, then 20 to 80 mg po q4 to 6 hr)
   - Inhibit peripheral T4 to T3 conversion with an oral iodinated contrast agent such as iopanoate (Telepaque, 1 g q8 hr po load, then 500 mg bid) and/or glucocorticoids such as dexamethasone (2 g IV/po q6 hr) or hydrocortisone (100 mg IV q8 hr); beta-blockers and PTU also block T4 to T3; the high iodine content in iopanoate may substitute for SSKI or Lugol solution
   - If intractable symptoms, consider dialysis, plasmapheresis, or enteric binding of thyroid hormone with cholestyramine (4 g po q6 hr)
3. Treat underlying illness such as occult infection, CHF, or diabetic ketoacidosis
4. General supportive care
   - Control hyperthermia with acetaminophen and cooling blankets
   - Fluid resuscitation and dextrose for diaphoresis, vomiting, diarrhea, and hypoglycemia
   - Parenteral vitamin supplements (such as B-complex)
   - Consider empiric glucocorticoids if adrenal insufficiency is suspected

Thyroid Function in Critical Illness[8]

Table M-1 Thyroid Function Tests

TSH	Free T4*	Free T3*	Interpretation
Normal	Normal	—	Thyroid disease is excluded
↓	Normal	↓ or normal	NTI (most common, especially if TSH >0.1 μU/ml) or subclinical hyperthyroidism (less common)
↓	↑	↓, ↑, or normal	NTI or primary thyrotoxicosis; NTI is more likely if free T3 is normal to low and symptoms are absent
↓	Normal	↑	T3 thyrotoxicosis
↓	↓	↓	Nonthyroid illness (most common) or central hypothyroidism (rare)
↑	Normal	↓ or normal	Recovery phase of NTI (common) or subclinical hypothyroidism (more likely if pattern found early in critical illness)
↑	↓	↓ to normal	Primary hypothyroidism
↑ to normal	↑	↑	Central hyperthyroidism (very rare)

*Direct measurement or calculated index.

Box M-1 Nonthyroid Causes of Abnormal TSH

Decreased TSH	Increased TSH
• Acute or chronic illness • Glucocorticoids • Caloric restriction • Dopamine or adrenergic agonists • Opiates • Phenytoin	• Recovery phase of acute illness • Cimetidine • Dopamine antagonists • Neuroleptics • Metoclopramide

Hyperglycemic Crisis[9,10]

Table M-2

Features	Diabetic Ketoacidosis (DKA)	Hyperosmolar Hyperglycemic State (HHS)
Type of diabetes	Type 1 more likely than type 2	Type 1 much less likely than type 2
Evolution	Hours to days	Days to weeks
Dehydration	Mild to moderate	Moderate to severe
Plasma glucose	>250; usually <800	>600; can be >1000
Arterial pH	Mild 7.25-7.3 Moderate 7.00-7.24 Severe <7.0	>7.3 (50% have mild anion gap)
Serum HCO_3^- (mEq/L)	Mild 15-18 Moderate 10-15 Severe <10	>15
Ketones	Positive	Trace
Serum osmolarity	Variable (usually <320 mOsm/kg)	>320 mOsm/kg
Stupor or coma	Variable, based on severity	Common (25% to 50% of cases)
Mortality	<5%	15%

Precipitating Factors

- Infection (30% to 60% of cases)
- New onset diabetes (20% to 25% of DKA)
- Noncompliance or inadequate treatment (15% to 20% of DKA)
- Stroke
- MI
- Pancreatitis
- Alcohol abuse
- Drugs (steroids, thiazide, sympathomimetics)
- Inadequate access to fluids (HHS)

Clinical Manifestations

- Symptoms
  - Polyuria/polydipsia
  - Weight loss
  - Nausea/vomiting
  - Abdominal pain (up to 50% of DKA)
  - Lethargy
  - Confusion
- Signs
  - Poor skin turgor
  - Kussmaul respiration (DKA)
  - Altered mental status (look for other cause if serum osmolality <320 mOsm/kg)
- Labs
  - ↑ anion gap (DKA)
  - ↑ serum osmolarity
  - ↑ WBC
  - ↑ amylase in absence of pancreatitis
  - Na^+ and K^+ are variable (Na^+ falls 12 mEq/L for every 40 to 60 mg/dl increase in glucose)

Management

- Seek the precipitating cause
- Fluids: The volume deficit averages 3 to 6 L in DKA and 8 to 10 L in HHS
  - Give 1 L NS within the first hour
  - Subsequent fluid therapy should be geared toward correction of volume deficit and volume expansion to enhance renal clearance of ketones (DKA); typical fluid rates are 500 ml/hr × 2 to 4 hr, then 250 ml/hr for mild to moderate deficit; give 750 to 1000 ml/hr × 2 to 4 hr, then 500 ml/hr for hypovolemic shock
  - After initial volume expansion, assess corrected serum sodium (add 1.6 × [glucose − 100] to measured sodium), serum osmolarity, and volume status; if corrected sodium is normal or elevated, change fluid to 0.45% NaCl; if corrected sodium is low or the patient is in hypovolemic shock, continue with 0.9% NaCl

- Insulin
  - Start with 10 units IV bolus followed by IV infusion at 0.1 unit/kg/hr
  - Rebolus and double the rate if glucose does not fall 100 to 500 mg/dl/hr
  - Continuous insulin is necessary to correct acidosis even after glucose normalizes; when glucose is <250 mg/dl (DKA) or <300 mg/dl (HHS), continue insulin at a lower rate (0.05 to 0.1 unit/kg/hr), but add D5 to the IV fluids to keep glucose 200 to 250 mg/dl
  - Subcutaneous short-acting insulin should be given at least 1 hour before the insulin infusion is discontinued
- Potassium: Total body depleted, but serum levels are variable
  - Add 20 to 40 mEq KCl to each liter IV fluids once serum K^+ <5 mEq/L, as long as urine output is adequate
  - If K^+ <4 mEq/L, add 40 to 60 mEq KCl to each liter of IV fluids
  - If K^+ <3.5 mEq/L, give KCl before insulin
- Bicarbonate: Indicated only for severe acidosis (pH <7) or symptomatic hyperkalemia
  - Give 50 to 100 mEq $NaHCO_3-$ diluted in 200 to 400 ml sterile water with the goal of raising the pH to 7.15 to 7.20
- Phosphate: Total body depletion, but serum levels are variable
  - There is no value in repletion unless cardiac dysfunction, respiratory depression, or serum levels <1 mg/dl
- Lab monitoring
  - Glucose every 1 to 2 hours
  - Electrolytes, PO_4, and venous pH (approximately 0.03 unit < arterial pH) every 2 to 6 hours

Complications

- Hypoglycemia (overdose of insulin) or rebound hyperglycemia (insulin discontinued too soon)
- Profound hypokalemia or hypophosphatemia
- Hyperchloremic (non-anion gap) acidosis following fluid resuscitation
- Noncardiogenic pulmonary edema from volume overload
- Cerebral edema: Common in first presentation of DKA or in HHS, especially if volume and sodium deficits are replaced too rapidly (>3 mOsm/kg/hr); mortality is >70% if early signs are not detected

Glycemic Control in Critical Illness[11,12]

Reduced morbidity and mortality are seen when intensive insulin therapy is used in postoperative patients, critically ill medical patients, and patients with acute MI. A possible mechanism includes tight glycemic control against the anabolic effects of insulin.

M

PEARLS

- *Mild ketosis is common in HHS and does not indicate DKA. However, ketoacidosis and hyperosmolar state may coexist in a patient.*
- *The goal of therapy is to eliminate acidosis (DKA) and restore normal volume and osmolarity, not to correct glucose.*
- *Urine and blood ketone levels fluctuate during illness and correlate poorly with response to treatment.*
- *Presenting K^+ levels vary, but total body K^+ depletion is the rule.*

Diabetic Ketoacidosis

Laboratory Diagnosis

- Blood glucose >300 mg/dl (DKA occasionally occurs with blood glucose below 300 mg/dl, especially in patients taking exogenous insulin)[13]
- Serum bicarbonate <15 mEq/L in the absence of chronic renal failure
- Serum acetone level >2:1 dilution
- Arterial pH <7.3 in the first 24 hours

Precipitants

- Recent change in insulin dose (40%)
- Infection (40%)
- Noncompliance (diet or medication) (23%)
- Trauma, injury, and stroke (10%)
- No previous diabetes (20%)

DKA Management

- Apply cardiac monitor and administer O_2 if altered mental status or shock
- Obtain labs and assess for DKA precipitants or complications
- IV fluids: Give IV NS until hypotension and orthostasis resolve
  - If corrected serum Na is normal or high, administer one-half NS at 4 to 14 ml/kg/hr, depending on hydration status
  - If corrected Na is low, administer NS at 4 to 14 ml/kg/hr, depending on hydration status
- Insulin
  - 0.15 U/kg (U) regular insulin IV, then 0.1 U/kg/hr IV
  - If serum glucose does not fall by 50 to 70 mg/dl in the first hour, double insulin infusion hourly until glucose falls 50 to 70 mg/dl in an hour

- When glucose falls to 250 mg/dl, change IV to D5 one-half NS at 150 to 250 ml/hr with adequate insulin (0.05 to 0.1 U/kg/hr) to keep glucose between 150 and 200 mg/dl until metabolic control is achieved.
- Change to SC, regular insulin once bicarbonate >15 mEq/L and there is no anion gap

• Replace potassium (first verify adequate urine output)
  - If initial K^+ is normal or low, add 10 to 40 mEq K^+/L to IV fluids; some recommend replacing K^+ with a 2:1 mixture of KCl and K_3PO_4; some recommend holding insulin until K^+ rises to >3.3 mEq/L
  - If initial K^+ is high, hold K^+, check levels q2 hr, then add potassium when it falls to normal
• Bicarbonate: Primarily indicated for hyperkalemia management, if needed

Hyperosmolar Hyperglycemic Nonketotic Coma

Diagnosis

• Plasma osmolarity >350 mOsm/L
• Glucose >600 mg/dl
• No ketosis (lactic acidosis may or may not be present)
• No history of diabetes in 50% to 65% of cases
• ↑ BUN with BUN/Cr ratio >30
• ↑ CK resulting from rhabdomyolysis

Precipitants

• Renal failure
• Pneumonia, sepsis
• GI bleed
• MI
• CNS bleed/stroke
• Pulmonary emboli
• Pancreatitis
• Burn
• Heat stroke
• Dialysis
• Recent surgery
• Medicines (thiazides, Ca^{2+} channel blocker, steroids, phenytoin, propranolol, furosemide, cimetidine, chlorthalidone, loxapine)

History

- Fever
- Thirst
- Polyuria
- Oliguria
- Polydipsia
- Confusion
- Seizures (focal)
- Hallucinations

Physical Examination

- ↓ consciousness
- Tachycardia, ↓ BP
- Fever
- Focal seizure
- Hemiparesis
- Myoclonus
- Quadriplegia
- Nystagmus

Management

- Admit to the ICU and consider placing a central line
- Obtain electrolytes, CK, UA, CXR, ECG, and cultures with or without head CT and spinal tap
- Fluids: The mean fluid deficit is 9 L. Start IV NS until BP and urine output are satisfactory; then change to one-half NS and replace 50% of the deficit over 12 hours and 50% over the next 12 to 24 hours
- Add dextrose (D5 one-half NS) once glucose falls ≤300 mg/dl
- Replace potassium (5 to 10 mEq/hr) when level is available and urine output is adequate
- Insulin may be unnecessary; consider single 0.1 U/kg IV dose with 0.05 U/kg/hr IV until glucose is 300 mg/dl
- Empiric phosphate repletion, subcutaneous heparin, and broad-spectrum prophylactic antibiotics may be needed depending on clinical circumstances

Hypothermia

Table M-3

Severity	Temperature °F (°C)	Features
Mild	91-95 (33-35)	Maximal shivering and slurred speech at 95° F
Moderate	85-90 (29-32)	Altered mental status, mydriasis, shivering ceases, muscles are rigid, incoordination, and bradypnea at 89° F
Severe	≤82 (≤28)	Bradycardia in 50%, Osborne waves on ECG, voluntary motion stops, pupils are fixed and dilated
	79 (26)	Loss of consciousness, areflexia, no pain response
	77 (25)	No respirations, appears dead, pulmonary edema
	68 (20)	Asystole

Management of Hypothermia

- Do not use vigorous manipulation or active external rewarming unless the patient has mild hypothermia
- Evaluate for cause (such as sepsis, hypoglycemia, CNS disease, or adrenal crisis)
- Mild hypothermia (>32° C): Administer humidified, warmed O_2; passive external rewarming and treatment of underlying disease is often the only treatment needed
- Moderate hypothermia (29° C to 32° C): Active internal rewarming
  - Drugs and cardioversion for cardiac arrest may be ineffective
  - Warm humidified O_2 with gastric or peritoneal lavage if temperature rise <1° C/hr
  - Give CPR and advanced life support prn
- Severe hypothermia (≤29° C)
  1. Warm humidified O_2, warm IV fluids.
  2. If nonarrested, warm peritoneal dialysis (41° C dialysate), or pleural irrigation (41° C).
  3. If core temperature <25° C, consider femoral-femoral bypass.
  4. Use open pleural lavage for direct cardiac rewarming if core temperature <28° C after 1 hour of bypass in an arrest rhythm. If there are signs of life and the patient is nonarrested, avoid CPR and ACLS. If the patient is in arrest, CPR and ACLS are appropriate.
  5. Do not treat atrial arrhythmias.
  6. Treat ↓ BP with NS first. Use pressors cautiously.
  7. Consider empiric D50, thiamine 100 mg IV, and naloxone (Narcan) 2 mg IV plus hydrocortisone 100 mg IV.

References

1. Orth DN, Kovacs WJ. The adrenal cortex. In Wilson JD, Foster DW, Kronenberg HM, et al, eds. Williams Textbook of Endocrinology, 9th ed. Philadelphia: WB Saunders, 1998.
2. Logcope CN, Aronin N. Hypoadrenal crisis. In Irwin RS, Rippe JM, eds. Intensive Care Medicine, 5th ed. Philadelphia: Lippincott Williams & Wilkins, 2003.
3. Dorin RI, Qualls CR, Crapo LM. Diagnosis of adrenal insufficiency. Ann Intern Med 139:194, 2003.
4. Annane D, Sébille V, Bellissant E, et al. Effect of treatment with low doses of hydrocortisone and fludrocortisone on mortality in patients with septic shock. JAMA 288:862, 2002.
5. Cooper MS, Stewart PM. Corticosteroid insufficiency in acutely ill patients. N Engl J Med 348:727, 2003.
6. Wartowsky L. Myxedema coma. In Braverman LE, Utiger RD, eds. Werner and Ingbar's the Thyroid: A Fundamental and Clinical Text, 8th ed. Philadelphia: Lippincott, 2000.
7. Safran MS, Abend SL, Braverman LE. Thyroid storm. In Irwin RS, Rippe JM, eds. Intensive Care Medicine, 5th ed. Philadelphia: Lippincott Williams & Wilkins, 2003.
8. Farwell AP. Sick euthyroid syndrome in the intensive care unit. In Irwin RS, Rippe JM, eds. Intensive Care Medicine, 5th ed. Philadelphia: Lippincott Williams & Wilkins, 2003.
9. Kitabchi AE, Umpierrez GE, Murphy MB, et al. Hyperglycemic crises in patients with diabetes mellitus. Diabetes Care 26(Suppl 1):S109, 2003.
10. Ennis ED, Kreisberg RA. Diabetic ketoacidosis and the hyperglycemic hyperosmolar syndrome. In LeRoith D, Olefsky JM, Taylor SI, eds. Diabetes Mellitus: A Fundamental and Clinical Text, 3rd ed. Philadelphia: Lippincott Williams & Wilkins, 2003.
11. Van den Berghe G, Wouters P, Weekers F, et al. Intensive insulin therapy in the critically ill patients. N Engl J Med 345:1359, 2001.
12. Krinsley JS. Association between hyperglycemia and increased hospital mortality in a heterogeneous population of critically ill patients. May Clin Proc 78:1471, 2003.
13. Faich GA, Fishbein HA, Ellis SE. The epidemiology of diabetic acidosis: a population-based study. Am J Epidemiol 117:551, 1983.

Appendix

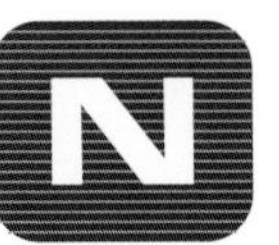

ELECTROLYTE DISORDERS

N

CALCIUM

- Hypocalcemia: Total calcium <8.5 mg/dl or ionized Ca^{2+} <2 mEq/L (1 mmol/L)
- Hypercalcemia: Total calcium >10.5 mg/dl or ionized Ca^{2+} >2.7 mEq/L (1.3 mmol/L)
- Hypoalbuminemia: Serum albumin ↓ of 1 g/dl will ↓ total serum Ca^{2+} 0.8 mg/dl

Hypercalcemia

Causes (PAM P SCHMIDT): Hyper**P**arathyroidism, **A**ddison's disease, **M**ilk-alkali syndrome, **P**aget's disease, **S**arcoidosis, **C**ancer, **H**yperthyroidism, **M**yeloma, **I**mmobilization, hypervitaminosis **D, T**hiazides

Clinical Features

- General: Weakness, polydipsia, dehydration
- Neurologic: Confusion, irritability, hyporeflexia, headache
- Skeletal: Bone pain, fractures
- Cardiac: Hypertension, QT shortening, wide T wave, arrhythmias
- GI: Anorexia, weight loss, constipation, ulcer, pancreatitis
- Renal: Polyuria, renal insufficiency, nephrolithiasis

Evaluation

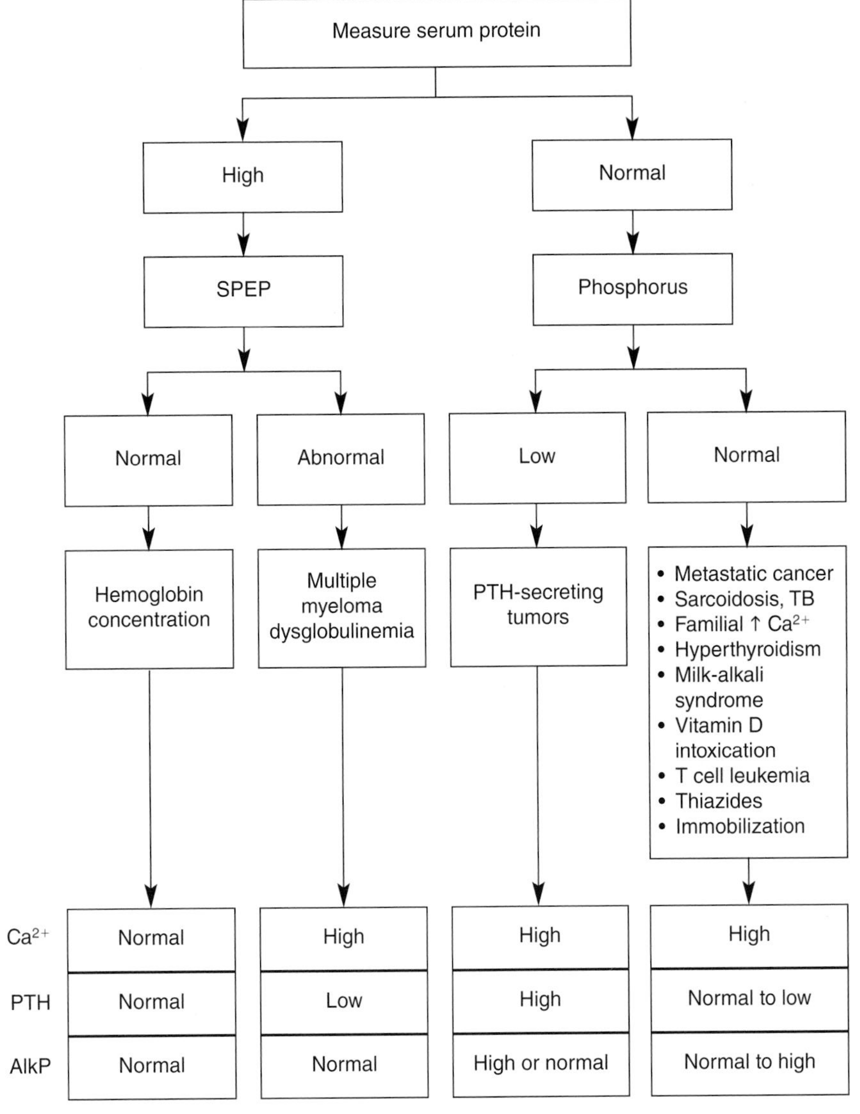

Fig. N-1

Management

- IV normal saline 1 to 2 L bolus, then 200 to 500 ml/hr
- Furosemide (Lasix) 10 to 40 mg IV q2 to 4 hr to keep urine output between 200 and 300 ml/hr
- Consider a central line, and watch closely for signs of heart failure or overload
- Follow urine Mg and K^+ losses, replacing prn or empirically administering 15 mg Mg per hour and ≤10 mEq K^+ per hour
- Consider dialysis with calcium-free dialysate if renal failure
- Give EDTA at 10 to 50 mg/kg IV over 4 hours only if there are life-threatening features
- Other adjuncts include calcitonin, mithramycin, gallium, and steroids

Hypocalcemia

Clinical Features

Table N-1

Symptoms	Physical Findings	Electrocardiogram
• Paresthesias, fatigue • Seizures, tetany • Vomiting, weakness • Laryngospasm	• Hyperactive reflexes • Chvostek sign/Trousseau sign* • Low blood pressure • Congestive heart failure	• Prolonged QT (especially Ca^{2+} <630 mg/dl) • Bradycardia • Arrhythmias

*Chvostek sign: Muscle twitch if facial nerve is tapped; Trousseau sign: Carpal spasm after forearm BP cuff is on for 3 minutes.

Evaluation

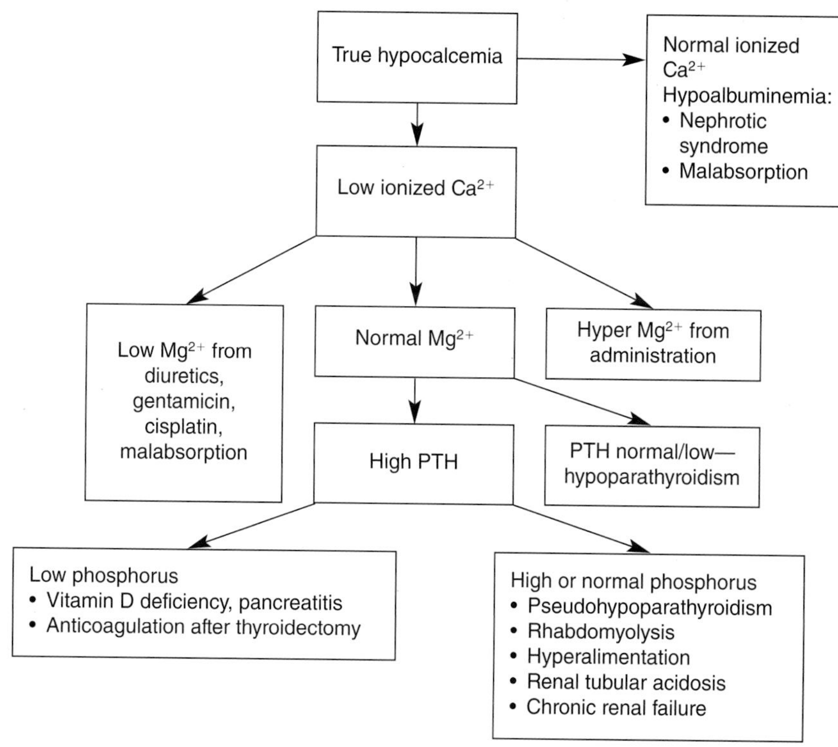

Fig. N-2

Drugs That Can Cause Hypocalcemia

- Cimetidine, cisplatin
- Citrate (transfusion)
- Dilantin, phenobarbital
- Gentamicin, tobramycin
- Glucagon, glucocorticoids
- Heparin
- Loop diuretics (furosemide)
- Magnesium sulfate
- Phosphates, protamine
- Norepinephrine
- Sodium nitroprusside
- Theophylline

N

Treatment

Table N-2

Drug	Preparation (Elemental Ca^{+})	Drug Dose*
Ca gluconate	10% solution—93 mg per 10 ml	15-30 ml IV over 3-5 min
Ca chloride	10% solution—273 mg per 10 ml	5 ml in 50 ml D5W IV over 10 min

*IV calcium may cause ↓ BP, tissue necrosis, ↓ HR, or digoxin toxicity. If possible, consider administration using a central line to prevent extravasation risk.

MAGNESIUM

- Hypomagnesemia (<1.5 mEq/L)
  - Caused by alcohol, diuretics, aminoglycosides, malnourishment
  - Clinical features: Irritable muscle, tetany, seizures
  - Treatment: $MgSO_4$ 5 to 10 mg/kg IV over 20 minutes
- Hypermagnesemia (>2.2 mEq/L)
  - Caused by renal failure, excess maternal Mg supplement, or overuse of Mg-containing medicine
  - Clinical features: Weakness, hyporeflexia, paralysis, and ECG with AV block and QT prolongation
  - Treatment: Ca gluconate (10%) 10 to 20 ml IV

POTASSIUM

Acute decreases in pH will increase K^+ (↓ pH of 0.1 will ↑ K^+ 0.3 to 1.3 mEq/L)

Hyperkalemia

Causes

- Pseudohyperkalemia: Blood sampling or hemolysis
- Exogenous: Blood, salt substitutes, potassium-containing drugs (such as penicillin derivatives), acute digoxin toxicity, beta blockers, succinylcholine
- Endogenous: Acidemia, trauma, burns, rhabdomyolysis, DIC, sickle cell crisis, GI bleed, chemotherapy (destroying tumor mass), mineralocorticoid deficiency, congenital defects (21-hydroxylase deficiency)

Evaluation

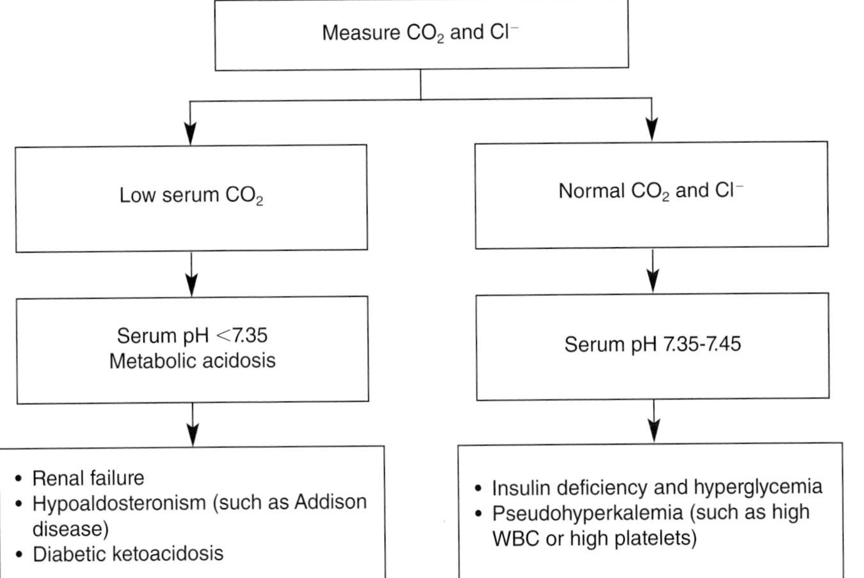

Fig. N-3

N

Clinical Features

- Paresthesias, weakness
- Ascending paralysis sparing the head, trunk, and respiration

ECG Findings (K^+ in mEq/L)

Table N-3

K^+	ECG Findings
>5.5-6	Peaked T waves
>6-6.5	↑ PR and QT intervals
>6.5-7	Flat or isoelectric P waves, ↓ ST segments
>7-7.5	↑ intraventricular conduction
>7.5-8	↑ QRS, ST and T waves merge
>10	Sine waves appear

Treatment of Hyperkalemia

- Calcium gluconate (10%) 5 to 30 ml IV over 2 to 5 minutes, then may repeat (contraindicated by digoxin toxicity; IV $CaCl_2$ can cause phlebitis) *or*
- $CaCl_2$ (10%) 5 to 10 ml IV over 5 to 10 minutes (contraindicated by digoxin toxicity; IV $CaCl_2$ can cause phlebitis)
- $NaHCO_3$ 1 mEq/kg IV, then repeat one-half dose q10 min pr (may worsen fluid overload—for example, congestive heart failure)
- Glucose/insulin—10 units regular insulin IV plus 1 amp D_{50} IV, then 10 to 20 units regular insulin in 500 ml D10W IV over 1 hour if needed
- Albuterol nebulizer 10 to 20 mg over 15 minutes; may repeat
- Furosemide 40 to 80 mg IV
- Kayexalate 15 to 60 g po or 50 g pr (may worsen fluid overload—for example, congestive heart failure)
- Dialysis

Hypokalemia

Causes

- Decreased K^+ intake
- Intracellular shift (normal stores): Alkalemia, insulin, pseudohypokalemia of leukemia, familial hypokalemic periodic paralysis (HPP)
- Increased excretion: Diuretics, hyperaldosteronism, penicillins (exchange Na^+/K^+), sweating, diarrhea (colonic fluid has high K^+), vomiting, binding in gut (clay ingestion, such as pica)

Evaluation

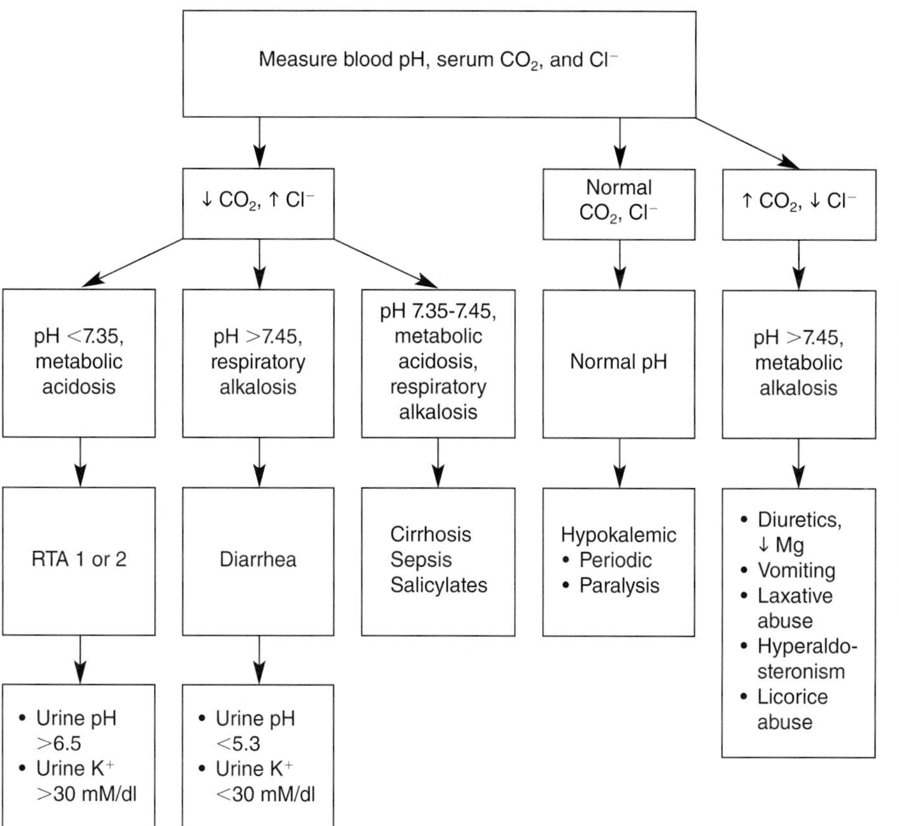

Fig. N-4

Clinical Features

- Lethargy, confusion, weakness
- Areflexia, difficult respirations
- Autonomic instability, low BP

ECG Findings

- K^+ ≤3.0 mEq/L: Low voltage QRS, flat Ts, ↓ ST, prominent P and U waves
- K^+ ≤2.5 mEq/L: Prominent U waves
- K^+ ≤2.0 mEq/L: Widened QRS

Treatment

- Ensure adequate urine output first
- If mild hypokalemia, replace orally only
- If severe ↓ K^+, use parenteral K^+ (such as cardiac, neuromuscular symptoms, or DKA)
- Administer K^+ at ≤10 mEq/hr using ≤40 mEq/L while the patient is on a cardiac monitor; 40 mEq raises serum K^+ by 1 mEq/L

SODIUM

- FENa is the fraction of Na^+ in urine filtered by the glomerulus and not reabsorbed

$$\text{FENa} = 100 \times \frac{\text{Urine Na}^+ \div \text{Plasma Na}^+}{\text{Urine creatinine} \div \text{Plasma creatinine}}$$

Hyponatremia

Na^+ falsely decreases by 1.6 mEq/L for each 100 mg/dl increase in glucose over 100 mg/dl.

Clinical Features

- Lethargy, apathy, cerebral edema
- Depressed reflexes, muscle cramps
- Seizures, hypothermia
- Pseudobulbar palsy

Evaluation

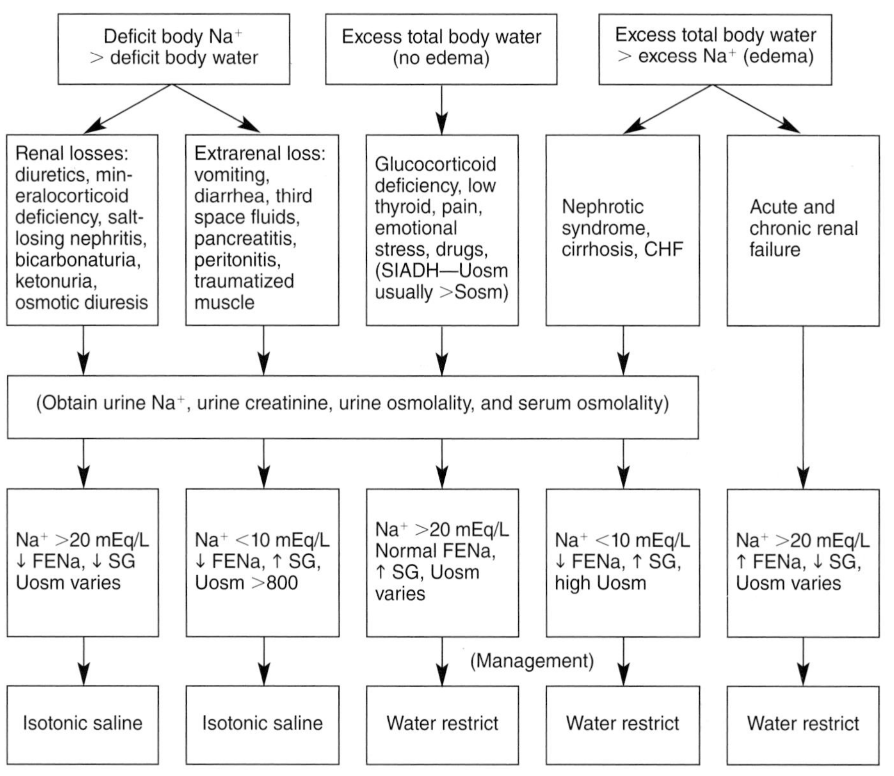

Fig. N-5

N

Hypertonic Saline Administration

Table N-4

Indication	Severe ↓ Na^+ with serious CNS manifestations (such as seizures)
Goal	Only ↑ Na^+ to 120-125 mEq/L acutely, with a maximum of 12 mEq/L/24 hr
Formula	Na^+ deficit = weight (kg) × 0.6 × (desired Na^+ [~125] − known Na^+) Infusion rate (ml/hr) that will increase Na^+ 1 mEq/L/hr: $\frac{\text{weight (kg)} \times 0.6}{0.513 \text{ mEq/L} \times 1 \text{ hr}}$
Rate	• 2-4 mEq/L/hr if active seizures or ↑ intracranial pressure over 1 hour or until seizures stop, then ↓ rate to 1-2 mEq/L/hr • 1-2 mEq/L/hr if patient is obtunded or showing other neurologic symptoms
Adjuncts	• Furosemide (Lasix) 40 mg IV; remember to check Na^+ q2 hr

Compiled from Fraser CL, Arieff AI. Epidemiology, pathophysiology, and management of hyponatremic encephalopathy. Am J Med 102:67, 1997.

APPENDIX

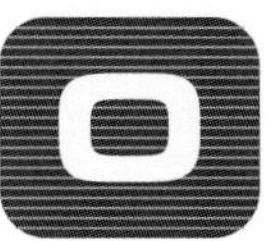

PHARMACOLOGY AND TOXICOLOGY

O

COMMON MEDICATIONS

Table O-1

Name	Trade Name	Class	Dosage
Acyclovir	Zovirax	Antiviral	Varies per viral infection
Albuterol	Proventil, Ventolin	Beta-2 agonist	2.5 mg in 2.5 ml NS nebulized
Alendronate	Fosamax	Bone stabilizer	10 mg qd or 70 mg q week
Allopurinol	Zyloprim	Uricosuric agent	400 mg qd (less for renal insufficiency)
Alprazolam	Xanax	Anxiolytic	0.25-0.5 mg qd
Amantadine	Symmetrel	Antiviral/ antiparkinson	100 mg bid
Amitriptyline	Elavil	Tricyclic antidepressant	30-100 mg/day hs (up to 300 mg)
Amlodipine	Norvasc	Ca^{2+} channel blocker	2.5-10 mg qd for HTN, angina
Amoxicillin	Amoxil	PCN antibiotic	250-500 mg tid (maximum dose of 2-3 g qd)
Amoxicillin and clavulanate	Augmentin	PCN antibiotic	250-500 mg tid or 875 mg bid
Amphotericin B	Amphocin	Antifungal	100 mg qid oral (other routes: IM, IV)
Ampicillin	Principen	PCN antibiotic	250-500 mg qid
Atenolol	Tenormin	Beta-1 blocker	50 mg qd up to 100 mg qd
Atorvastatin	Lipitor	Hypolipidemic	10-80 mg qhs
Atropine		Anticholinergic	See ACLS
Azithromycin	Zithromax	Macrolide antibiotic	500 mg first day, then 250 mg qd × 2-5 days
Bacitracin	AK-Tracin	Topical antibiotic	Topical 1-5 ×/day (IM available)
Beclomethasone dipropionate	Beclovent	Inhaled corticosteroid	MDI 2 puffs 3-4 ×/day 16 puffs/ day to start for severe asthmatics
Benazepril	Lotensin	ACE inhibitor	10-40 mg qd
Benzocaine	Americaine, Anbesol	Local ester anesthetic	Topically as needed

Table O-1—cont'd

Name	Trade Name	Class	Dosage
Benztropine	Cogentin	Antiparkinson	0.5-2 mg qd
Betamethasone	Celestone	Corticosteroid	2.4-4.8 mg/day in 2-4 doses
Bethanechol	Urecholine	Cholinergic	10-50 mg tid-qid po
Bisacodyl	Dulcolax, Bisco-Lax	Stimulant laxative	5-15 mg po prn
Bismuth subsalicylate	Pepto-Bismol	Antidiarrheal	2 tablets 4 ×/day
Bisoprolol	Zebeta	Beta-1 blocker	5-20 mg qd
Bretylium	Bretylol	Antiarrhythmic	Follow ACLS protocol
Bromocriptine	Parlodel	Antiparkinson	1.25 mg qd to start, then titrate by 2.5 mg
Bupropion	Wellbutrin, Zyban	Antidepressant	Depression: 100 mg tid Smoking: 150 mg qd × 3 weeks, then 150 mg bid × 4-9 weeks
Buspirone	BuSpar	Anxiolytic	5 mg tid to start (maximum of 60 mg/day)
Butorphanol	Stadol	Opioid	2 mg IM or 1 mg IV q4 hr
Calcitonin	Miacalcin	Antiosteoporotic	200 IU qd nasal spray
Captopril	Capoten	ACE inhibitor	12.5-25 mg tid for HTN start dose
Carbamazepine	Tegretol	Anticonvulsant	200 mg bid to start (800-1200 qd normal)
Carbidopa	Lodosyn	Antiparkinson	70-100 mg qd (maximum of 200 mg qd)
Carisoprodol	Soma	Muscle relaxant	350 mg 3-4 ×/day
Carvedilol	Coreg	Beta blocker and alpha blocker	3.125-25 mg bid
Cefaclor	Ceclor	2nd generation cephalosporin	250-500 mg tid
Cefadroxil	Duricef	1st generation cephalosporin	1-2 g/day in two doses
Cefazolin sodium	Ancef	1st generation cephalosporin	500-1000 mg q12 hr

Continued

Table O-1—cont'd

Name	Trade Name	Class	Dosage
Cefdinir	Omnicef	3rd generation cephalosporin	300 mg bid or 600 mg qd × 10 days
Cefepime hydrochloride	Maxipime	4th generation cephalosporin	0.5-2 g IV q12 hr
Cefixime	Suprax	3rd generation cephalosporin	200 mg bid or 400 mg qd
Cefmetazole sodium	Zefazone	2nd generation cephalosporin	2 g q6-12 hr IV
Cefonicid sodium	Monocid	2nd generation cephalosporin	0.5-1 g q24 hr IV
Cefoperazone	Cefobid	3rd generation cephalosporin	2-4 g q24 hr IV
Cefotaxime sodium	Claforan	3rd generation cephalosporin	1-2 g q8-12 hr IV
Cefotetan disodium	Cefotan	2nd generation cephalosporin	1-2 g q12-24 hr IV
Cefoxitin sodium	Mefoxin	2nd generation cephalosporin	1-2 g q6-8 hr IV
Cefpodoxime proxetil	Vantin	3rd generation cephalosporin	100-200 mg q12 hr
Cefprozil	Cefzil	2nd generation cephalosporin	250 mg bid × 10 days
Ceftazidime sodium	Fortaz	3rd generation cephalosporin	250-500 mg q8-12 hr IV
Ceftibuten	Cedax	3rd generation cephalosporin	400 mg qd po
Ceftizoxime sodium	Cefizox	3rd generation cephalosporin	1-2 g q8-12 hr IM, IV
Ceftriaxone	Rocephin	3rd generation cephalosporin	1-2 g q12-24 hr
Cefuroxime	Ceftin	2nd generation cephalosporin	250-500 mg bid (125-250 bid for UTI)
Cephalexin	Keflex	1st generation cephalosporin	250-1000 mg qid (maximum of 4 g/day)

Table O-1—cont'd

Name	Trade Name	Class	Dosage
Cephalothin sodium	Keflin	1st generation cephalosporin	500 mg—1 g q4-6 hr IV
Cephapirin sodium	Cefadyl	1st generation cephalosporin	500 mg—1 g q4-6 hr IV
Cephradine	Velosef	1st generation cephalosporin	250-500 mg q6-12 hr
Cetirizine hydrochloride	Zyrtec	Antihistamine	5-10 mg qd
Chlordiaz-epoxide	Librium	Anxiolytic	5-25 mg tid or qid
Chlorothiazide	Diuril	Thiazide diuretic	250-1000 mg bid
Chlorphenir-amine maleate	Chlor-Trimeton	H1 blocker, antihistamine	4 mg q4-6 hr (maximum of 24 mg/day)
Chlorpropamide	Diabinese	Hypoglycemic	100-250 mg qd
Cholestyramine	Questran	Lipid lowering agent	2-4 g bid initially, then 8-16 g/day maintained
Cimetidine	Tagamet	H2 blocker	300 mg qid, 400 mg bid, or 800 mg qd
Ciprofloxacin	Cipro	Quinolone antibiotic	250-500 mg bid × 7-10 days
Clarithromycin	Biaxin	Macrolide antibiotic	250-500 mg q12 hr × 7-14 days
Clemastine fumarate	Tavist	H1 blocker, antihistamine	1.34 mg bid or 2.68 mg tid (maximum of 8 mg/day)
Clindamycin	Cleocin	Antibiotic	150-450 mg q6-8 hr
Clonazepam	Klonopin	Antiepileptic	0.5-1 mg tid (maximum of 20 mg)
Clonidine	Catapres	Alpha adrenergic agonist	0.1 mg bid po to start
Clotrimazole	Lotrimin	Antifungal	Apply cream bid-tid
Clozapine	Clozaril	Antipsychotic	25 mg qd-bid to start (maximum of 300-450 mg qd)
Colchicine		Antigout	0.5 mg qd
Colestipol	Colestid	Hypolipidemic	2-16 g qd

Continued

Table O-1—cont'd

Name	Trade Name	Class	Dosage
Cortisone	Cortone	Corticosteroid	25-300 mg/day
Cotrimoxazole, sulfamethoxazole, trimethoprim	Bactrim	Sulfa antibiotic	1 DS tablet q12 hr × 10-14 days
Cromolyn sodium	Intal, NasalCrom	Mast cell stabilizer	MDI 2 puffs 2-4 ×/day Nasal spray qid
Cyclobenzaprine	Flexeril	Muscle relaxant	10 mg tid
Cyclosporine	Sandimmune	Immuno-suppressant	5-10 mg/kg/day
Cyproheptadine	Periactin	Antihistamine	4 mg tid
Dalteparin sodium	Fragmin	Low molecular weight heparin	2500 units qd 5-10 days postoperatively
Dantrolene sodium	Dantrium	Muscle relaxant	25-100 mg qd
Dapsone		Leprostatic	100 mg qd
Desipramine HCl	Norpramin	TCA	75-300 mg/day
Dexamethasone	Decadron	Corticosteroid	Look up for each disorder
Diazepam	Valium	Anxiolytic/anticonvulsant	2-10 mg IM, IV
Diazoxide	Proglycem	Hyperglycemic agent	3-8 mg/kg po divided into bid or tid dosing
Diclofenac	Voltaren	NSAID	100-200 mg qd
Dienestrol	Ortho Dienestrol	Estrogen cream	Apply qd-bid
Diethylstilbestrol	Stilphostrol	Estrogen cream	Look up for prostate/breast cancer
Diltiazem HCl	Cardizem	Ca^{2+} channel blocker	Angina: 30 mg qid
Dimenhydrinate	Dramamine	Antiemetic	50-100 mg q4-6 hr
Diphenhy-dramine	Benadryl	H1 blocker, antihistamine	25-50 mg q6-8 hr

Table O-1—cont'd

Name	Trade Name	Class	Dosage
Dipyridamole	Persantine	Antiplatelet, vasodilator	75-400 mg/day given in three to four doses
Dirithromycin	Dynabac	Macrolide antibiotic	500 mg qd × 7-14 days
Disulfiram	Antabuse	Antialcoholic	Maximum of 500 mg qd × 1-2 weeks
Divalproex sodium	Depakote	Antiepileptic	15 mg/kg/day to start to a maximum of 60 mg/kg/day
Docusate calcium	Surfak	Stool softener	240 mg qd
Docusate sodium	Colace	Stool softener	50-200 mg qd
Donepezil	Aricept	Antialzheimer	5-10 mg qd
Doxazosin mesylate	Cardura	Alpha-1 blocker	1 mg qd; titrate up to a maximum of 16 mg qd for HTN and 8 mg qd for BPH
Doxepin	Sinequan	Anxiolytic	75-150 mg qd
Doxycycline	Vibramycin	Tetracycline antibiotic	100-200 mg/day in one or two doses
Econazole	Spectazole	Antifungal	Apply topically qd-bid
Enalapril	Vasotec	ACE inhibitor	2.5-5 mg/day, then titrate to a maximum of 40 mg
Enoxaparin	Lovenox	Anticoagulant	30 mg SC qd-bid
Epinephrine	Adrenalin	Sympathomimetic	See Chapter 35
Erythromycin	Erythrocin	Macrolide antibiotic	250-500 mg q6-12 hr
Estradiol	Estrace	Estrogen	1-2 mg qd
Estrogen, conjugated	Premarin	Estrogen	0.3-1.25 mg qd
Ethacrynic acid	Edecrin	Loop diuretic	50-200 mg/day given in one to two doses
Etodolac	Lodine	NSAID	200-400 mg q6-8 hr (maximum of 1200 qd)

Continued

Table O-1—cont'd

Name	Trade Name	Class	Dosage
Famciclovir	Famvir	Antiviral	Differs per infection
Famotidine	Pepcid	H2 blocker	20-40 mg qd-bid
Felodipine	Plendil	Ca^{2+} channel blocker	2.5-10 mg qd
Ferrous gluconate	Fergon, Ferralet	Iron salt (anemias)	60 mg 2-4 ×/day; 60 mg qd for maintenance
Ferrous sulfate	Feratab, Slow FE	Iron salt (anemias)	300 mg 2-4 ×/day; 300 qd for maintenance
Fexofenadine	Allegra	Antihistamine	60 mg bid
Finasteride	Proscar, Propecia	Androgen inhibitor	1-5 mg qd
Flecainide	Tambocor	Antiarrhythmic	100 mg q12 hr, then titrate up by 50 mg
Fluconazole	Diflucan	Systemic antifungal	Differs per infecting fungus
Flumazenil	Romazicon	Benzodiazepine antidote	1-3 mg using 0.2 mg at 1-minute intervals
Flunisolide	AeroBid	Corticosteroid	2 puffs 2-8 ×/day
Fluoxetine	Prozac, Sarafem	SSRI antidepressant	10-80 mg qd
Flurazepam	Dalmane	Hypnotic	15-30 mg qhs
Flurbiprofen	Ansaid	NSAID	200-300 mg/day given in two, three, or four doses
Fluticasone	Flonase, Flovent	Inhaled steroid	2 sprays/puffs bid
Fluvastatin	Lescol	Hypolipidemic	20-40 mg qhs
Fluvoxamine	Luvox	Antidepressant	50-300 mg qd
Folic acid	Folvite	Vitamin	0.15-0.2 mg/day
Fosinopril	Monopril	ACE inhibitor	10-40 mg qd
Furosemide	Lasix	Loop diuretic	20-80 mg/day
Gabapentin	Neurontin	Antiepileptic	300-1800 mg qd in divided doses
Gatifloxacin	Tequin	Quinolone antibiotic	200-400 mg qd

Table O-1—cont'd

Name	Trade Name	Class	Dosage
Gemfibrozil	Lopid	Hypolipidemic	1200 mg qd divided into two doses
Gentamicin	Garamycin	Aminoglycoside	1 mg/kg IV q18 hr
Glimepiride	Amaryl	Hypoglycemic	1-4 mg qd
Glipizide	Glucotrol	Hypoglycemic	2.5-40 mg qd divided into two doses
Glyburide	DiaBeta, Micronase	Hypoglycemic	1.25-5 mg to start, then ↑ to 20 mg qd
Glycopyrrolate	Robinul	Anticholinergic	1 mg qd-tid
Griseofulvin	Fulvicin	Antifungal	500 mg qd × 7-14 days
Guaifenesin	Robitussin	Expectorant	200-400 mg q4 hr
Haloperidol	Haldol	Antipsychotic	0.5-5 mg bid-tid
Heparin		Anticoagulant	Varies, but usually 5000-10,000 units SC
Hydralazine HCl	Apresoline	Antihypertensive	10 mg qid × 4 days, then ↑ to 25 mg qid
Hydrochloro-thiazide	HCTX/Esidrix	Diuretic	25-100 mg qd divided into two doses
Hydrocortisone	Cortef	Steroid	2.5 mg qd or 80 mg qid, depending on the patient
Hydromorphone	Dilaudid	Opioid	2-4 mg q4-6 hr
Hydroxyurea	Hydrea	Antineoplastic	20-30 mg/kg qd
Hydroxyzine	Atarax, Vistaril	Antihistamine	25-100 mg qid
Hyoscyamine	Levsin	Anticholinergic	0.125-0.25 mg q4 hr
Ibuprofen	Advil, Motrin	NSAID	400-800 mg tid/qid (3.2 g maximum/day)
Imipramine HCl	Tofranil	TCA	25 mg tid-qid (300 mg/day maximum)
Indinavir sulfate	Crixivan	Protease inhibitor	800 mg q8 hr
Indomethacin	Indocin	NSAID	25-50 mg bid-tid (200 mg/day maximum)
Ipratropium	Atrovent	Bronchodilator	MDI 2 puffs qid

Continued

O

Table O-1—cont'd

Name	Trade Name	Class	Dosage
Isoniazid	Nydrazid, Laniazid	Antituberculosis	TB: 5-10 mg/kg/day
Isosorbide dinitrate	Isordil	Antianginal	5-40 mg qid
Isosorbide mononitrate	Imdur	Antianginal	20 mg bid
Isotretinoin	Accutane	Acne	0.5-2 mg/kg/day divided into two doses
Itraconazole	Sporanox	Antifungal	200-400 mg qd
Ketoconazole	Nizoral	Antifungal	200-400 mg/day
Ketoprofen	Orudis	NSAID	50-75 mg tid-qid
Ketorolac	Toradol	NSAID	30-60 mg IM/IV
Labetalol	Trandate	Beta-blocker and alpha-blocker	100-400 mg bid po
Lactulose	Chronulac	Laxative	15-30 ml qd
Lamivudine	Epivir	Reverse transcriptase inhibitor	150 mg bid
Lansoprazole	Prevacid	Proton pump inhibitor	15-30 mg qd
Latanoprost	Xalatan	Antiglaucoma	1 drop qd
Levobunolol	Betagan	Antiglaucoma	1 drop qd
Levodopa	Atamet	Antiparkinson	500-1000 mg/day
Levofloxacin	Levaquin	Quinolone antibiotic	250-500 mg qd
Levothyroxine sodium	Synthroid	Thyroid hormone	12.5-50 μg/day to start
Lidocaine HCl	Xylocaine	Antiarrhythmic	See Chapter 35
Lindane	Kwell	Scabicide	Apply to skin q8-12 hr
Liothyronine	Cytomel	Thyroid hormone	25-75 μg qd
Lisinopril	Prinivil, Zestril	ACE inhibitor	5-40 mg qd

Table O-1—cont'd

Name	Trade Name	Class	Dosage
Lithium carbonate	Eskalith	Antimaniacal	300 mg tid-qid
Loperamide	Imodium	Antidiarrheal	4-8 mg
Loracarbef	Lorabid	2nd generation cephalosporin	200-400 mg/day × 7 days
Loratadine	Claritin	H1 blocker, antihistamine	10 mg qd
Loratadine and pseudoephedrine	Claritin-D	H1 blocker, decongestant	1 tablet q12 hr
Lorazepam	Ativan	Anxiolytic	2-4 mg divided bid-tid
Losartan potassium	Cozaar	Angiotensin receptor blocker	25-100 mg qd
Lovastatin	Mevacor	Hypolipidemic	20-80 mg qd
Mebendazole	Vermox	Antihelmintic	100 mg qd-bid
Meclizine	Antivert	H1 blocker/vertigo	12-25 mg/day
Medroxy-progesterone	Provera, Cycrin	Progestin	5-10 mg qd
Megestrol acetate	Megace	Progestin/appetite stimulant	800 mg qd
Meperidine hydrochloride	Demerol	Narcotic analgesic	50-150 mg q3-4 hr
Meropenem	Merrem	Carbapenem antibiotic	1 g q8 hr IV
Metaproterenol sulfate	Alupent	Beta-2 bronchodilator	2.5 mg in 3 ml saline
Metaxalone	Skelaxin	Muscle relaxant	800 mg tid-qid
Metformin	Glucophage	Hypoglycemic	500-2500 mg divided qd-bid
Methicillin	Staphcillin	Penicillin antibiotic	4-12 g IV qd divided tid-qid
Methimazole	Tapazole	Antithyroid	5-60 mg qd divided tid
Methocarbamol	Robaxin	Muscle relaxant	1000-1500 mg qid

Continued

Table O-1—cont'd

Name	Trade Name	Class	Dosage
Methyldopa	Aldomet	Alpha blocker	500-2000 mg qd divided bid-qid
Methylpredni-solone acetate	Depo-Medrol	Corticosteroid	20-80 mg IM
Methylpredni-solone sodium	Solu-Medrol	Corticosteroid	30 mg/kg IV
Metoclopramide	Reglan	GI motility	10-15 mg qid
Metoprolol	Lopressor	Beta blocker	100-450 mg/day in two to three doses
Metronidazole	Flagyl	Antiprotozoal/ antibiotic	Trichomoniasis: 250 mg q8 hr × 7 days
Miconazole	Monistat	Antifungal/ vaginal yeast	Topically
Midazolam hydrochloride	Versed	Sedative/ hypnotic	0.07-0.08 mg/kg IM (~5 mg)
Minocycline	Minocin	Tetracycline antibiotic	200-400 mg/day
Minoxidil	Loniten	Antihypertensive	50-40 mg qd
Mirtazapine	Remeron	Antidepressant	15 mg qd or qhs
Misoprostol	Cytotec	Prostaglandin	200 μg qid
Moexipril	Univasc	ACE inhibitor	7.5-30 mg qd
Mometasone	Elocon	Corticosteroid	Topically qd-bid
Montelukast	Singulair	Leukotriene inhibitor	10 mg qd
Mupirocin	Bactroban	Topical antibiotic	Apply topically 2-5 ×/day
Nabumetone	Relafen	NSAID	1000 mg/day
Nadolol	Corgard	Beta blocker	40 mg/day to start (maximum of 240 mg/day)
Nafcillin sodium	Nafcil, Unipen	PCN antibiotic	250-500 mg q4-6 hr
Naloxone	Narcan	Opioid antagonist	0.4-2 mg IV
Naproxen	Naprosyn, Anaprox	NSAID	250 mg q6-8 hr (maximum of 1250 mg/day)

Table O-1—cont'd

Name	Trade Name	Class	Dosage
Nedocromil sodium	Tilade	Inhaled antihistamine	MDI 2 puffs qid
Nefazodone	Serzone	Antidepressant	300-600 mg qd divided bid
Niacin (nicotinic acid)	Vitamin B3, Niaspan	Anticholesterol	Start 250 mg qd-bid, then titrate to a maximum of 6 g/day (usually 2 g/day)
Nicardipine HCl	Cardene	Ca^{2+} channel blocker	20-40 mg tid
Nicotine	Nicotrol	Smoking deterrent	Depends on delivery device; refer to appropriate device information
Nifedipine	Procardia	Ca^{2+} channel blocker	10-30 mg po tid
Nisoldipine	Sular	Ca^{2+} channel blocker	20-40 mg qd-bid
Nitrofurantoin	Furadantin, Macrobid	Miscellaneous antibiotic	50-100 mg q6 hr
Nitroglycerin	Nitrostat, Nitro-Dur	Vasodilator	Depends on patient; consult protocols
Norfloxacin	Chibroxin	Quinolone antibiotic	800 mg 3-4 ×/day UTI or GC
Norgestrel	Ovrette	Oral contraceptive	1 tablet qd
Nortriptyline	Pamelor	TCA	25 mg 3-4 ×/day (maximum of 150 mg)
Nystatin	Mycostatin	Antifungal	400,000-600,000 units qid
Ofloxacin	Floxin	Quinolone antibiotic	400 mg qd
Olanzapine	Zyprexa	Antipsychotic	2.5-10 mg qd/qhs
Omeprazole	Prilosec	Proton pump inhibitor	20 mg qd
Orphenadrine	Norflex	Muscle relaxant	100 mg bid po
Oxacillin sodium	Bactocill	Penicillin antibiotic	500-1000 mg q4-6 hr IM/IV

Continued

Table O-1—cont'd

Name	Trade Name	Class	Dosage
Oxandrolone	Oxandrin	Anabolic steroid	2.5 mg bid-qid × 2-4 weeks
Oxybutynin chloride	Ditropan	Urinary antispasmodic	5 mg bid-tid
Oxycodone hydrochloride	OxyContin	Opioid analgesic	10 mg q12 hr
Oxytocin	Syntocinon	Hormone	1 spray per nostril 2-3 minutes before breastfeeding or pumping breasts
Paroxetine	Paxil	SSRI	20-50 mg qd
Penicillin G	Bicillin	PCN antibiotic	1.2 million units IM
Penicillin V	V-cillin K	PCN antibiotic	125-500 mg q6-8 hr
Pentoxifylline	Trental	Decreases blood viscosity	400 mg tid with meals
Permethrin	Elimite	Scabicide	Apply to body for 8-14 hr
Phenazopyridine	Pyridium	Urinary analgesic	200 mg tid × 2-3 days
Phenelzine	Nardil	MAOI	15 mg tid to start, then titrate by 15 mg
Phenylephrine	Neo-Synephrine	Alpha-1 agonist	prn
Phenytoin	Dilantin	Anticonvulsant	200 mg bid to start, then 300 mg qd
Pilocarpine HCl	Adsorbocarpine	Cholinergic	1-2 drops (maximum of 6 ×/day)
Pindolol	Visken	Beta blocker	10-60 mg qd divided bid
Pioglitazone	Actos	Hypoglycemic	15-45 mg qd
Piperacillin sodium	Pipracil	Penicillin antibiotic	100-125 mg/kg/day IM/IV divided q6-12 hr
Pirbuterol	Maxair	Bronchodilator	2 puffs q4-6 hr
Piroxicam	Feldene	NSAID	10-20 mg qd
Polymyxin B	Neosporin	Topical antibiotic	Topically
Potassium chloride	K-Dur	K^+ supplement	Start 10 mEq qd, then titrate to serum potassium levels
Pravastatin	Pravachol	Hypolipidemic	10-20 mg qhs
Prazosin	Minipress	Alpha-1 blocker HTN	3-15 mg/day divided, 2-4 ×/day

Table O-1—cont'd

Name	Trade Name	Class	Dosage
Prednisone	Sterapred	Steroid	5-60 mg qd (must taper after course)
Primaquine		Antimalarial	15 mg qd × 14 days
Probenecid	Benemid	Antigout/PCN adjunct	Gout: 250-500 mg bid; adjunct: 1 g bid
Procainamide	Pronestyl	Antiarrhythmic	See Chapter 35
Progesterone	Crinone	Progestin derivative	5-10 mg/day × 6 days
Promethazine	Phenergan	Antiemetic/ sedative	Emesis: 12.5-25 mg q4 hr prn
Propoxyphene hydrochloride	Darvon	Opioid analgesic	65 mg q4 hr prn
Propranolol	Inderal	Beta blocker	1 mg IV over 1 minute q5 min to maximum of 5-8 mg
Propylthiouracil		Antithyroid	100-300 mg qd divided into three doses
Protamine sulfate		Heparin antagonist	1 mg/90-115 units heparin (maximum of 50 mg)
Pseudo-ephedrine	Actifed, Sudafed	Decongestant	30-60 mg q4-6 hr (maximum of 240 mg)
Quinapril	Accupril	ACE inhibitor	10-80 mg qd
Ramipril	Altace	ACE inhibitor	2.5-20 mg qd
Ranitidine	Zantac	H2 blocker	150 mg bid or 300 mg hs
Repaglinide	Prandin	Hypoglycemic	0.05-4 g 15-30 minutes before meal
Reserpine	Serpalan	Antihypertensive	0.1-0.25 mg qd
Rifampin	Rifadin, Rimactane	Miscellaneous antibiotic for TB and flu	TB: varies; flu: 600 mg qd × 4 days
Risperidone	Risperdal	Antipsychotic	1-3 mg bid
Ritonavir	Norvir	Protease inhibitor	600 mg bid with food
Rivastigmine	Exelon	Antialzheimer	1.5-3 mg bid

Continued

Table O-1—cont'd

Name	Trade Name	Class	Dosage
Rizatriptan	Maxalt	Antimigraine	10 mg at onset of headache
Rosiglitazone	Avandia	Hypoglycemic	4-8 mg qd
Salmeterol	Serevent	Bronchodilator	2 puffs bid
Scopolamine HBr (oral)	Isopto	Anticholinergic	0.3-0.65 mg q4-6 hr
Scopolamine transdermal	Transderm Scop	Anticholinergic	1 disk behind ear 2-3 hours before needed
Selenium sulfide	Selsun	Antifungal	Apply topically qd-bid
Senna	Senokot	Irritant laxative	10-15 ml qd
Sertraline	Zoloft	SSRI	50-200 mg qd
Simvastatin	Zocor	Hypolipidemic	Start 5-10 mg/day hs
Sodium nitroprusside		Antihypertensive	0.3-10 mg/kg/min IV
Sotalol hydro-chloride	Betapace	Antiarrhythmic	80 mg bid, then titrate to a maximum of 320 mg qd
Spironolactone	Aldactone	K1 sparing diuretic	25-200 mg/day in one to two divided doses
Stavudine	Zerit	Antiviral (NRTI)	30-40 mg bid
Sucralfate	Carafate	Antiulcer agent	1 g bid-qid on empty stomach
Sulfacetamide sodium	Sulamyd	Topical antibiotic	One to two drops q2-4 hr
Sulfamethox-azole	Gantanol, Urobak	Sulfonamide antibiotic	2 g, then 1g 2-3 3/day (maximum of 3 g/day)
Sulfasalazine	Azulfidine	Bowel antiinflam-matory	2-4 g qd
Sulindac	Clinoril	NSAID	150-200 mg bid (maximum of 400 mg/day)
Sumatriptan succinate	Imitrex	Antimigraine	25 mg po with fluids (maximum of 300 mg/day); intranasally: 5, 10, or 20 mg per nostril
Tacrine hydro-chloride	Cognex	Antialzheimer	10-40 mg qid

Table O-1—cont'd

Name	Trade Name	Class	Dosage
Tacrolimus	Prograf	Immuno-suppressant	0.15-0.3 mg/kg/day po
Tamoxifen citrate	Nolvadex	Antineoplastic	10-20 mg q12 hr
Temazepam	Restoril	Hypnotic	7.5-30 mg qhs
Terazosin	Hytrin	Alpha-1 blocker that decreases HTN	1-5 mg/day (maximum of 20 mg/day)
Terbinafine	Lamisil	Antifungal	Topically bid
Terbutaline sulfate	Brethine	Beta-2 bronchodilator	5 mg po q6 hr (maximum of 5 mg/day)
Testosterone	Androderm	Androgen	2 patches qd
Tetracaine	Pontocaine	Ester anesthetic	1-2 qtt in eyes
Tetracycline HCl	Achromycin	Topical antibiotic	Apply lotion 1-4 ×/day
Theophylline	Theo-Dur, Slo-bid	Bronchodilator	100-300 mg bid to start (check serum levels)
Thyroid	Thyroid extract	Thyroid hormone	Start with 15-30 mg, then ↑ by 15 mg q2-4 weeks
Thioridazine	Mellaril	Antipsychotic	200-800 mg qd divided bid-qid
Ticarcillin disodium	Ticar	Penicillin antibiotic	150-300 mg/kg/day divided q4-6 IV
Ticlopidine hydrochloride	Ticlid	Platelet inhibitor	250 mg bid
Timolol maleate	Blocadren	Beta blocker that decreases HTN	10 mg bid to start (maximum of 60 mg/day)
Timolol (ophthalmic)	Timoptic	Beta blocker that decreases glaucoma	1 qtt bid of 0.25% solution
Tioconazole	Vagistat	Antifungal	Intravaginally qhs
Tizanidine	Zanaflex	Muscle relaxant	4-12 mg tid
Tobramycin	Tobrex	Topical antibiotic	1-2 qtt q4 hr to affected eye
Tolazamide	Tolinase	Hypoglycemic	100-500 mg qd

Continued

Table O-1—cont'd

Name	Trade Name	Class	Dosage
Tolbutamide	Orinase	Hypoglycemic	250-2000 mg qd
Torsemide	Demadex	Loop diuretic	5-20 mg qd
Tramadol hydrochloride	Ultram	Central analgesic	50-100 mg q4-6 hr (maximum of 400 mg/day)
Trandolapril	Mavik	ACE inhibitor	1-2 mg qd
Trazodone HCl	Desyrel	Antidepressant	150 mg/day divided into three doses (maximum of 600 mg)
Tretinoin	Retin-A	Antiacne	45 mg/m^2 body surface area/day; very teratogenic
Triamcinolone	Azmacort	Steroid	One to two puffs 3-4 ×/day
Triamterene	Dyrenium	K^+ sparing diuretic	100-300 mg/day in one to two divided doses
Triamterene/ HCTZ	Dyazide, Maxzide	Diuretic	One to two tablets qd
Triazolam	Halcion	Benzodiazepine	Sedation: 0.125-0.25 mg qhs
Trihexyphenidyl	Artane	Anticholinergic	1-10 mg qd
Trimetho-benzamide	Tigan	Antiemetic	250 mg tid-qid po or 200 mg tid-qid IM
Trimethoprim	TMP, Trimpex	Antibiotic	100 mg q12 hr or 200 mg qd
Trimethoprim and sulfameth-oxazole	Bactrim	Antibiotic	UTI: 1 DS q12 hr × 10-14 days
Triple sulfa	Sultrin Triple Sulfa	Sulfonamide antibiotic	Lotion 10%
Valacyclovir hydrochloride	Valtrex	Antiviral	500 mg bid × 5 days (genital herpes)
Valproic acid	Depakote	Anticonvulsant	10-15 mg/kg/day in one to three divided doses
Venlafaxine	Effexor	Antidepressant	75-225 mg/day divided bid-tid
Verapamil	Calan	Ca^{2+} channel blocker	80-120 mg tid (differs for extended release [ER and SR] formulas)
Warfarin	Coumadin	Anticoagulant	2-10 mg qd (monitor PT/INR)

Table O-1—cont'd

Name	Trade Name	Class	Dosage
Zafirlukast	Accolate	Leukotriene inhibitor	20 mg bid
Zidovudine	AZT	Antiviral	100 mg q4 hr for HIV
Zidovudine and lamivudine	Combivir	Antiviral	One tablet bid
Zileuton	Zyflo	Leukotriene inhibitor	600 mg qid with meals and at bedtime
Zolmitriptan	Zomig	Antimigraine	2.5 mg q2 hr (maximum of 10 mg/day)
Zolpidem	Ambien	Hypnotic	10 mg qhs

PHARMACOLOGY EQUATIONS

Elimination constant: $K_{el} = \ln \frac{(\text{Peak})}{(\text{Trough})} \div (\text{Time}_{peak} - \text{Time}_{trough})$

Clearance: $Cl = V_d \times K_{el}$

Half-life: $T_{1/2} = \frac{0.693}{K_{el}} = 0.693 \times \frac{V_d}{Cl}$

Loading dose: $V_d \times$ Target peak

Dosing interval: $\frac{1}{K_{el}} \times \frac{(\text{Desired peak})}{(\text{Desired trough})} + \text{Infusion time}$

Ideal body weight (male): 50 kg + (2.3 kg/in over 5 ft)

Ideal body weight (female): 45 kg + (2.3 kg/in over 5 ft)

O

BEDSIDE ANALGESIA OPTIONS

Mild Pain

- Acetaminophen (650 mg po/pr q4 to 6 hr prn)
- Aspirin (650 mg po q4 to 6 hr prn)
- Ibuprofen (400 to 800 mg po q6 to 8 hr prn)

Moderate Pain

- Acetaminophen and codeine (Tylenol #3) (1 to 2 tablets po q4 hr prn)
- Acetaminophen and oxycodone (Percocet) (1 to 2 tablets po q4 hr prn)
- Oxycodone (5 mg po q4 hr prn)
- Tramadol (50 to 100 mg po q4 to 6 hr up to 400 mg/day)

Severe Pain

- Morphine (10 to 30 mg po q3-4 hr or 0.1 to 0.2 mg/kg IV up to 15 mg q4 hr)
- Fentanyl (0.1 mg IV q1-3 hr)
- Hydromorphone (2 to 4 mg po q4-6 hr or 1 to 4 mg IV q4-6 hr)
- Oxymorphone (1 mg IV q3-4 hr)
- PCA pump (patient-controlled administration of analgesia)

TOXINS THAT AFFECT VITAL SIGNS AND PHYSICAL EXAMINATION

All agents that cause decreased BP, fever, hypoglycemia, and CNS bleeding can cause seizures.

Hypotension

- ACE inhibitors
- Alpha and beta antagonists
- Anticholinergics
- Arsenic (acutely)
- Ca^{2+} channel blockers
- Clonidine
- Cyanide
- Antidepressants
- Disulfiram
- Ethanol
- Methanol
- Iron
- Isopropanol
- Mercury

- GHB
- Nitrates
- Nitroprusside
- Opioids
- Organophosphates
- Phenothiazines
- Sedatives
- Theophylline

Hypertension
- Amphetamines
- Anticholinergics
- Cocaine
- Lead
- MAOIs
- Phencyclidine
- Sympathomimetics

Tachycardia
- Amphetamines
- Anticholinergics
- Arsenic (acutely)
- Antidepressants
- Digitalis
- Disulfiram
- Ethylene glycol
- Iron
- Organophosphates
- Sympathomimetics
- PCP
- Phenothiazines
- Theophylline

Bradycardia
- Antidysrhythmics
- Alpha and beta antagonists
- Ca^{2+} channel blockers
- Digitalis
- Opioids
- GHB
- Organophosphates

Tachypnea

- Ethylene glycol
- Methanol
- Nicotine
- Organophosphates
- Salicylates
- Sympathomimetics
- Cocaine
- Theophylline

Bradypnea

- Barbiturates
- Botulism
- Clonidine
- Ethanol
- Isopropanol
- Opioids
- Organophosphates
- Sedatives

Hyperthermia

- Amphetamines
- Anticholinergics
- Arsenic (acutely)
- Cocaine
- Antidepressants
- LSD
- Phencyclidine
- Phenothiazines
- Salicylates
- Sedative-hypnotics
- Theophylline
- Thyroxine

Hypothermia

- Carbon monoxide
- Ethanol
- Hypoglycemic agents
- Opioids
- Phenothiazines
- Sedative-hypnotics

Mydriasis (Pupil Dilation)

- Anticholinergics
- Antihistamines
- Antidepressants
- Anoxia (any cause)
- Amphetamines
- Cocaine
- Sympathomimetics
- Drug withdrawal

Miosis (Pupilloconstriction)

- Anticholinesterase
- Opioids
- Nicotine
- Pilocarpine
- Clonidine
- Coma from barbiturates, benzodiazepines, ethanol

Seizures

- Antidepressants
- Beta blockers
- Cocaine
- Camphor
- Ethanol withdrawal
- INH
- Lead
- Lithium
- PCP
- Theophylline
- Organophosphates
- Sympathomimetics

Lithium

Lithium absorption leads to peak serum levels 0.5 to 3 hours after ingestion. Significant delayed absorption/symptom onset may occur up to 72 hours later. Therapeutic serum concentration for acute mania is 0.6-1.2 mEq/L; maintenance is 0.5-0.8 mEq/L.

Table O-2 Clinical Features of Lithium Toxicity Based on Serum Levels

Lithium Level (mEq/L)	Clinical Features*
<1.2	Fine tremor, dry mouth, thirst, polyuria, nausea (not toxic signs)
1.2-2.0	Vomiting and diarrhea
2.0-2.5	Blurred vision, muscle weakness/fasciculations, dizziness, vertigo, ataxia, confusion, slurred speech, ↑ DTRs, transient scotomas
2.5-3.0	Myoclonic twitches, choreoathetoid movements, incontinence, stupor, ECG: flat/inverted Ts, U wave, SA/AV block, prolonged QT
3.0-4.0	Seizures, cardiac arrhythmias (ventricular tachycardia, PVCs, ventricular fibrillation)
≥4.0	Hypotension, peripheral vascular collapse

*Serum levels do not always correlate with features; toxicity can occur with normal levels (especially with acute or chronic ingestion).

Lithium may cause diabetes insipidus (↑ Na^+), ↓ anion gap, ↑ K^+ (displacement of K^+ by intracellular lithium), ECG changes similar to ↓ K^+, and hypothyroidism.

Treatment

- Monitor
  - Apply cardiac monitor and pulse oximeter, obtain ECG and serum electrolytes, and observe for neurologic or cardiac deterioration
  - Obtain serum lithium 2 hours after acute ingestion and 6 to 12 hours after chronic ingestion; repeat lithium levels q4 hr until a peak is reached
- Decontamination
  - Use gastric lavage if recent ingestion (charcoal is ineffective)
  - Give sodium polystyrene sulfonate (Kayexalate) 1 g/kg po or pr
  - Use whole-bowel irrigation (especially if sustained release)
- Fluids and electrolytes
  - Restore fluid and electrolyte deficits (NS administration supplies Na^+ ions, which may increase renal lithium excretion)
  - Controversy exists regarding the use of $NaHCO_3$, acetazolamide, and osmotic diuretics; contact poison center for direction

- Indications for hemodialysis
  - Signs of severe poisoning (such as seizures, altered mental status, ventricular arrhythmias)
  - Decreasing urine output or renal failure
  - Lithium level ≥4 mEq/L regardless of symptoms
  - Repeat dialysis is often needed 6 to 12 hours later because of slow distribution
  - Check levels q4 hr after dialysis for 12 to 24 hours

Aminoglycoside Dosing in Renal Failure

- Loading dose: Administer the same loading dose regardless of renal function
- Estimate creatinine clearance: $\text{CLcr} = \dfrac{(140 - \text{age [years]}) \times \text{weight (kg)}}{\text{serum creatinine (mg/dl)} \times 72}$
- Multiply calculated CLcr by 0.85 for women

Maintenance Dose for Traditional Dosing Based on Creatinine Clearance

Table O-3

Creatinine Clearance	Dose to Administer or Interval Alteration
>50 ml/min	• Administer 60%-90% of traditional dose q8-12 hr, or • Increase interval alone to q12-24 hr
10-50 ml/min	• Administer 30%-70% of traditional dose q12 hr, or • Increase interval alone to q24-48 hr
<10 ml/min	• Administer 20%-30% of traditional dose q24-48 hr, or • Increase interval alone to q48-72 hr

Maintenance Dose for Once-Daily Aminoglycosides (First Maintenance Dose Timing)

Table O-4

Creatinine Clearance	Timing of Maintenance Dose (Gentamicin Is Used as an Example)
>60 ml/min	Normal time for recommended interval (q24 hr)
40-59 ml/min	At 1.5 × the recommended dosing interval (q36 hr)
20-39 ml/min	At 2 × the recommended dosing interval (q48 hr)

Check 12-hour level with this regimen. For subsequent doses, if 12-hour gentamicin or tobramycin level is ≤3μg/ml, widen the dosing interval to q24 hr; if it is 3 to 5 μg/ml, administer q36 hr; if it is 5 to 7 μg/ml, administer q48 hr.

Treatment of Digoxin Toxicity

- Use multi-dose charcoal ± lavage
- Give atropine 0.5 mg for decreased HR
- For ventricular arrhythmia, give lidocaine 1 mg/kg IV ± $MgSO_4$ 20 mg/kg IV
- For increased K^+, do not use calcium
- Avoid cardioversion if possible (predisposes ventricular fibrillation)
- Digoxin-specific Fab fragments (Digibind)

Indications for Digibind

- Ventricular arrhythmias
- Symptomatic bradyarrhythmias unresponsive to medication
- Ingestion of >0.1 mg/kg
- Digoxin level of >5 ng/ml
- Consider if K^+ >5 to 5.5 mEq/L

Total Body Load of Digoxin (TBLD) Estimates

- $\text{TBLD (mg)} = \dfrac{\text{Digoxin level (ng/ml)} \times \text{Weight (kg)}}{100}$

  (Chronic ingestions may have normal to mildly elevated digoxin levels.)
- Acute ingestion—total mg ingested, if digoxin capsules or elixir are ingested
- Acute ingestion—total mg ingested × 0.8, if digoxin tablets (because of 80% bioavailability)

Digibind Dosing

- $\text{Number of vials to administer} = \dfrac{\text{TBLD (mg)}}{\text{0.5 (mg/vial)}}$

- If the ingested quantity is unknown, consider empiric administration of 10 vials
- One 40 mg Digibind vial can bind 0.5 mg of digoxin if amount ingested is known
- Dilute Digibind to 10 mg/ml and administer IV over 30 minutes
  - Consider using 0.22 micron filter for infusion
  - Serum levels are useless after administration, because assay measures bound plus unbound digoxin
  - Once bound, digoxin-Fab complex is renally excreted

Acetaminophen

Ingestion of ≥140 mg/kg is potentially toxic. Obtain acetaminophen level ≥4 hours after acute ingestion and plot on the Rumack-Matthews nomogram. A 4-hour level ≥140 μg/ml indicates the need for N-acetylcysteine. If time from ingestion is unknown, obtain level at time 0 and 4 hours later to calculate half-life. If half-life is >4 hours, administer antidote.

Acetaminophen Toxicity

Table O-5

Phase	Time After Ingestion	Signs and Symptoms
1	30 minutes to 24 hours	Asymptomatic or minor GI irritant effects
2	24-72 hours	Relatively asymptomatic, GI symptoms resolve, possible mild elevation of LFTs, or renal failure
3	72-96 hours	Hepatic necrosis with potential jaundice, hepatic encephalopathy, coagulopathy, and renal failure
4	4 days to 2 weeks	Resolution of symptoms or death

Management

- Decontamination
  - Charcoal is indicated only if toxic coingestants are present
  - Increase oral N-acetylcysteine dose by 20% if charcoal is given
- N-acetylcysteine (NAC) (Mucomyst; Acetadote [IV formulation])
  - Assess toxicity based on nomogram
  - If the drug level will return sooner than 8 hours after ingestion, treatment can be delayed until the level is known. NAC prevents 100% of toxicity if it is administered <8 hours after ingestion. If the level will return later than 8 hours and if ≥140 mg/kg were ingested, administer the first dose. NAC is definitely useful ≤24 hours after ingestion, and possibly ≤72 hours after ingestion
  - Oral dose: 140 mg/kg po, then 70 mg/kg q4 hr × 17 doses
    - A shorter course (36 hours) may be effective if there is no liver toxicity at 36 hours; contact a poison center for short protocol specifics
  - IV dose: 150 mg/kg IV (in 200 ml D5W) over 15 minutes, then 50 mg/kg (in 500 ml D5W) over 4 hours, then 100 mg/kg (in 1000 ml D5W) over 16 hours
    - Up to 18% of patients develop anaphylactoid reaction (especially if asthmatic or if previous NAC reaction); if this happens, discontinue and manage symptoms (using antihistamines, epinephrine, inhaled beta agonists, IV fluids); if symptoms stop and were mild, consider restarting NAC; otherwise, do not restart

Poison Antidotes and Treatments

Table O-6

Toxin	Antidote/Treatment	Other Considerations
Acetaminophen	N-acetylcysteine (See page 456 for dose)	• Very effective if used within 8 hours • May be helpful if used within 72 hours
Beta blockers	Glucagon 1-5 mg IV/SC/IM (drip may be required)	Glucagon may help reverse ↓ pulse and ↓ BP
Ca^{2+} channel blockers	$CaCl_2$ (10%) 10 ml IV, glucagon 1-5 mg IV/SC/IM	Glucagons may help reverse ↓ pulse and ↓ BP
Cyanide	Lilly cyanide kit (amyl nitrate, sodium nitrite, and sodium thiosulfate)	• Treatment induces methemoglobinemia and ↓ BP • Sodium thiocyanate is excreted in urine
Digoxin	Digoxin-specific Fab fragments	See page 455 for dose
Ethylene glycol	Fomepizole (Antizol)	If fomepizole is not available, give ethanol; the goal is a level of 0.1 g/dl
Isoniazid	Pyridoxine 4 g IV, then 1 g IM q30 min if needed	Reverses seizures
Methanol	Fomepizole, ethanol, dialysis	Also thiamine and folate
Nitrites	Methylene blue (0.2 ml/kg of 1% solution IV over 5 minutes)	Consider exchange transfusion if severe methemoglobinemia
Opiates	Naloxone 0.4-2 mg IV	Diphenoxylate and propoxyphene may require higher doses
Organophosphates, carbamates	Atropine 0.05 mg/kg IV pralidoxime (PAM)	• Exceptionally high atropine doses may be necessary • PAM does not work for carbamate toxicity
Salicylates	Dialysis or sodium bicarbonate 1 mEq/kg IV	Goal of alkaline diuresis is a serum pH of 7.50-7.55
Tricyclic antidepressants	Sodium bicarbonate 1 mEq/kg IV	Goal is a serum pH of 7.5-7.55 to alter protein binding

O

Radiopaque Ingestions (CHIPES)

- **C**hloral hydrate, chlorinated hydrocarbon
- **H**eavy metals (such as arsenic, lead, mercury)
- Health food (such as bone meal, vitamins)
- **I**odides, iron
- **P**otassium, psychotropics (such as phenothiazines, antidepressants)
- **E**nteric coated tablets (such as KCl, salicylates)
- **S**olvents (such as chloroform, CCl_4)

Drugs Cleared by Hemodialysis

Consult a local poison center for more details concerning the latest indications.

- Bromide
- Salicylates
- Lithium
- Methanol
- Isopropyl alcohol
- Chloral hydrate
- Ethylene glycol

Drugs Cleared by Hemoperfusion

Consult a local poison center for more details concerning the latest indications.

- Barbiturates (such as phenobarbital)
- Theophylline, phenytoin
- Possibly digoxin

Identification of Abused Drug Based on Street Name

Table O-7

Street Name	Drug	Street Name	Drug
Acid	LSD	Dishrag	Heroin
Angel dust	LSD	Dollies	Methadone
Apples	Marijuana	Dust (Dusted)	PCP
Bam	Heroin + Preludin	Eve	Ecstasy
Bazooka	Cocaine	4 and doors	Codeine + glutethimide
Bazooka paste	Marijuana + procaine	Footballs	Amphetamines
Bennies	Amphetamines	Girl	Cocaine
Black beauty	Caffeine PPA	Green	Ketamine
Black molly	Look-alike amphetamines	Happy dust	Cocaine
Blue angels	Amphetamines	Happy sticks	Marijuana + PCP
Boat	PCP	Hawaiian wood rose	PCP
Breakin'	Heroin	Jamestown	Jimsonweed
Brick	Marijuana	Jet	Ketamine
Butt naked	PCP	John Hinckley	PCP
Chiva	Heroin—Mexican brown	Joy stick	Marijuana + PCP
Christmas trees	Depressant or stimulant	Juice	PCP
Clickers	Marijuana + PCP	Junk	Heroin
Coast	Methylphenidate IV	Ketamine green/purple	LSD
Coke (Cola)	Cocaine	Lady	Cocaine
Crack	Rock cocaine	Loads	Codeine + glutethimide
Crank	Amphetamines, heroin, or methamphetamines	Love (Lovely)	PCP
Crystal	Methamphetamines	Love boat	Marijuana + PCP
Disco hits	PCP	Mauve	Ketamine
		Maze	Fentanyl
		Mexican maid	Heroin

Continued

O

Table O-7—cont'd

Street Name	Drug
Mickey Mouse	LSD
Monster	Methamphetamines
Mr. Natural	LSD
Mud	Heroin/molasses
NASA	Heroin
New boy	Heroin
Nose candy	Cocaine
One and one	Pentazocine + tripelennamine; pentazocine + methylphenidate; methylphenidate + diazepam
Packs	Codeine + glutethimide
Pasta	Cocaine
Perks	Oxycodone (Percodan/ Percocet)
Persia white	Fentanyl
Peruvian white	Cocaine
Pink and grey	Propoxyphene
Pink hearts	Look-alike amphetamines
President	Heroin
Purple	Ketamine
Risking high	Heroin
Robin's egg	Look-alike amphetamines
Rock	Amphetamines or methamphetamines
Roofies	Flunitrazepam
Scat/Skag	Heroin
Shermans/Sherms	PCP + marijuana or formaldehyde
Shrooms	Psilocybe
Silent partner	Heroin
Sinsemilla	Marijuana
Smack	Heroin
Snow candy	Cocaine
Snort/Snuff	Cocaine
Special LA	Ketamine
Speckled bird	Look-alike amphetamines
Speed	Amphetamines or methamphetamines
Speedball	Heroin + cocaine
Stardust	Cocaine
Stuff	Heroin
Super C or Super K	Ketamine
Super grass	PCP
Syrup and bean	Codeine + diazepam
Ts and blues	Pentazocine + tripelennamine
Ts and purple	Pentazocine/ tripelennamine/ naloxone
Tar	Opium
Thriller	Heroin
Tic and Tac	PCP
Tolley	Toluene
Toot	Cocaine
Tootsie roll	Heroin—Mexican brown

Table O-7—cont'd

Street Name	Drug
Unicorn	LSD
USDA	Heroin
Vitamin C	Cocaine
Wack	PCP
WACs	Marijuana/Black Flag roach killer
Watergate	Heroin
West Coast	Methylphenidate IV
Whippet	Nitrous oxide
White (white dust)	Cocaine
White, China	Fentanyl
Window pane	LSD
Wizard	LSD
Yo Yo	Yohimbine

Appendix

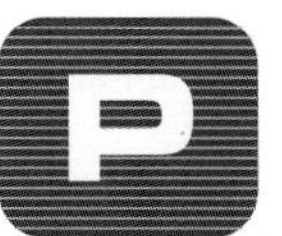

OTHER USEFUL INFORMATION

P

ABSORBABLE SUTURES

Table P-1

Suture	Use	Architecture	Tissue Reaction Generated	50% Tensile Strength Loss
Polyglyconate (Maxon)	Muscle, fascia, GI tract	Monofilament	Mild	4 weeks
Polydioxanone (PDS)	Muscle, fascia, GI tract	Monofilament	Mild	4 weeks
Polyglactic acid (Vicryl)	Muscle, fascia, GI tract	Braided	Medium	2-3 weeks
Polyglycolic acid (Dexon)	GI tract	Braided	Medium	2-3 weeks
Poliglecaprone (Monocryl)	Skin, subcutaneous tissue	Monofilament	Mild	1 week
Chromic gut	Mucosa, viscera	Twisted	High	2 weeks
Plain gut	Mucosa	Twisted	High	1 week
Fast gut	Facial lacerations in children	Twisted	High	4 days

NONABSORBABLE SUTURES

Table P-2

Suture	Use	Architecture	Tissue Reaction Generated	Tensile Strength
Silk	GI tract, vessel ligation	Braided	High	Good
Nylon (Ethilon, Dermalon)	Skin, draining stitches, vasculature	Monofilament	Mild	High
Nylon (Nurolon, Surgilon)	Neurosurgery, dural closure	Braided	Medium	High
Polypropylene (Prolene, Surgilene)	Cardiac, vessels, skin, tendons	Monofilament	Mild	Good
Polyester (Ethibond, Tycron)	Cardiac, vessels, tendons	Braided	Medium	High
Stainless steel	Sternal closure, orthopedics	Monofilament	Mild	High

SUTURE NEEDLES

Table P-3

Needle	Shape	Use	Advantages
Blunt point	Tapered body, blunt point	Visceral organs, GI tract	Less bleeding
Taper point	Tapers to sharp point, no cutting edges	Biliary tree, dura, peritoneum, pleura, GI tract	Smallest needle hole with decreased leakage around suture
Conventional cutting	Three cutting edges, needle tip concavity	Cosmetic surgery	Penetrates tissue easily but with risk of cutout
Reverse cutting	Three cutting edges, needle tip convexity	Skin, cosmetic surgery, ENT	Penetrates tissue easily but with lesser risk of cutout

BURN THERAPY

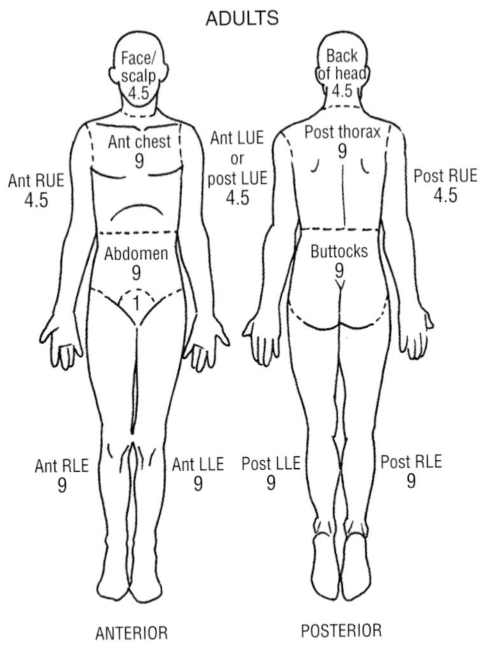

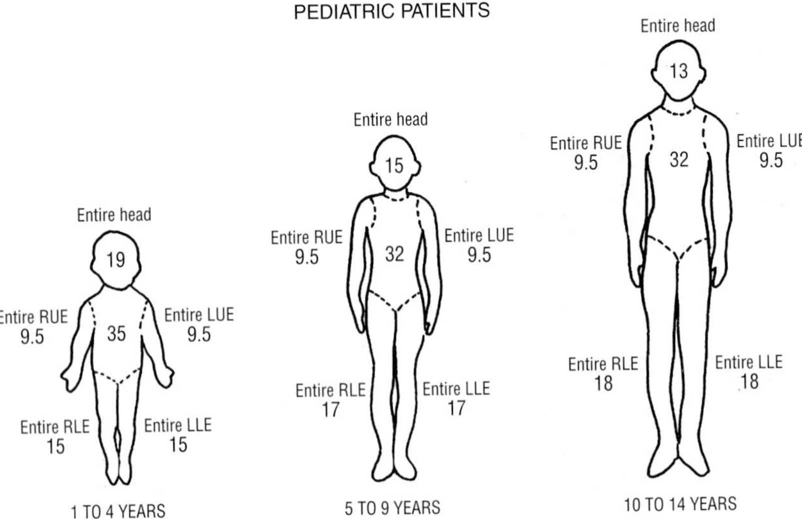

Fig. P-1 Estimated total body surface area burned. Numbers are % for anterior only and posterior only for adults, and anterior and posterior combined for pediatric patients. The size of the patient's palm can be used in all age groups to approximate 1% TBSA.

Admission Criteria

- 2nd and 3rd degree burns on ≥10%-15% TBSA
- 3rd degree burns on ≥5% TBSA
- Burns to hands, feet, face, or perineum
- Circumferential burns anywhere on body (concern for compartment syndrome)
- Minor chemical burns
- Significant electrical burns
- Inhalation injury (elevated blood carbon monoxide levels, singed nasal hairs, soot in mouth or nose, and/or decreased oxygenation)
- Social issues preventing adequate outpatient treatment or follow-up
- Any suspicion of abuse
- Significant medical comorbidities affecting wound healing such as poorly controlled diabetes or renal disease

FLUID RESUSCITATION IN BURN VICTIMS

Parkland Formula

- For significant burns (≥10%-15% TBSA), use Parkland formula to calculate the amount of fluid resuscitation for the first 24 hours (given in addition to maintenance fluids)
- Total fluid resuscitation in first 24 hours (lactated Ringer's solution) = 4 ml/kg/% TBSA burned
- Give half of resuscitation fluids over first 8 hours, then second half over next 16 hours

Alternatives

- Amended Parkland formula (for ED stays <8 hours)

$$\text{IV rate over maintenance (ml/h)} = \frac{\text{Weight (kg)} \times \text{Burn TBSA \%}}{4}$$

- Carvajal's formula: Carvajal's solution 5000 ml/m^2 of burn plus maintenance of 2000 ml/m^2 in the first 24 hours, with one half over the first 8 hours and one half over the subsequent 16 hours.

$$\text{BSA (m}^2) = \sqrt{(\text{Height [cm]} \times \text{Weight [kg]}) \div 3600}$$

$$\text{BSA (m}^2) = \sqrt{(\text{Height [in]} \times \text{Weight [lb]}) \div 3131}$$

P

SPINAL METASTASES

Spinal metastases occur most often because of lymphoma, lung, breast, or prostate cancer. Sixty-eight percent are thoracic, 19% are lumbosacral, and 15% are cervical spinal. Steroids and radiation may be necessary if cancer is the cause of compression.

Clinical Features

- Back pain: 95%
- Weakness (usually symmetric): 75%
- Autonomic or sensory symptoms: 50%
- Inability to walk: 50%
- Flaccidity, hyporeflexia (early)
- Spasticity, hyperreflexia (late)
- Bowel/bladder incontinence

Diagnosis

- Plain radiographs show abnormalities in 60% to 90% of cases
- MRI, CT scan, or myelography

Management

- Dexamethasone 25 mg IV q6 hr
- Radiation therapy
- Surgery may be needed for epidural abscess or bleeding, or disc herniation

SUPERIOR VENA CAVA SYNDROME

Superior vena cava syndrome occurs in 3% to 8% of patients with lung cancer and lymphoma. Symptoms are caused by venous hypertension in areas drained by the superior vena cava. Death occurs from cerebral edema, airway compromise, or cardiac compromise.

Clinical Features

- Thoracic distention or neck vein distention: 65%
- Shortness of breath: 50%
- Tachypnea: 40%
- Upper trunk or extremity edema: 40%
- Cough/dysphagia/chest pain: 20%
- Periorbital or facial edema
- Stokes' sign (tight shirt collar)

Diagnosis

- Chest radiographs show a mediastinal mass or a parenchymal lung mass in 10% of the lung
- CT scans are diagnostic

Management

- Furosemide 40 mg IV
- Methylprednisolone 1 to 2 mg/kg IV
- Mediastinal radiation

TUMOR LYSIS SYNDROME

Tumor lysis syndrome occurs within 1 to 2 days of starting chemotherapy or radiation therapy for rapidly growing tumors (especially leukemias and lymphomas). Clinical features are a result of hyperuricemia (renal failure), increased K^+ (arrhythmias), increased phosphate (renal failure), and decreased Ca^{2+} (causing cramping, tetany, confusion, and seizures).

Management

- Hydration with NS
- Allopurinol 100 to 200 mg/day po
- Alkalinize serum with $NaHCO_3$ to urine pH ≥7
- Dialysis

Criteria for Hemodialysis

- K^+ >6 mEq/L
- Creatinine >10 mg/dl
- Uric acid >10 mg/dl
- Symptomatic hypocalcemia
- Serum phosphorus >10 mg/dl

MANAGEMENT OF SUSPECTED TESTICULAR TORSION

- In men younger than 40 with a painful testicle, assume torsion until proven otherwise.
- Contact a urologist immediately, because early surgical detorsion offers the best chance of saving the testicle.
- An attempt to manually detorse the testicle may restore blood flow. To manually detorse, rotate the anterior aspect of the testicle toward the ipsilateral thigh (like opening a book). The testicle will need to be torsed at least 360 degrees. If successful, the patient will experience a marked relief of pain, and the testicle will develop a normal lie (position in scrotum).

LIFE-THREATENING RASHES

Table P-4

Epidemiology	Manifestations	Diagnosis	Prognosis/ Treatment
Rocky Mountain Spotted Fever (RMSF)			
• *Rickettsia rickettsii* • Tick-borne • Occurs in almost all U.S. states, but most cases occur in the southeast • Most cases occur in spring/ summer	• Fever, myalgia, headache • Rash: Typically starts on day 4 on wrists/ankles and spreads to palms/soles then centrally; initially pink-red macules that blanch; it evolves to petechiae, purpura, and gangrene of digits, nose, and genitals • 10% of patients are spotless • Atypical rash can occur in deeply pigmented patients	• Clinical diagnosis • No early laboratory clues • Triad of fever, rash, and tick bite in only 60%-70% of cases • Late serology is confirmatory • DFA of skin biopsy is 70% sensitive, 100% specific	• Mortality is 5%-25% (higher with delayed diagnosis) • Treatment: Doxycycline (IV or po); chloramphenicol for pregnant women or young children

Compiled from Drage L. Life-threatening rashes: dermatologic signs of four infectious diseases. Mayo Clin Proc 74:68, 1999.

Table P-4—cont'd

Epidemiology	Manifestations	Diagnosis	Prognosis/ Treatment
MENINGOCOCCAL SEPSIS			
• *Neisseria meningitides* • Transmission through respiratory droplets (close contact) • Most cases occur in winter/spring • Patients are usually <20 years old	• Fever, headache, N/V, confusion, meningeal signs • Rash: Petechial, scattered on trunk/ extremities; evolves to palpable purpura ("gun-metal gray" with necrotic center); petechiae are clustered at pressure points • Purpura fulminans: Cutaneous DIC with hemorrhagic bullae	• Gram stain/culture of blood, CSF, skin • Gram stain of petechiae 70% sensitive • Culture of skin biopsy may remain positive after antibiotics are given	• Mortality rate is 10%-20% • Treatment: PCN G IV • Contacts: Rifampin, ciprofloxacin, or ceftriaxone
STAPHYLOCOCCAL TOXIC SHOCK SYNDROME (STSS)			
• *Staphylococcus aureus* (toxin-producing) • Most cases are nonmenstrual • Associated with flu, childbirth, tracheitis, wound infection, nasal packing • 40% recurrence	• Fever, malaise, myalgia, N/V, diarrhea • Prominent confusion • Rash: Sunburn-like, diffuse macular erythroderma, followed by desquamation of hands and feet in 5-14 days; also causes conjunctival injection, oral-genital hyperemia, mucosal hyperemia, and strawberry tongue	• Isolation of *Staphylococcus aureus* from blood is unusual • Diagnostic criteria: Fever or ↓ BP, typical rash, exclusion of other causes	• Mortality rate is 10%-15% (5% in menstrual cases) • Treatment: Antistaphylococcal antibiotic, supportive care, removal of source • Concurrent clindamycin may reduce toxin release • Possible role for IVIG

Continued

Table P-4—cont'd

Epidemiology	Manifestations	Diagnosis	Prognosis/ Treatment
STAPHYLOCOCCAL TOXIC SHOCK SYNDROME (STSS)—CONT'D			
• Group A *Streptococcus* • Soft tissue infections most common • Most patients are 20-50 years old and otherwise healthy	• Fever, hypotension, severe local pain • Rash: Highly variable, localized erythema, diffuse erythroderma, or violaceous bullae • Pain is a prominent symptom • Can occur after blunt trauma or muscle strain	• Bacteremia in 60% of cases, but open biopsy is often necessary • Diagnostic criteria: Isolation of group A *Streptococcus,* ↓ BP, and multi-organ involvement	• Mortality rate is 30%-70% • Treatment: PCN G plus aggressive surgical exploration and debridement • Concurrent clindamycin may reduce toxin release

GLOSSARY OF ABBREVIATIONS

5-HIAA	5-hydroxyindoleacetic acid
5′-NT	5′ nucleotidase
ABG	Arterial blood gas
AC	Assist-control
ACE	Angiotensin converting enzyme
ACE-I	Angiotensin converting enzyme inhibitor
ACLS	Advanced cardiac life support
ACTH	Adrenocorticotropic hormone
ADH	Antidiuretic hormone
AF	Atrial fibrillation
AG	Aminoglycoside
AlkP	Alkaline phosphatase
ALT	Alanine aminotransferase
aPTT	Activated partial thromboplastin time
ARDS	Acute respiratory distress syndrome
ASA	Acetylsalicylic acid
ASCVD	Atherosclerotic cardio-vascular disease
ASD	Atrial septal defect
AST	Aspartate aminotransferase
ATN	Acute tubular necrosis
A-V	Arteriovenous
AV	Atrioventricular
$AVDO_2$	Arteriovenous oxygen difference
aVF	Augmented volt foot
aVL	Augmented volt left
AVM	Arteriovenous malformation
aVR	Augmented volt right
BBB	Bundle branch block
Beta-hCG	Human chorionic gonadotropin
bid	Twice per day (bis in die)
BiPAP	Bilevel positive airway pressure
BMI	Body mass index
BP	Blood pressure
BPH	Benign prostatic hyperplasia
BSA	Body surface area
BT	Bleeding time
BUN	Blood urea nitrogen
CA-125	Cancer antigen 125
Ca^{2+}	Calcium
CABG	Coronary artery bypass graft
CBC	Complete blood count
CEA	Carcinoembryonic antigen
CHF	Congestive heart failure
CI	Cardiac index
CK	Creatine kinase
Cl^-	Chloride ion
CML	Chronic myelogenous leukemia
CMV	Cytomegalovirus
CNS	Central nervous system
CO	Cardiac output
COPD	Chronic obstructive pulmonary disease
Cp	Cephalosporins
CPAP	Continuous positive airway pressure
CPK	Creatine phosphokinase
Cr	Creatinine
CRNA	Certified registered nurse anesthetist

CSF Cerebrospinal fluid
CV Cardiovascular
CVP Central venous pressure
CXR Chest radiograph (x-ray)

D&C Dilation and curettage
D10W 10% dextrose in water
D5W 5% dextrose in water
DA Dopamine
DBP Diastolic blood pressure
DDAVP Desmopressin
DFA Direct fluorescent antibody
DIC Disseminated intravascular coagulation
DIP Distal interphalangeal joint
DKA Diabetic ketoacidosis
DNR Do not resuscitate
DPL Diagnostic peritoneal lavage
DTR Deep tendon reflex
DVT Deep vein thrombosis

EBL Estimated blood loss
EBV Epstein-Barr virus
ECG Electrocardiogram
ED Emergency department
EDTA Ethylenediaminetetraacetic acid
ELISA Enzyme linked immunosorbent assay
ENT Ear, nose, and throat
ERCP Endoscopic retrograde cholangiopancreatography
ERV Expiratory reserve volume
ESBL Extended spectrum beta lactamase
ESR Erythrocyte sedimentation rate
EtOH Ethyl alcohol
ETT Endotracheal tube

F Female
FDP Fibrinogen degradation product
$FEF_{25\% \text{ to } 75\%}$ Forced expiratory flow from 25% to 75%
FENa Fractional excretion of sodium
FET Forced expiratory time
FEV_1 Forced expiratory volume in 1 second
FFP Fresh frozen plasma
Fio_2 Fraction of inspired oxygen
FRC Functional residual capacity
FSH Follicle stimulating hormone
FSP Fibrin split product
FT4I Free T4 index
FVC Forced vital capacity

G6PD Glucose-6-phosphate dehydrogenase
GC Cervical gonorrhea
GFR Glomerular filtration rate
GGT Gamma glutamyl transferase
GHB Gamma hydroxybutyrate
GhC A protein
GI Gastrointestinal
GP Glycoprotein
gtt Drops (guttae)
GU Genitourinary

H2 Histamine2
HACEK A group of gram-negative bacteria that includes *Haemophilus* spp., *Actinobacillus actinomycetemcomitans, Cardiobacterium hominis, Eikenella corrodens,* and *Kingella kingae.*
HAV Hepatitis A virus
Hb Hemoglobin
Hb S Sickle hemoglobin
HBe Hepatitis B envelope
HBs Hepatitis B surface
HBV Hepatitis B virus
Hct Hematocrit
HCTX Hydrochlorothiazide
HCV Hepatitis C virus
HELLP Hemolysis, elevated liver enzymes, low platelet count

HHNC Hyperosmolar hyperglycemic nonketotic coma
HHS Hyperosmotic hyperglycemic state
HIT Heparin-induced thrombocytopenia
HITTS Heparin-induced thrombocytopenia with thrombosis syndrome
HPP Hypokalemic periodic paralysis
HR Heart rate
hs At bedtime (hora somni)
HTLV Human T-cell leukemia virus
HTN Hypertension
HUS Hemolytic uremic syndrome

I/O Input/output
IABP Intraaortic balloon pump
IBD Inflammatory bowel disease
IC Inspiratory capacity
ICP Intracranial pressure
ICU Intensive care unit
IDSA Infectious Diseases Society of America
IE Infective endocarditis
IgA Immunoglobulin A
IgG Immunoglobulin G
IgM Immunoglobulin M
IM Intramuscular
IMV Intermittent mandatory ventilation
INH Isonicotinyl hydrazine
INR International normalized ratio
ITP Idiopathic thrombocytopenic purpura
IU International units
IVDA Intravenous drug abuse
IVDU Intravenous drug use
IVF Intravenous fluids
IVIG Intravenous immunoglobulin
IVP Intravenous pyelogram

JVP Jugular venous pressure

K Potassium
KCl Potassium chloride

LA Left atrium
LAC Lupus anticoagulant
LAD Left axis deviation
LBBB Left bundle branch block
LDH Lactate dehydrogenase
LFT Liver function test
LGV Lymphogranuloma venereum
LH Luteinizing hormone
LMA Laryngeal mask anesthesia
LMWH Low-molecular-weight heparin
LR Lactated Ringer's solution
LSD d-Lysergic acid diethylamide
LV Left ventricle
LVEDP Left ventricular end diastolic pressure
LVH Left ventricular hypertrophy

M Male
MAC Mycobacterium avium complex
MAOI Monoamine oxidase inhibitors
MAP Mean arterial pressure
MB Myoglobin
MCH Mean corpuscular hemoglobin
MCHC Mean corpuscular hemoglobin concentration
MCP Metacarpal phalangeal joint
MCV Mean corpuscular volume
MDI Metered dose inhaler
MDRD Modification of diet in renal disease
mEq Milliequivalents
Mg^{2+} Magnesium
$MGSO_4$ Magnesium sulfate
MI Myocardial infarction
MR Mitral reflux
MRCP Magnetic resonance cholangiopancreatography

MRSA Methicillin-resistant *S. aureus*
MSSA Methicillin-sensitive *S. aureus*
MVI Multivitamin infusion

N/V Nausea/vomiting
NA Sodium
NAC N-acetylcysteine
NaCl Sodium chloride
NG Nasogastric
NPO Nothing by mouth (nil per os)
NPPV Noninvasive positive pressure ventilation
NRTI Nucleoside reverse transcriptase inhibitor
NS Normal saline
NSAID Nonsteroidal antiinflammatory drug
NTI Nonthyroidal illness

P Plasma, *or* pressure
PA Pulmonary artery
$Paco_2$ Arterial carbon dioxide partial pressure
$PAco_2$ Alveolar carbon dioxide partial pressure
PAD Pulmonary artery diastolic pressure
PAM Pulmonary arterial mean pressure, *or* pulmonary alveolar macrophages
Pao_2 Arterial oxygen partial pressure
PAo_2 Alveolar oxygen partial pressure
PAWP Pulmonary artery wedge pressure
PC Platelet concentrate
PCI Percutaneous coronary intervention
PCN Penicillin
PCN G Penicillin G
pCO_2 Partial carbon dioxide pressure
PCP Phencyclidine
PCR Polymerase chain reaction
PCV Pressure control ventilation
PCWP Pulmonary capillary wedge pressure
PDA Patent ductus arteriosus
PE Pulmonary embolism
PEEP Positive end expiration pressure
PEFR Peak expiratory flow rate
PID Pelvic inflammatory disease
PIH Pregnancy-induced hypertension
PIP Peak inspiratory pressure, *or* proximal interphalangeal joint
PMN Polymorphonuclear neutrophil
PNGT Per nasogastric tube
po By mouth (per os)
PPA Phenylpropanolamine
pr Per rectum
PRBC Packed red blood cell
prn As needed (pro re nata)
PSA Prostate-specific antigen
PSV Pressure support ventilation
PT Prothrombin time
PTCA Percutaneous transluminal coronary angioplasty
PTH Parathyroid hormone
PTP Posttransfusion purpura
PTT Partial thromboplastin time
PTU Propylthiouracil
PUD Peptic ulcer disease
PVC Premature ventricular contraction
PVR Pulmonary vascular resistance

qd Daily (quaque die)
qhs Every night (quaqua hora somni)
qid Four times a day (quater in die)
QRS An ECG wave measurement
QT An ECG wave measurement

RA Rheumatoid arthritis, *or* right atrium
RAD Right axis deviation
RAH Right atrial hypertrophy
RAP Right atrial pressure
RBBB Right bundle branch block
RBC Red blood cell
RDW Red blood cell distribution width
RFI Renal failure index
RhIG Rh immune globulin
RIA Radioimmunoassay
rPA Reteplase
RR Respiratory rate
RSBI Rapid shallow breathing index
RTA Renal tubular acidosis
RUQ Right upper quadrant
RV Residual volume, *or* right ventricle
RVEDP Right ventricular end diastolic pressure
RVH Right ventricular hypertrophy

SAAG Serum-ascites albumin gradient
SB tube Sengstaken-Blakemore tube
SBP Systolic blood pressure
SC Subcutaneous
SDP Single-donor platelet
SG Specific gravity
SGPT Serum glutamic pyruvic transaminase
SIADH Syndrome of inappropriate antidiuretic hormone
SIRS Systemic inflammatory response syndrome
SK Streptokinase
SLE Systemic lupus erythematosus
Sosm Serum osmolality
SPEP Serum protein electrophoresis
SSKI Super saturated potassium iodide
SSRI Selective serotonin reuptake inhibitor
ST An ECG wave measurement
Stat Immediately (statim)
ST-T An ECG wave measurement
SV Stroke volume
SVC Superior vena cava
SVR Systemic vascular resistance
SVT Supraventricular tachycardia

TB Tuberculosis
TBG Thyroid binding globulin
TBSA Total body surface area
TCA Angiotensin converting enzyme
TIA Transischemic attack
TIBC Total iron binding capacity
tid Three times a day (ter in die)
TLC Total lung capacity
TNKase Tenecteplase
tPA Tissue plasminogen activator
TPN Total parenteral nutrition
TRALI Transfusion-related acute lung injury
TSH Thyroid stimulating hormone
TT Thrombin time
TTKG Transtubular K^+ gradient
TTP Thrombotic thrombocytopenic purpura
TV Tidal volume

UA Urinalysis
UOP Urinary output
Uosm Urine osmolality
US Ultrasound
UTI Urinary tract infection

V Volume
V/Q Ventilation/perfusion
VC Vital capacity
VF Ventricular fibrillation
VSD Ventricular septal defect
VWF von Willebrand factor

WBC White blood cell

INDEX

A

B

Q

R

S

W